EPIDEMICS AND PANDEMICS

Epidemics and Pandemics

Philosophical Perspectives

MICHELE NICOLETTI AND ALESSANDRO PALAZZO

BREPOLS

The research leading to these results has received funding from the Department of Humanities of the University of Trento as part of the "Departments of Excellence – Law 232/216 art. 1 p. 314-338

D/2024/0095/189
ISBN 978-2-503-59892-5
DOI 10.1484/M.STPH-EB.5.127756
ISSN 2566-0683
eISSN 2566-0691

Printed in the EU on acid-free paper.

Contents

Concepts and Theories

NAOMI ZACK

Epidemics and Pandemics: Philosophical Perspectives

What's Philosophy Got to Do with It?

Pandemics and epidemics are kinds of disaster and like disaster, generally, can be viewed through many lenses, including history, art, medicine, economics, sociology, literature, journalism, psychology, biology, and philosophy. And the lenses themselves are multi-focal, allowing for subfields within professions and practices. One can scan the approaches through a broad perspective, such as ethics, which is itself multidisciplinary, or as a philosopher, just zero in, without announcing one's academic ID.[1] But the subtitle of this book, *Philosophical Perspectives*, seems to up the ante by requiring justification or demonstration of a specifically philosophical approach. I am not interested in the aspect of 'proving' that a subject is or is not philosophical, but I think that demonstration, or the practice of philosophical method seems to be announced in the subtitle. So this book should show what philosophy has to do with pandemics and epidemics. I believe it does accomplish that, in both directions — pandemics and epidemics as part of philosophical studies of disaster, and philosophy as a contribution to studies of pandemics and epidemics in other fields.

The first part of the book is a history of ideas about pandemics and epidemics and the second part offers 'theory' that brings us up through the COVID-19 pandemic. In both the past and present, pandemics and epidemics raise the same urgent questions: What is the disease agent? How does it spread? What, or who caused it? Answers to these questions depend on prior epistemological commitments and whether or not modern science is accepted. Before the acceptance and development of science, there could not be scientific commitments and acceptance, although we can discern a rough distinction between natural and supernatural posits in answers to all three questions. Looking back, even the natural posits, such as *miasma* or bad air, have non-scientific, speculative aspects, while the notion of *contagion* that illness is "catching", has a magical component in its model of automatic disease replication that did not take development or different effects on different people into account. For contemporary studies of disaster, E.L. Quarantelli's (1924–2017) insistence that the effects of a

1 I did the first in my *Ethics for Disaster* (Lanham, Md.: Rowman & Littlefield, 2009, 2010–11) and the second in *The American Tragedy of COVID-19: Social and Political Crises of 2020* (Lanham, Md.: Rowman & Littlefield, 2021).

Epidemics and Pandemics, ed. by Michele Nicoletti and Alessandro Palazzo (Turnhout: Brepols, 2024), pp. 7–12
BREPOLS PUBLISHERS 10.1484/M.STPH-EB.5.136403

disaster are part of a disaster makes it possible to consider pandemics as societal phenomena, because they affect human populations as they have already developed, with social hierarchies, pre-existing vulnerabilities, and complex dependencies on human-made products. Quarantelli's main example was psychological depression as an effect of disaster that should be counted as part of the disaster.[2]

Thucydides provided the original anchor for Quarantelli's idea in the fifth century BCE, through naturalistic analyses of "plague". But Thucydides who was schooled in both medicine and disease itself, did not base his insights on what we would call psychological responses to disaster, but human nature. As Mauro Bonazzi explicates in 'Thucydides and the Politics of the Plague', he focused on the anti-social, antagonistic, and politically anarchic responses to disaster. Jean-Jacques Rousseau was to explain the devastation of the Lisbon earthquake of 1755, in a similar way. Rousseau blamed the arrogance of seven-story human architecture and graspingness in returning to devastated buildings to save possessions.[3] While blaming human victims of natural disaster was a way to block recourse to religious explanations, it was a moral focus on causes, rather than examination of the mechanisms or reverberations of epidemics and pandemics.

From the Middle Ages through the nineteenth century, ideas of the plague were debated both medically and philosophically through the posits of contagion versus miasma. Alessandro Palazzo, Concetta Pennuto, and Mariangela Priarolo take up these arguments and scholarship in Europe, which reaches an interesting humanistic culmination in Fabrizio Meroi's interpretation of Henri Bergson's thought. Meroi reads Bergson as using the idea of contagion in intellectual and psychological, as well as biological spheres of life. If plausible, this would be an instance of the contagion of contagion from the physical to the psychic world, but the issue is more likely the model of biological contagion as a model for psychic influence among humans. Also in the first part of this collection, Marco Di Branco expands the discussion of contagion to Islamic scholarship and Diana Di Segni considers Latin-into-Hebrew treatises on the Black Death.

Of course, we would not be interested in this intellectual history but for the COVID-19 pandemic. The writers in Part II view the COVID-19 pandemic as an occasion to call for something more from philosophers. Indeed, the widespread imposition of scientific surveillance and public prescription, together with renewed rejection of the content of science, has created what in earlier ages would be considered a spiritual vacuum. In 'Zoonosis', Carlo Brentari reminds us that we humans

2 Quarantelli emphasized psychological depression as an effect of disaster that should be viewed as part of the event. See Enrico L. Quarantelli, 'What Is Disaster? The Need for Clarification in Definition and Conceptualization in Research', in Disaster Research Center, *University of Delaware*, Article 177 (repr. from Barbara Sowder [ed.], *Disasters and Mental Health Selected Contemporary Perspectives* [Washington, D.C.: U.S. Government Printing Office, 1985], pp. 41–73) available at http://udspace.udel.edu/handle/19716/1119 (last accessed 08/06/2022) quotation p. 13.

3 John R. Mullin, 'The Reconstruction of Lisbon Following the Earthquake of 1755: A Study in Despotic Planning', in *Journal of the International History of City Planning Association*, 45 (1992), available at https://scholarworks.umass.edu/larp_faculty_pubs/45/ (last accessed: 08/06/2022).

are animals, part of the biological ecosystems that connect us to other animals and make us susceptible to their diseases. Michele Nicoletti strives for a universal idea of identity in the face of world-scale illness and death, based on the dignity and "self-possession" of all individuals. Nidesh Lawtoo, working with *mimesis* as imitation in both viral reproduction and the spread of conspiracy theories calls for new understandings of crowd behaviour. Ľudmila Lacková examines the loss of real contact and communication in our new age of digitization, post-COVID. Federico Laudisa interrogates the representational role of scientific models, raising questions about their underlying realities and reliability for prediction. Finally, Pejman Abdolmohammadi considers the instabilities wrought by the pandemic in the Middle East and North Africa.

Putting the scholarship from Parts I and II of this volume together, readers may enter an intellectual respite from both the individual and societal crises they have recently experienced. The historical and geographical breadth in the volume affords whatever detachment is possible, because it expands subjective perspectives. We can see how the long and somewhat stagnant history of contagion debates followed by the accelerated and immediate need to re-question fundamentals of human orientation capture the unique rupture to reality that the COVID-19 pandemic has wrought. The net effect is indeed existential, without either supernatural or scientific reassurance and little that collectives can count on for confidence going forward.

This history and apprehension of our current world circumstances create situations of extreme freedom for both individuals and collectives. This is moral freedom as Jean-Paul Sartre described, because a whole moral system must be chosen before concrete decisions can be made by applying its principles. And there is always ambivalence in choosing a moral system, since they are all plausible in their own ways. Thus, we are continually confronted with the arbitrary nature of such choices, before we commit to them by action.[4]

To conclude, the philosophical history of ideas and analyses of leading concepts presented herein are, as Michele Nicoletti and Alessandro Palazzo intended, an important antidote to the starkness of contemporary scientific information and the conspiracy theories it attracts in the public auditorium. There were analogues to conspiracy theories in earlier ages —we need think only of the age of witchcraft persecution, and before then more robust demonology.[5] Present democratic practices allow conspiracy thought to flourish autonomously and propagate (especially through electronic 'contagion'), but on the other side, there is also freedom to contemn and dismiss it. It would greatly enrich public thought about pandemics, particularly COVID-19, if both science and conspiracies could be balanced by philosophical reflection and analyses, in the same public auditorium. Again, the main contribution exemplified in *Epidemics and Pandemics: Philosophical Perspectives* is *how* we think

4 Jean-Paul Sartre, *L'existentialisme est un humanisme* (Paris: Nagel, 1946) (Translated as *Existentialism is a Humanism*, ed. by John Kulka, trans. by Carol Macomber [New Haven, CT: Yale University Press, 2007]).

5 See Carl Sagan, *The Demon-Haunted World: Science as a Candle in the Dark* (New York: Random House, 1995).

about these ills, which is both intrinsically interesting and our best defense against them. The biggest rhetorical and political problem of our time is that people think, speak, and act, without considering the nature of their thought. If more in an age with a surfeit of influential talking heads and shared opinions could pause to consider how they are thinking about disasters and pandemics — and also climate change — we could all be more optimistic about the global future. Thinking about how we collectively think, and have thought, produces new ideas. In the desperation of our time, there is an eager hunger for new ideas. Some of the fabulation in conspiracy thought dulls that appetite, but the kind of reflection offered in this book can be recognized as more substantial fare by probably more people than easily apparent.

Bibliography

Mullin, John R., 'The Reconstruction of Lisbon Following the Earthquake of 1755: A Study in Despotic Planning', in *Journal of the International History of City Planning Association*, 45 (1992), https://scholarworks.umass.edu/larp_faculty_pubs/45/

Quarantelli, Enrico L., 'What Is Disaster? The Need for Clarification in Definition and Conceptualization in Research', in Disaster Research Center, *University of Delaware*, Article 177 (repr. from Barbara Sowder [ed.], *Disasters and Mental Health Selected Contemporary Perspectives* [Washington, D.C.: U.S. Government Printing Office, 1985], pp. 41–73), https://udspace.udel.eduhandle/19716/1119

Sagan, Carl, *The Demon-Haunted World: Science as a Candle in the Dark* (New York: Random House, 1995).

Sartre, Jean-Paul, *L'existentialisme est un humanisme* (Paris: Nagel, 1946) (trans. as *Existentialism is a Humanism*, ed. by John Kulka, trans. by Carol Macomber [New Haven, CT: Yale University Press, 2007]).

Zack, Naomi, *Ethics for Disaster* (Lanham, Md.: Rowman & Littlefield, 2009, 2010–11).

———, *The American Tragedy of COVID-19: Social and Political Crises of 2020* (Lanham, Md.: Rowman & Littlefield, 2021).

MICHELE NICOLETTI, ALESSANDRO PALAZZO

Introduction

Despite all the progress made by the biomedical sciences in the identification of pathogens, development of vaccines, and discovery of cures, contagious diseases remain a major threat to contemporary societies. Before the outbreak of the COVID-19 pandemic, the twentieth century and the first two decades of the current century had already seen a long series of epidemics and pandemics hit populations worldwide with different morbidity and mortality rates (influenza, AIDS/HIV, MERS, SARS, swine flu, and Ebola). The growth of crowded urban environments, more frequent traveling, and emigration waves are all factors contributing to the outbreak and spread of contagious diseases.

In such a global and interconnected world, epidemics and pandemics generate, today more than in the past, extremely complex health crises impacting almost every area of human life: they endanger economies, determine government decisions, affect individual psychologies, and stimulate cultural reactions. Scientific research and biomedical management of diseases are only two among many aspects of this phenomenon.

Many studies have been produced on epidemics, pandemics, contagion, and related concepts. The multilevel relevance of these phenomena has led, in many cases, to the adoption of a multidisciplinary perspective involving different approaches and methods (historical, socio-political, medical, cultural-historical, literary, etc.).[1]

In most of these studies, however, the philosophical outlook, when there is one at all, tends to be marginal. The purpose of this book is to give a philosophical treatment of epidemics and pandemics. In particular, the book will address a range

1 See, e.g., *Epidemics and Ideas: Essays on the Historical Perception of Pestilence*, ed. by Terence Ranger and Paul Slack (Cambridge: Cambridge University Press, 1992); *Contagion. Historical and Cultural Studies*, ed. by Alison Bashford and Claire Hooker (London-New York: Routledge, 2001); Saul Jarcho, *The Concept of Contagion in Medicine, Literature, and Religion* (Malabar: Krieger, 2000); *Imagining Contagion in Early Modern Europe*, ed. by Claire L. Calrin (Basingstoke: Palgrave Macmillan, 2005); *Tracés. Revue de Sciences humaines*, 21 (*Contagions*) (2011); *Contagion: Perspectives from Pre-Modern Societies*, ed. by Lawrence I. Conrad and Dominik Wujastyk (London-New York: Routledge, 2017 [1st ed. 2000]); Frank M. Snowden, *Epidemics and Society: From the Black Death to the Present* (New Haven: Yale University Press, 2019); *Die Corona-Gesellschaft. Analysen zur Lage und Perspektiven für die Zukunft*, ed. by Michael Volkmer and Karin Werner (Bielefeld: Transcript Verlag, 2020); *Le Medical Humanities al tempo del Covid-19. Temi, Problemi, Prospettive*, ed. by Stefano Scioli (Bologna: Emil di Odoya, 2021).

Epidemics and Pandemics, ed. by Michele Nicoletti and Alessandro Palazzo (Turnhout: Brepols, 2024), pp. 13–22
BREPOLS PUBLISHERS 10.1484/M.STPH-EB.5.136404

of longstanding issues (the notion of contagion, its meanings and its applications; the explanatory models for contagious and epidemic diseases; public authorities' reactions; the global nature of pandemics; practices of social control; the rationality of social and individual behaviours; the knowability of contagion and the forecasting of its spread; the role of the biomedical sciences; the struggle against superstitious and irrational beliefs; etc.).

The first part of the volume ('History of a Problem') explores the significance of these topics in philosophical and medical debates from classical Antiquity to the twentieth century. The seven contributions in this part deal with the issues of contagion and disease causation. Plague outbreaks feature as a main focus. The reading of all these papers in a historical sequence provides striking evidence that explanatory models based on miasmas and air corruption remained key to understanding the etiology of contagious diseases until the emergence of the germ theory and the discoveries of bacteriology. Neither Gerolamo Fracastoro's theory of seeds of contagion nor mechanism undermined the preeminence of the Galenic miasma theory. However, the historical reconstructions offered in this first section of the volume problematize this picture, calling attention to the existence, from ancient times onward, of contagionist models, describing their interactions with the miasma theory, and highlighting the ancient roots of the idea of contagion, its evolution during the Middle Ages and Modern Times, and its conceptual reconfiguration in contemporary philosophy.

The second section of the volume ('Concepts and Theories') gathers six papers providing a philosophical assessment of the cultural and social relevance of the epidemics and contagious diseases in today's societies. This relevance is assessed through an in-depth analysis of some concepts which characterized the public discourse during the COVID-19 crisis (zoonosis, contagion, immunization, conspiracy, fear, and emergency), and an investigation on the role of communication and science in the era of pandemic. Philosophical anthropology, ethics, social and political philosophy, semiotics, and philosophy of science offer a multifaceted interpretation of the radical challenges which pandemics pose to human life, identifying elements of discontinuity and continuity between the past and the present age. This multidisciplinary approach is enriched by the presence of an essay in the field of the Islamic Studies, which concludes this second part of the volume.

Though focusing on Western thought and society, the volume is open to other cultural areas; in particular, two contributions deal with medieval plague literature in Arabic and Hebrew, while another is dedicated to the impact of the Covid-19 pandemic on the political regimes of Middle Eastern countries.

It is also important to add that each paper in the volume provides not only a substantial contribution to the topic it discusses, but also an analytical recapitulation of previous specialist literature. As a consequence, the volume consolidates philosophical scholarship on epidemics and pandemics, laying the groundwork for future research.

Needless to say, the health crisis the world has been going through since 2019 had an influence on the choice of the subject of the volume. Since its outbreak, the

Covid-19 pandemic has been at the centre of a public debate marked by a variety of discourses and approaches. Different narratives have interacted, mixed, and interfered with each other. The constant appeal of newspapers and news broadcasts to stick to the results of medical and scientific research has failed to prevent the proliferation of antiscientific misinterpretations and online manipulation, with baseless conspiracy theories sometimes becoming viral or influential. In this context, the philosophical point of view has been largely underrepresented or badly represented. But in this very situation we strongly believe that a philosophical framework is needed to achieve a deeper understanding of the events that have already occurred and those still to come, and to fully grasp the overall impact of the pandemic. In our opinion, philosophical analysis has an important political value, as it allows one to comprehend the past in critical ways and get rid of the superficial judgements, emotional interpretations, and fake news that distort the perception of the present.

Mauro Bonazzi's paper ('Thucydides and the Politics of Plague') is dedicated to Thucydides' description of the 'plague' (today there is a consensus among scholars that the epidemic so vividly described by the Greek historian was not the contagious disease caused, as we know today, by the bacterium *Yersinia Pestis*) that ravaged Athens for two years, in 430–429 BCE. The paper contrasts Thucydides' account with analyses contained in coeval works of the Hippocratic *corpus*, highlighting similarities and divergences. On the one hand, Bonazzi argues on the basis of a meticulous linguistic analysis that Thucydides was acquainted with medical tradition and its methods. On the other, the Thucydidean account was not primarily aimed at a medical understanding of the disease. Rather, Thucydides' purpose was to explore the social consequences of the epidemic. From his account it emerges that the plague brought to light the unsocial and anti-political aspect of human nature, which remains hidden in peaceful times. By insisting on this point, Thucydides was able to oppose the belief prevailing in fifth-century Athens that human society had progressed from an unsecure and violent past.

Many other works written in subsequent centuries were to portray, more or less effectively, the impact of epidemics on moral laws, family ties, and social rules — e.g., Procopius' *Persian War*, Petrus Diaconus' *Historia Langobardorum*, or Boccaccio's *Decameron*. Still, Thucydides' description can be considered the seminal text in the Western tradition on plague and epidemic diseases.

Marco Di Branco ('Between Religion and Science. The Debate on the Concept of Contagion in the Medieval Islamic World and Its Western Parallels') analyzes the contribution that two fourteenth-century Arab Andalusian intellectuals, Ibn Ḫātima, d. 1369 *c.*, and Ibn al-Ḫaṭīb, 1313–1374, made to the notion of contagion, understood as disease transmission through direct contact or by proximity. After briefly outlining the key steps in the history of the concept of contagion, from classical Antiquity to the Black Death, Di Branco remarks that the notion of contagion was looked upon with suspicion in the Arabic medical tradition. Medieval Islamic theologians generally ascribed epidemics to the will of God, denied contagion, and believed that an epidemic disease was to be accepted as a fatality, or even a blessing for the believer, as dying of plague could be regarded as a form of martyrdom that granted direct access to paradise.

By contrast, in the works of Ibn Ḫātima and Ibn al-Ḫaṭīb we find clear clinical evidence of the contagious nature of the pandemic. The two disagreed on important points, though. While Ibn Ḫātima traced the phenomenon back to a law of nature established by God, Ibn al-Ḫaṭīb directly accused theologians of causing the deaths of countless people by denying the reality of contagion.

Alessandro Palazzo ('Pestilences and Contagious Diseases in the Middle Ages. Albert the Great and the Fourteenth-Century Plague Treatises') explores Albert the Great's views on pestilences and contagious diseases. Albert (1200–1280), a Dominican theologian and a commentator on the Aristotelian corpus, was also an important authority on medicine who addressed the key issues of the late-medieval medical debates and was acquainted with the chief sources in this field (Aristotle, Galen, and Avicenna).

Even though Albert did not dedicate a specific work or part of a work to these topics, pestilences are given careful attention in his oeuvre. Despite objective limitations (he did not experience any plague outbreaks during his lifetime, and — for this reason as well as others — in his works the terms *pestis* and *pestilentia* are vague, lumping together a large variety of different sicknesses), Albert's investigation of the causes of pestilential and contagious diseases is worthy of consideration for at least two reasons. One is that he explained these phenomena in scientific terms and not as a result of God's will, which in the Middle Ages was often invoked as the cause of natural calamities. The other is that, as a consequence, his explanatory models provided the basis for the late medieval discourse on plague. In his works, the fourteenth-century treatises on plague, the so-called *Pestschriften*, found some of the conceptual tools they used to construct the etiological and nosological identity of this devastating disease.

Diana Disegni ('Latin-into-Hebrew Treatises on the Black Death') focuses on the reaction of medieval medicine to the mid-fourteenth-century plague outbreak, the so-called Black Death. Whereas scholars have so far mainly dealt with the Latin and vernacular medical literature on plague, Disegni investigates a so far less studied part of that vast corpus, namely, medical manuals written in Hebrew. Some of these were original works by Jewish physicians, while others were translations into Hebrew of Arabic and Latin works. Among these works were some by the most renowned Western physicians of the time, including Gentile da Foligno, Francesco Zanelli of Bologna, John of Burgundy, Petrus de Tossignano, Antonio Guaineri of Pavia, and Valescus de Taranta.

Disegni's paper offers a general overview of all these texts, correcting, completing, and expanding on the incomplete or erroneous accounts currently available in scholarship. Moreover, by focusing on Hebrew plague treatises, the paper sheds light on the phenomenon of Latin-into-Hebrew translation, which has long been dismissed as a marginal aspect of the intercultural exchanges between Mediterranean cultures in the Middle Ages, especially compared to Arabic-into-Hebrew translation.

Concetta Pennuto ('Contagion and Pandemics. Plague in Early Modern Medical Thought') deals with early modern sources, and specifically with the evolution of the notion of contagion. The plague outbreaks that struck Europe on a regular basis from the mid-fourteenth century until the eighteenth century led physicians and public officials to take steps to counter the spread of the disease. In particular, the extreme danger practitioners were exposed to impelled them to adopt means to protect themselves. Moreover, while the recurring outbreaks stimulated medical and philosophical reflections on the concept of contagion, assistance to the sick foregrounded the physician's relationship with his patients and his own responsibilities. Thus, the paper also explores the interaction between medical theory and practice by shedding light on the practitioners' social and ethical engagement and analyzing the evolution of ideas regarding the cure of plague-afflicted patients.

Mariangela Priarolo ('New Sciences and Old Diseases: Seventeenth-Century Readings of the Causes of the Plague') investigates the persistence of the miasmatic explanation of the plague until the nineteenth century. It is claimed that one of the reasons for this persistence is that the Galenic model of explanation was reinforced by mechanism, the new dominant scientific paradigm in the seventeenth century. One should notice that early modern criticism of Galenism, especially that coming from mechanist philosophers, was indeed concerned more with the notion of natural faculties than with Galen's concrete descriptions of specific diseases, such as plague.

Through a reinterpretation of Fracastoro's notion of seeds of contagion, the seventeenth-century corpuscular version of mechanism made it possible to see Galenic (putrid) exhalations, or 'effluvia', as (very tiny) parts of matter in motion that could be described, analyzed, and quantified, and hence rightfully included within the new view of the world.

Fabrizio Meroi ('Contagion and Epidemics in Twentieth-Century Thought. A Hypothesis About Bergson') addresses the issues of epidemics and contagion in late modern philosophy and culture. In particular, he investigates the discussion of these topics in the fields of literature, philosophy, and the human sciences in general. The main focus of his essay, however, is Henri Bergson. Meroi argues that the concept of contagion is ubiquitous in Bergson's works, albeit in a very peculiar form. Bergson often resorts to terms and concepts such as influence, diffusion, propagation, and transmission when dealing with psychological and gnoseological issues, the evolution of life, and anthropological, ethical, and religious themes. According to Meroi, in Bergson's work contagion is not a mere metaphor, but underpins an original theoretical model of interpretation of reality based on a dynamic of interaction and transfer that constitutes a conceptual structure characteristic of his thought.

The second part of the volume is opened by an analysis of the concept of 'zoonosis'. The COVID-19 pandemic has forced humans to confront fundamental questions of identity. Carlo Brentari ('Zoonosis') argues that the species identity — namely that humans should consider the fact that they belong to the species *Homo sapiens* within a larger ecosystem — should be brought to the fore in light of the pandemic. This identity of humans as biological runs up against other kinds of identities, for example of humans as fundamentally religious beings, with accompanying rituals that might need to be altered or ceased during the pandemic. Since the pandemic affected the entire globe, the author also suggests this fact could encourage humans to think of themselves as part of a larger collective, given the common experience of all. The pandemic also calls into question understandings of nature as apart from civilization; climate change shows that human activity impacts the environment beyond the narrow confines of what happens in 'islands of civilization'. In the end, there is no escape from the fact that humans are animals and are part of nature, and thinking of humans' ability to modify the environment also holds out hope that they could yet re-balance it in the face of climate change.

But the pandemic has also represented the return of 'large-scale death' on the public scene of the world. This is the starting point of Michele Nicoletti's essay ('Fear and Dispossession') which analyzes the nexus between fear, society, and politics in general terms and, more specifically, in the time of pandemics. This chapter identifies the fear of self-dispossession as a feature common to contemporary societies. The COVID-19 crisis has emphasized this fear and has limited the opportunities for enjoying personal liberties and rights. Within this context, the author maintains that an important role can be played by a vigorous re-proposal of the principle of 'self-belonging', understood as, on the one hand, the aspiration that one's dignity be respected, and, on the other, that the irreducibility and inviolability of the Self be recognized. This principle can serve as the foundation for not only an existential perspective of the liberty and relationality of the individual, but also a vision of society based upon respect for basic universal rights and a democratic practice which extends from the local to the global level. The principle of self-belonging is seen as an alternative to the authoritarian and paternalistic approaches to the pandemic crisis.

Nidesh Lawtoo ('The Mimetic Faculty Reloaded. Contagion, Immunization, Conspiracies in the Age of Viral Reproduction') takes as his starting point the idea of humans as mimetic beings, in the sense that they represent the world around them, but also imitate others. This fact takes on particular relevance in the pandemic, since as the virus literally creates copies of itself and spreads, conspiracy theories arise in an analogical fashion, and in turn the two contagions mutually amplify each other. As with vaccination against the coronavirus, the author calls us to rethink what a 'vaccination' might look like for the affective contagion of rumours and conspiracy theories. The author traces the genealogy of the concept of mimesis in Plato and Nietzsche, both of whom speak of 'mimetic pathos' which 'has the (will to) power to take possession of spectators, dispossess them of their rational faculty, or logos, and generate mimetic pathologies that are constitutive of the *vita mimetica*'. In the twenty-first century, with the rise of conspiracy theories around COVID, a new understanding of mimesis and crowd psychology is needed. The solution cannot be in *logos*, or scientific discourses, since this is what the *pathos* of the conspiracy theories contradicts. The answer might instead be 'balancing diagnostic operations that account for the role of *pathos* in reloading the mimetic faculty in the digital age — and perhaps turn[ing] the mimetic faculty to *patho*-logical use by relying on the power of positive models or examples to promote the importance of vaccination and preventive measures more generally via both logical and affective means'.

The crisis of the subject is the main focus of L'udmila Lacková's chapter ('Crisis of the Subject in Mediated Communication'). The author explores how the pandemic has changed communication. With face-to-face communication — unmediated communication — much less possible during the pandemic, we are forced to turn to various forms of new media. The author highlights how the seeming freedom offered by new media can actually be limiting, since it imposes limits onto the subject and mediates the ways in which they interact with others. Thus, it is not simply that new media creates an intermediary between the addressor and addressee, the media fundamentally changes the communication itself. The increased popularity of visual media, for example, made it easier to display and spread emotive messages than in purely verbal media. In some ways, mediated communication might allow us to express ourselves better than in unmediated forms of communication, and simplistic fears of new technology for its own sake are often unfounded. In any case, the pandemic has created new conditions for communication, the results of which we are still reckoning with.

But the COVID-19 crisis also affected the role of science. Federico Laudisa ('The Epistemology of Models in the Era of Pandemic') explores the philosophical issues of modelling in the sciences, something that gained particular importance during the pandemic. What, the author asks, are models actually representing? And what should we do with these models? The author investigates different types of models — for example, scale models that offer a scaled down representation of a specified target, or toy models that strip away irrelevant factors to give an isolated representation of a target. When it comes to pandemic modelling, compartmental models show the relative numbers of susceptible people, infected people, and so on, while agent-based models assign greater importance to capturing behaviour at the individual level. Both kinds of model, however, face various issues with collecting, measuring, and analyzing data. All these models furthermore suffer from the well-known problem of induction. While the author offers potential solutions to this problem, nonetheless, the pandemic and the subsequent response by scientists and the general public suggests that a new epistemology of science may be necessary.

The last chapter ('The COVID-19 Pandemic. An Exogenous Shock into Political Systems in the Middle East and North Africa?') aims at including the area of Islamic Studies in this rich and plural overview. Pejman Abdolmohammadi examines the effects of the pandemic on countries in the Middle East and North Africa, a region already suffering from a range of crises. Economically, the pandemic will contribute to instability and economic downturns. While wealthy oil states can weather this economic instability to some extent, and already war-torn countries simply have less to lose since they began with so little, the economic changes will particularly hit developing countries, like Iran and Turkey. Nonetheless, in all cases, the resulting instability could lead to further sectarian tensions and violence on an everyday level, as well as bolster recruitment efforts by terrorist groups. Furthermore, people across the region may become increasingly disillusioned with traditional narratives that elites use to justify keeping themselves in power, thus creating an even more unstable situation. As a new global competition between Western nations and countries like Russia and China emerges in the wake of the pandemic, the strategic role of the region becomes that much more important.

Bibliography

Bashford, Alison, and Hooker, Claire (eds.), *Contagion. Historical and Cultural Studies* (London-New York: Routledge, 2001).

Calrin, Claire L. (ed.), *Imagining Contagion in Early Modern Europe* (Basingstoke: Palgrave Macmillan, 2005).

Conrad, Lawrence I., and Wujastyk, Dominik (eds.), *Contagion: Perspectives from Pre-Modern Societies* (London-New York: Routledge, 2017 [1st ed. 2000]).

Jarcho, Saul, *The Concept of Contagion in Medicine, Literature, and Religion* (Malabar: Krieger, 2000).

Scioli, Stefano, (eds.), *Le Medical Humanities al tempo del Covid-19. Temi, Problemi, Prospettive* (Bologna: Emil di Odoya, 2021).

Snowden, Frank M., *Epidemics and Society: From the Black Death to the Present* (New Haven: Yale University Press, 2019).

Terence, Ranger, and Slack, Paul (eds.), *Epidemics and Ideas: Essays on the Historical Perception of Pestilence* (Cambridge: Cambridge University Press, 1992).

Tracés. Revue de Sciences humaines, 21 (*Contagions*) (2011).

Volkmer Michael, and Werner, Karin (eds.), *Die Corona-Gesellschaft. Analysen zur Lage und Perspektiven für die Zukunft* (Bielefeld: Transcript Verlag, 2020).

History of a Problem

MAURO BONAZZI

1. Thucydides and the Politics of Plague

▼ **ABSTRACT** The paper analyses Thucydides' description of the plague which ravaged Athens for two years, in 430–429 BC. In the first part of the paper, a detailed comparison with the medical, Hippocratic, *corpus* is provided, proving that the historian was familiar with that tradition and its methods. The second part of the paper, however, argues that the relationship with the medical tradition does not play a prominent role in the Thucydidean account. What matters most for him is the exploration of the social consequences of the pandemic. The plague uncovers a more violent and greedy dimension, an unsocial and anti-political aspect of human nature which remains hidden in peaceful times. By insisting on this point, Thucydides can thus oppose the common belief that human society had progressed from an unsecure and violent past which was dominant in fifth-century Athens.

1.

Plagues were common occurrences in the Ancient world, and they often make their appearance in literary texts, from the very beginning. The *Iliad*, the first and most influential poem, opens with the description of an epidemic in the Achaean camp. Indeed, the plague triggers all action in the poem. What is interesting, for the present analysis, is the 'ordinariness' of such experience. Unfortunate yet possible events like an epidemic could happen, and the problem is to find a solution. In Homer, this occurs in a divine context. The cause of the plague is traced back to a god (Apollo) who has been offended — nobody doubts that the plague has been unleashed by the god — and the priority is how to placate him. Once an explanation is offered (Apollo's wrath was caused by the treatment which the Achaean reserved to his priest Chryses) and a solution is found (to return the daughter to the priest), the plague disappears, and the real problems of the *Iliad* begin, with the confrontation between Achilles and Agamemnon. The situation is no different when we turn to another masterpiece, Sophocles' *Oedipus Tyrannus*. As in the *Iliad*, the tragedy begins with a plague which has been unleashed by Apollo, and the problem is again to placate his wrath and end the plague — a more difficult task, in this case, given that it will take

Epidemics and Pandemics, ed. by Michele Nicoletti and Alessandro Palazzo (Turnhout: Brepols, 2024), pp. 25–36
BREPOLS PUBLISHERS 10.1484/M.STPH-EB.5.136405

much more time for the person in charge, Oedipus, to discover that he is also the indirect cause of the pandemic. Again, events like plagues happen, they are part of the common experience of the Greeks living in those centuries, and do not receive special attention. They remain in the background, so to say.

The opposite is the case with another writer, the historian Thucydides. In his book, known as *The Peloponnesian War*, there is not a fictional account, but rather an effort to reconstruct an episode that actually took place, the plague which ravaged Athens for two years, in 430–29 BC. at the beginning of the war against Sparta.[1] What is remarkable, in his case, is the fact that the plague is no longer relegated to the background, as a tragic experience which was all too common, yet not particularly relevant, for the Greeks. Unlike other authors, Thucydides offers a detailed analysis of the plague, which turns out to be highly original from a variety of perspectives, as I will try to show in the present paper. I will first explore Thucydides' relationship with the medical tradition, and I will then underline what is really distinctive about his account. Thucydides does not limit himself to providing the reader with a careful account of the problem from a medical perspective, but also explores the social consequences of the pandemic in Athens. Such interest in social and political consequences is not accidental. For Thucydides the plague has a heuristic potential, because it helps us to better understand human civilization and human nature. In other words, the event of the plague conveys a political lesson, which needs to be brought to light.

2.

Thucydides tells us that he himself suffered and recovered from the disease and saw others who did so (2. 48. 3).[2] As one who survived the plague, he can thus present himself not only as a reliable witness, but also as an authority on a subject which, as a consequence of its radical nature, remained inexplicable even for doctors. 'For neither were physicians able to cope with the disease, since they at first had to treat it without knowing its nature, the mortality among them being greatest because they were exposed to it'.[3] This brief remark reveals Thucydides' ambition to compete with doctors and their explanations. This relation with the medical tradition has been the object of an intense debate in the scholarly literature and plays an important

1 See Thucydides, 2. 47–54; see also 1. 23. 3; 2. 57. 1; 2. 58. 1; 3. 3. 1; 3. 87. 1–2 (informing us about a second outburst, 426 BC); 6. 12. 1 and 26. 2.

2 On Thucydides' description of the plague and his relationship with Hippocratic literature in general, see Charles Lichtenthaeler, *Thucydide et Hippocrate vus par un historien-medecin* (Droz: Geneve, 1965); Georg Rechenhauer, *Thukydides und die hippokratische Medizin* (Hildesheim: Olms, 1991); Rosalind Thomas, 'Thucydides Intellectual Milieu and the Plague', in *Brill's Companion to Thucydides*, ed. by Antonios Rengakos and Antonis Tsamakis (Leiden: Brill, 2006), pp. 87–108.

3 Thucydides, 2. 47. 4; translations are from Thucydides, *History of the Peloponnesian War*, with an English Translation by Charles F. Smith (Cambridge, Mass.: Harvard University Press, 1959). Despite many attempts, the identification of the disease remains an insoluble problem: see A. J. Holladay and J. F. C. Poole, 'Thucydides and the Plague of Athens', *Classical Quarterly* 29 (1979), pp. 282–300 and Simon Hornblower, *A Commentary on Thucydides* (Oxford: Clarendon Press, 1991), vol. 1, p. 316.

role in our appreciation of Thucydides' self-presentation as a rigorous historian, working in the footsteps of the scientific tradition, best represented by the writings collected under the name of Hippocrates.[4] Indeed, the image of Thucydides as a close affiliate of the Hippocratic school of medicine enjoyed great popularity in the past,[5] but is no longer attractive for many readers who underline the rhetorical and dramatic dimension of his style.[6] To discuss this problem in all of its complexity would require much more space than is available here. For the sake of the present paper, what is important to remark is that Thucydides possesses good knowledge of medical terminology and practices, as was already shown by Page in his seminal paper in 1953.[7] Even those scholars who have underlined the rhetorical and dramatic aspects of Thucydides' style agree that he belongs to the same intellectual context as the doctors and, more generally, to the new world of sophists and philosophers. The problem is thus to understand how Thucydides uses this tradition for his own purposes.

A superficial reading of the description is sufficient to see the proximity between the historian and the doctors, and his knowledge of their theories. To begin with, Thucydides shares with the Hippocratic doctors a naturalistic approach, which leaves aside religious or supernatural explanations (2. 47. 4). In his account, the disease is no longer understood in terms of divine retribution for some offense, nor is there any room for the Homeric Calchas, the seer who saved the Achaean camp by revealing the cause of Apollo's anger in the *Iliad* ('and the supplications made at sanctuaries, or appeals to oracles and the like, were all futile, and at last men desisted from them, overcome by calamity', 2. 47. 4). The methodology is also similar, because Thucydides too begins by setting out the provenance of the disease (Ethiopia, 2. 48. 1), the atmospheric conditions (1. 23. 3), the general state of health in the year in question (2. 49. 1), and even considers what the Hippocratics called critical days by observing that most people died on the seventh or ninth day (2. 49. 6).[8] The first two elements are especially relevant. Also other texts from the Hippocratic

4 An important problem, which cannot be discussed here with the attention it deserves, is the degree of uniformity in the Hippocratic collection. As has become clear by now, this *corpus* contains essays by different authors covering the late fifth and fourth centuries: see for instance Thomas, 'Thucydides Intellectual Milieu', pp. 93–95. Interestingly, later physicians such as Galen read Thucydides carefully, thus filling up the gaps in the Hippocratic treatises: see Galenus, *De difficultate respirationis*, ed. Karl Gottlob Kühn, vol. 7 (Leipzig: 1824, repr. Hildesheim: Georg Olms Verlagsbuchhandlung, 1965), II. 7, pp. 850–51 and Rebecca Fleming, 'Galen and the Plague', in *Galens'* peri alypias *and the History of the Roman Empire*, ed. by Caroline Petit (Leiden: Brill, 2019) pp. 219–44.

5 The most famous proponent of such a reading probably remains Charles Norris Cochrane, *Thucydides and the Science of History* (Oxford University Press: London, 1929).

6 Hornblower, *A Commentary on Thucydides*, vol. 1, p. 317 and especially W. Robert Connor, *Thucydides* (Princeton: Princeton University Press, 1984).

7 Denys Lionel Page, 'Thucydides' Description of the Great Plague at Athens', *Classical Quarterly*, 47 (1953), pp. 97–119; *contra*, with some valuable comments, see Adam Parry, 'The Language of Thucydides' Description of the Plague', *Bulletin of the Institute of Classical Studies*, 16 (1969), pp. 106–18 (pp. 111–14).

8 Geoffrey Ernest Richard Lloyd, *In the Grip of Disease. Studies in Greek Imagination* (Oxford: Oxford University Press, 2003), p. 124.

collection underline the importance of air as the cause of the outbreak of diseases.[9] Thucydides tacitly agrees, and by adding the reference to Ethiopia further confirms the importance of the combination between atmospheric and geographical factors. As the plague brings a strong fever about, it is reasonable to assume a relation between the plague and extreme dryness, which is typical of that region.[10] In tracing this connection, Thucydides also tacitly refutes the idea that the plague exclusively depends on Athenian atmospheric conditions and their worsening through the arrival of people from the countryside (2. 52. 1).[11]

No less relevant, from a methodological perspective, is the search for an external, triggering cause (*prophasis, aitia*), which in this specific case is not found (2. 48. 3, 2. 49. 2); the absence of any *prophasis* is also noted in several Hippocratic treatises.[12] Since no *prophasis* is found, Thucydides proceeds with a full account of signs and symptoms. The description is very accurate: after a period of incubation, the sick were first hit by violent fevers (*ischurai thermai*), eye inflammation (*eruthemata*), redness of the throat and tongue, hoarseness, coughing, vomiting, and insomnia. This was the acute phase of the disease, lasting between 6 and 8 days. The disease would then affect the abdominal part, with ulcerations, diarrhea, and weakness ending in most cases in death. Many of the few who survived lost the use of their extremities (genitals, hands, feet; sometimes eyes), and in some cases also suffered from memory loss and mental disorder. Even though it is difficult to establish in all cases whether a given term belongs to the medical jargon or to ordinary parlance, the extent of the parallels — and 'the very idea of setting out the symptoms in this extraordinary detail' — certainly proves that Thucydides was familiar with the Hippocratic tradition.[13] Interestingly, his physiology too presents remarkable affinities with medical

9 See for instance *Airs, waters, places*, 9.3, and 5; *Breaths* 6; Anon. Lond. 7.15–23. See also Herod., 2. 77 and Plat. *Symp.* 188b. Thucydides also acknowledges the importance of this factor at 7. 87. 1, when talking about the Athenian prisoners in Syracuse. As we will see in chapters 2 to 6 of this volume, the idea that air was a main factor in causing pandemics would have a long life.

10 On Ethiopia as the land of incubation for such diseases, see Strabo, *Geogr.*, 17. 3. 10.

11 This is also confirmed by that fact that that year 'happened to be unusually free from disease as far as it regards the other maladies (2. 49. 1 and 50. 1)'. On the hypothesis of an Athenian origin, see Diodorus 12. 45. 2 and Plut., *V. Pericl.*, 34. 5; Id., *V. Nic.*, 6. 3 with Paul Demont, 'Notes sur le récit de la pestilence athénienne chez Thucydide et sur ses rapports avec la médecine grecque de l'époque classique', in *Formes de la pensée dans la Collecion Hippocratique* ed. by François Lasserre and Philippe Mudry (Drosz: Genève, 1983), pp. 341–53 (pp. 348–52), who further observes that the idea of an Athenian origin was also polemically used in an anti-Periclean context (2. 59. 2).

12 Lloyd, *In the Grip of Disease*, p. 124; in general, on the notion of *prophasis* in the Hippocratic texts and in other authors, see Hunter R. Rawlings, *A Semantic Study of* prophasis *to 400 BC.* (Wiesbaden: Hermes, 1975).

13 An interesting example is the mention of 'all kinds of purging of bile (*apokatharsesi choles*) named by the doctors'. Parry (Parry, 'The *Language of Thucydides*, p. 113) used this as an example of Thucydides' unwillingness to follow the doctors too strictly, and as a proof of his aristocratic disdain for technical terminology — which is partly true. And yet, Thucydides clearly shows that he was aware of the medical jargon and that he was unwilling to distance himself completely from it, see Thomas, 'Thucydides Intellectual Milieu', p. 98.

theories.[14] By describing the progress of the plague in the body in a clear sequence, from the head to the feet, Thucydides does indeed adopt the Hippocratic theory of bodily flux: the body is viewed as roughly consisting of a set of hollow tubes of various kinds and the progress of the disease seems to depend on an unbalance of the humors present in it. More precisely, this leads Thucydides to suspect that there are two routes taken by the plague — through the trachea to the lungs, and through the oesophagus to belly — thereby affecting two different areas, the chest and the belly. This description of the human body presents clear parallels with the medical texts.[15]

Some scholars have also argued that Thucydides was developing his own medical theory, in some cases at least, in an attempt to prove his superiority.[16] Allegedly, he seems to be the only one to have understood that the plague spread by contagion,[17] and he also outlined what in modern medicine would be called immunity.[18] This is an intriguing hypothesis, but it risks being too speculative. As a matter of fact, Thucydides merely records some details, but he does not develop any generally applicable theories.[19]

More importantly, these parallels must not lead us to overlook significant differences,[20] the most notable one being that Thucydides does not seem to be interested in what probably matters most for the doctors, that is diagnosis in view of treatment.[21] In the Hippocratic treatises the collection of data is intended to be used by the doctor to deduce what the course of the disease might be and to decide how to intervene. Thucydides did not intend his account to be a guide for the future treatment of the

14 Elizabeth M. Craik, 'Thucydides on the Plague: Physiology of Flux and Fixation', *Classical Quarterly*, 51 (2001), pp. 102–08.

15 Craik, 'Thucydides on the Plague', p. 107.

16 Another element confirming that he was somehow engaging with the doctors is his remark on dogs and birds (2. 50). As Demont, 'Notes sur le récit de la pestilence', pp. 341–47, brilliantly observed, this seems to be an objection against the widespread assumption that the plague was a purely human disease. More generally, on the competition with other intellectuals — for instance the sophists, the doctors' rivals — see Mauro Bonazzi, *The Sophists* (Cambridge University Press: Cambridge, 2020), pp. 138–40.

17 See Thucydides, 2. 47. 4: doctors were the most exposed; Id., 2. 50. 1–2: the disease spread to other species and animals no longer approached corpses; Id., 2. 58. 3: Hagnon's expedition to Chalcis brought the disease to the soldiers stationed there. See Thomas, 'Thucydides Intellectual Milieu', pp. 102–3 and Paul Demont, 'The Causes of the Athenian Plague and Thucydides', in *Thucydides between History and Literature*, ed. by Antonis Tsakmakis and Melina Tamiolaki (Berlin: De Gruyter, 2013), pp. 73–87 (pp. 75–77). The idea is paralleled by what we find in some Hippocratic treatises (see *Breaths* 6, and *On the Nature of Man* 9; see above note 9), where *miasma* — understood as airborne pathogenic elements — are considered the possible cause of the plague. The use of this notion, dependent as it is on a religious context, is rare but significant: see Jacques Jouanna, 'Air, Miasma, Contagion in the Time of Hippocrates and the Survival of Miasmas in Post-Hippocratic Medicine (Rufus of Ephesus, Galen and Palladius)', in *Greek Medicine from Hippocrates to Galen. Selected Papers*, ed. by Jacques Jouanna (Leiden: Brill, 2012), pp. 121–37.

18 Those who survived were not struck by the disease again, or only caught a very mildly case of it.

19 Craik, 'Thucydides on the Plague', p. 103.

20 Besides, we should also take account of certain inaccuracies: see Thomas E. Morgan, 'Plague or Poetry? Thucydides on the Epidemic at Athens', *Transactions of the American Philological Association*, 124 (1994), pp. 197–209 (p. 204).

21 Parry, 'The Language of Thucydides', pp. 108–10; Jonathan J. Price, *Thucydides and Internal War* (Cambridge: Cambridge University Press, 2001), p. 18; See also Page, 'Thucydides' Description of the Great Plague', pp. 98–99 on the importance of *prognosis*.

plague, given the exceptional nature of this disease. The implicit competition with the doctors, however, seems to suggest that Thucydides did not exclude that his description could also be of some practical use, not in terms of treatment but at least of diagnostics.[22] A possible goal of Thucydides' account is to offer a diagnosis that may be useful in the future, by helping his readers recognize the disease, should it strike again (2. 48. 3). Most importantly, this diagnostic analysis is not limited to the disease, as in the case of the Hippocratic treatises. The medical description is only one part of Thucydides' account, leading up to a different kind of exploration, one focused no longer on the disease but on its psychological and social effects. A correct understanding of what happened in Athens is propaedeutic to a better understanding of the dynamics governing human society and human nature. In so doing Thucydides can thus claim his superiority over the medical tradition.

3.

The plague was a significant factor in the war.[23] Therefore, it is hardly surprising that Thucydides devotes so much space in his history to a detailed reconstruction of it. But there is more. Thucydides' interest does not depend only on his desire to give a diagnostic account which might prove useful in the future, as we have seen in the last section; nor does it depend only on the need to provide the reader with an accurate reconstruction of an event that played an important role in the war between Athens and Sparta. The plague has a much bigger heuristic potential, because it helps us to understand history dynamics and therefore reveals the real nature of the protagonists and creators of history — human beings.

The key expression occurs midway through Thucydides' description, where he underlines that the pandemic was too extreme to bear 'for human nature', *kata ten anthropeian physin* (2. 50. 2). A similar expression, with a reference to human nature, also occurs in another strategic and well-known section of the text, namely at the beginning of the analysis of the civil war (*stasis*) in Corcyra: 'while human nature is always the same (3. 82. 1)'. The starting point is the idea of the regularity of human nature, the assumption of an unchanging human nature that always remains the same; and the goal of Thucydides' historical investigation is apparently to reach a proper understanding of what this human nature precisely consists in. Within this context, the pandemic and the civil war, or indeed war in general (including the Peloponnesian war),[24] play a decisive role for those who are interested in understanding human nature. War, civil war and plagues constitute extremes cases which by robbing 'men

22 Hornblower, *A Commentary on Thucydides*, vol. 1, pp. 320–21.

23 See also Thucydides, 3. 87: 'no fewer than four thousand four hundred of those enrolled as hoplites died and also three hundred cavalry, and of the populace a number that cannot be ascertained'.

24 Unlike for us moderns, war, *polemos*, and civil war, *stasis*, were two different things for the Ancient Greeks: see for instance Price, *Thucydides and Internal War*, p. 70. One of the many provocative moves in Thucydides' account is the attempt to prove that they are actually identical: see Colin MacLeod, 'Thucydides on Faction', *Proceedings of the Cambridge Philological Society*, 205 (1979), pp. 52–68 and Nicole

of the easy supply of their daily wants' (3. 82. 2) reveal what remains obscure to the non-expert eye: certain social and psychological dynamics that are otherwise difficult to grasp.[25] It is also for this reason Thucydides is so interested in a careful analysis of these events.

In other words, the parallel with medicine returns at a deeper level, and the potential of the disease becomes clear. As Enzo Paci brilliantly remarked, Thucydides is interested in 'the pathology of history'.[26] Just as the doctor starts from a specific state, that is disease, in order to gain an overall understanding of the human body, so Thucydides starts from these specific and extreme situations (war, the plague, civil war) in order to gain a proper understanding of the dynamics of history and of human nature in general. And it is by virtue of this understanding, insofar as he makes visible what would otherwise remain obscure, that Thucydides can claim that his work is 'a possession for always' (1. 22, where mention is made again of an unchanging human nature, *kata to anthropinon*). Taken in itself, the plague is an extraordinary event, not susceptible to rational explication. And yet, despite this exceptionality (or perhaps because of it), it also turns out to be revelatory, a real guide for those who are interested in the dynamics of the human world.

4.

In light of all this, it is possible to appreciate the strategic importance of the second part of Thucydides' account (2. 51–53), where he explores the social consequences of the pandemic, the upheaval it brought about in Athens. As has been rightly remarked, Thucydides puts 'such emphasis and intellectual power into charting these effects that the physical, medical description of the plague pales beside it'.[27] Indeed, this is one of the most remarkable pages in Thucydides' remarkable work. More precisely, this second part can be further divided into two sections and can be compared with two other sections of Thucydides' book, Pericles' epitaph, which immediately precedes the account about the plague (2. 35–46), and the above-mentioned description of the civil war in Corcyra (3. 82–83).

In the first section (2. 51), where Thucydides begins his description of the social and psychological effects of the plague, he offers a complex picture, made up of different and contrasting elements. The recurrent element is human weakness,

---

Loraux, 'Thucydide et la sédition dans les mots', in Ead., *La tragédie d'Athènes. La politique entre l'ombre et l'utopie* (Paris: Seuil, 2005), pp. 84–87.

25 'La *stasis* n'apparait pas tant comme la venue brutale d'un irrationel caché qui activerait des principes maléfiques que comme la radicalisation des mécanismes déjà en jeu dans le reste du déroulement des événements, y compris le long processus de civilisation': Pierre Ponchon, *La rationalité tragique. Essai sur la constitution d'une forme de pensée d'Héraclite à Thucidyde et sur sa critique platonicienne*, Ph.D. thesis, Clermont-Ferrand, p. 686. The terms used by Thucydides for these disrupting events is *kinesis*: see Mario Bonazzi, 'Il Movimento reale. Tucidide sulla guerra e l'uomo', in *Guerra e pace. Storia e teoria di un'esperienza filosofica e politica*, ed. by Carlo Altini (Bologna: Il Mulino, 2015), pp. 35–49.

26 Enzo Paci, *Storia del pensiero presocratico* (Rome: ERI, 1957), p. 313.

27 Thomas, 'Thucydides' Intellectual Milieu', p. 106.

man's inability to deal with a disease which exceeds his capacities — whether a sick person would die or not was unpredictable, for no human art (neither medicine nor religious practices) could prevent it.[28] Such uncertainty engenders two alternative attitudes. On the one hand, this sense of impotence predictably leads to despondency (*athymia*) and despair (*anelpiston*), not only in the case of the sick persons themselves, by now resigned to die, but also in the case of their relatives, who are unable to bear the groans of the sick. On the other hand, however, a new sense of solidarity emerges, at least in some persons, who 'made it a point of honour (*aischyne*) to visit their friends without sparing themselves'.

In the second part (2. 52–53) the perspective is not longer focused on individual choices and behaviours, but rather concerns the city as a whole. In this case, what Thucydides observes is the progressive affirmation of *anomia*, the breaking down of laws or customs, which results from despondency (2. 53. 1)[29] — 'No fear of gods or law of men restrained anyone' (2. 53. 4). The first example is the upheaval of funerary traditions (*nomoi*), which are now fulfilled without *aischyne* ('and many resorted to shameless modes of burial', 2. 53. 4). As the plague becomes more and more oppressive, the first type of behaviour, out of the two just mentioned, appears to become predominant and soon affects other aspects (*ta alla*, 2. 53. 1) of societal life too. Interpersonal attachments and communal bonds collapse. In the context of growing confusion,[30] people no longer seem interested in respecting the rules and moral codes of societal life, and apparently nothing can curb these unsocial tendencies. Fear of the gods[31] or of human laws are no longer a sufficient bridle, as new priorities take the lead: the pursuit of immediate pleasure and gain outweighs respect for the *kalon* (the honourable, noble or fine; this is another term belonging to the sphere of moral values). As a consequence, any kind of moral uprightness somehow present at the beginning quickly seems to disappear once the pandemic begins to ravage the city. In short, this is what Thucydides observes. A comparison with some other important passages from his book will help us to better understand the strategic importance of this description.

As several scholars have noted, the fact that the account of the plague occurs right after Pericles' funeral speech adds to its dramatic force.[32] Right before his description of the outbreak of the plague, Thucydides reports Pericles' speech in honour of those who had died in battle the previous year (2. 35–47). This is probably the most famous

28 On the unpredictability of death in pandemics and its social effects, see chapter 9 of this volume.

29 For a parallel in medical literature see *Epid.* III, 1, case 11, and *Sacr. Dis.*, 4.

30 In consequence of some military decisions, the inhabitants of the countryside moved to the city, causing overcrowding, 2. 52. 1.

31 It is interesting to observe that Thucydides' remarks about the collapse of religious belief and practice seems to contrast with the theories of several modern historians, who see the experience of the plague as the traumatic event *par excellence* which led to a religious revival: see William D. Furley, 'Thucydides and Religion', in *Brill's Companion to Thucydides*, ed. by Antonios Rengakos and Antonis Tsamakis (Leiden: Brill, 2006), pp. 415–38 (pp. 431–32) for an analysis of this problem.

32 See, for instance, Arnold Wycombe Gomme, *A Historical Commentary on Thucydides* (Oxford: Clarendon Press, 1945), vol. 2, p. 161 and especially Eirene Visvardi, *Emotion in Action. Thucydides and the Tragic Chorus* (Leiden: Brill, 2015), pp. 49–56.

part of his book, thanks to its magnificent celebration of democratic Athens as the ideal human community, projected towards success and glory.[33] The contrast with the description of the plague, which immediately follows, is clearly intentional and could hardly have been stronger.[34] The greatness of Pericles' virtuous Athenians depends on a combination of intelligence and audacity, *logos* and *tolma*; their confidence in human resourcefulness, in human *logos*, is fueled by the ambition, *tolma*, to always move further (2. 43. 1). The experience of the plague reveals the fragility of this combination. Reason, *logos*, turns out to be much weaker than Pericles and his Athenians could possibly have imagined.[35] Equally importantly, the new situation created by the plague also shows what audacity — a central motif in Pericles' speech — really means. *Tolma* now appears in a new, negative, light (2. 53. 1). It is not that positive spirit of enterprise which always pushes the Athenians to act bravely; it is rather a selfish impulse to pursue one's own interest and pleasure. The plague, in other words, brings out a more violent and greedy dimension, an unsocial and anti-political aspect of human nature that Pericles' speech had kept artfully hidden. What is more, this extreme event also reveals how superficial and weak any sense of morality was: celebrated as an essential component of social life in the epitaph (2. 37. 3), it quickly disappears during the pandemic, leaving the field open to the selfish pursuit of pleasure and interest (2. 53. 3: 'the pleasure of the moment and whatever was in any way conducive to it came to be regarded as at once honourable and expedient, *kalon kai chresimon*').[36]

Unsurprisingly, the same dynamics also emerge in the description of the *stasis* in Corcyra.[37] The moment 'the supply of daily wants' is cut off (3. 82. 2), citizens' behaviour in Corcyra comes to resemble that of the Athenians hit by the plague (see, for instance, 3. 81. 5).[38] Passions dominate the human mind and reason, leading citizens to embark on daring and bold undertakings (3. 83); parental bonds, moral duties and respect for the divine (3. 82. 6) all fail to prevent increasingly bestial actions, and the result is the triumph of *anomia*, the progressive collapse of society. Indeed, events in Corcyra are even more dramatic than in Athens: *stasis*, civil war, is the most radical event, and as a consequence the most revealing, especially with respect to political dynamics. But the anthropological model remains the same, with the impossible combination of reason on the one hand and audacity and greed on

33 See Connor, *Thucydides*, pp. 68–69; Mauro Bonazzi, *Atene la città inquieta* (Torino: Einaudi, 2017), pp. 91–99, with further bibliography.

34 See also 2. 34. 1, with the emphatic reference to the *patrios nomos* that governs funeral practices.

35 Parry, 'The Language of Thucydides', p. 116: 'The plague offers the most violent challenge to the Periclean attempt to exert some kind of rational control over the historical process'.

36 See also the implicit opposition between the emphasis on *patrios nomos* at 2. 34. 1 (introducing Pericles' speech) and the reference to *nomoi* at 2. 52. 4 ('the shameless modes of burial').'The narrative of the plague exposes the instability of Athenian *gnome* as this was presented in the funeral oration, namely an effortless ability to judge and choose ethical behavior that consolidates individual independence and collective cohesion': Visvardi, *Emotion in Action*, p. 54.

37 For a detailed comparison, see Clifford Orwin, '*Stasis* and Plague: Thucydides on the Dissolution of Society', *Journal of Politics*, 50 (1988), pp. 831–47.

38 Connor, *Thucydides*, pp. 99–102.

the other.[39] Using a memorable expression, Thucydides describes *stasis* as the violent teacher (*biaios didaskalos*) that taught the Greeks not only how to become violent but also, and more importantly, how to reflect on their own violent nature.[40] The lesson of the plague, which is described as advancing like a military attack,[41] is no different. These radical experiences reveal that there is an ongoing conflict between reason and irrational desires, resulting in the victory of the latter, and in ever-greater audacity, which can potentially lead to the collapse of the political community.[42] Which is precisely what happened to Athens.

Indeed, in the context of Athenian intellectual debates, Thucydides' analysis stands out for its originality. One of the most hotly debated topics was progress and the origins of human civilization. The common belief being that human society had progressed from an unsecure and violent past, the discussion was about the causes of such progress: whether it depended on the development of *technai* such as medicine and agriculture or on political skills.[43] Against this background, Thucydides' remarks about the powerlessness and ignorance of doctors in the face of the plague cannot but sound extremely polemical with respect to the optimism implicit in these theories. But this implicit polemic does not mean that he was siding with those thinkers who laid emphasis on the importance of politics as the real factor responsible for human progress. On the contrary, an analysis of special events such as war and the plague reveals just how unstable human society is. In a city such as Athens, which had made *nomos* its watchword, the emphasis on *anomia* emerged in all its paradoxical and provocative complexity. Perhaps somewhat surprisingly, the scientifically minded and rigorous Thucydides turns out to be much closer to the traditional world of poets such as Homer and Sophocles than one would have expected — although he does not share their religious beliefs and therefore leaves human beings in an even more precarious condition.[44]

39 One clear and predictable difference between the description of Corcyra and that of the plague is that the former is more focused on political actions, whereas the latter is more focused on individual behaviour.

40 McLeod, 'Thucydides on Faction', p. 53.

41 Parry, 'The Language of Thucydides', p. 116.

42 See Connor, *Thucydides*, pp. 100–01, Michael Mittelstadt, 'The Thucydidean Tragic View: The Moral Implications', *Ramus*, 14 (1985), pp. 59–73 (p. 67) and Price, *Thucydides and Internal War*, pp. 50–57. As correctly remarked by Visvardi, *Emotion in Action*, p. 55, the predominance of passion does not so much mean the disappearance of reason as its subordination.

43 For a reconstruction of these debates, I refer the reader to Mauro Bonazzi, 'Political, all too Political: Again on Protagoras' Myth in its Intellectual Context', *Polis. The Journal for Ancient Political Thought*, 39 (2022), 425-45; a useful collection of these sources is in William Keith Chambers Guthrie, *The Sophists* (Cambridge: Cambridge University Press, 1971), pp. 79–84. With regard to medicine, see *On ancient medicine* 3.

44 As Paul Demont, 'The Causes of the Athenian plague', pp. 74–75, brilliantly remarked, Thucydides reverses the causal order of the tradition — it is not *anomia*, understood as the lack of respect due to the gods, that brings about the disease, but the disease that brings about *anomia*.

Bibliography

Galenus, *De difficultate respirationis*, ed. Karl Gottlob Kühn, vol. 7 (Leipzig: 1824, repr. Hildesheim: Georg Olms Verlagsbuchhandlung, 1965).

Herodotus, *Historiarum libri IX*, ed. Heinrich Rudolf Dietsch (Leipzig: Teubner, 1926–).

Hippocrates, *Ancient Medicine*, in Hippocrates. Volume 1, trans. by W.H.S. Jones (Cambridge, Mass.: Harvard University Press, 1923).

———, *Airs, waters, places*, in Hippocrates. Volume 1, trans. by W.H.S. Jones (Cambridge, Mass.: Harvard University Press, 1923).

———, *Epidemics 1 and 3*, in Hippocrates. Volume 1, trans. by W.H.S. Jones (Cambridge, Mass.: Harvard University Press, 1923).

———, *Breaths*, in Hippocrates. Volume 2, trans. by W.H.S. Jones (Cambridge, Mass.: Harvard University Press, 1923).

———, *The Sacred Disease*, in Hippocrates. Volume 2, trans. by W.H.S. Jones (Cambridge, Mass.: Harvard University Press, 1923).

———, *Nature of Man*, in Hippocrates. Volume 4, trans. by W.H.S. Jones (Cambridge, Mass.: Harvard University Press, 1931).

Plato, *Symposium*, in Platonis *Opera*, ed. J. Burnet, vol. II (Oxford: Clarendon, 1899).

Strabo, *Geographica*, ed. August Meineke (Leipzig: Teubner: 1895–1899).

Thucydides, *History of the Peloponnesian War*, with an English Translation by Charles F. Smith (Cambridge, Mass.: Harvard University Press, 1959).

***

Bonazzi, Mauro, 'Il Movimento reale. Tucidide sulla guerra e l'uomo', in *Guerra e pace. Storia e teoria di un'esperienza filosofica e politica*, ed. by Carlo Altini (Bologna: Il Mulino, 2015), pp. 35–49.

———, *Atene la città inquieta* (Torino: Einaudi, 2017).

———, *The Sophists* (Cambridge University Press: Cambridge, 2020).

———, 'Political, all too Political: Again on Protagoras Myth in its Intellectual Context', *Polis. The Journal for Ancient Political Thought*, 39 (2022), 425-445.

Cochrane, Charles Norris, *Thucydides and the Science of History* (Oxford University Press: London, 1929).

Connor, W. Robert, *Thucydides* (Princeton: Princeton University Press, 1984).

Craik, Elizabeth M., 'Thucydides on the Plague: Physiology of Flux and Fixation', *Classical Quarterly*, 51 (2001), pp. 102–8.

Demont, Paul, 'Notes sur le récit de la pestilence athénienne chez Thucydide et sur ses rapports avec la médecine grecque de l'époque classique', in *Formes de la pensée dans la Collecion Hippocratique* ed. by François Lasserre and Philippe Mudry (Drosz: Genève, 1983), pp. 341–53.

———, 'The Causes of the Athenian Plague and Thucydides', in *Thucydides between History and Literature*, ed. by Antonis Tsakmakis and Melina Tamiolaki (Berlin: De Gruyter, 2013), pp. 73–87.

Fleming, Rebecca, 'Galen and the Plague', in *Galens'* peri alypias *and the History of the Roman Empire*, ed. by Caroline Petit (Leiden: Brill, 2019), pp. 219–44.
Furley, William D., 'Thucydides and Religion', in *Brill's Companion to Thucydides*, ed. by Antonios Rengakos and Antonis Tsamakis (Leiden: Brill, 2006), pp. 415–38.
Gomme, Arnold Wycombe, *A Historical Commentary on Thucydides*, vol. 2 (Oxford: Clarendon Press, 1945).
Guthrie, William Keith Chambers, *The Sophists* (Cambridge: Cambridge University Press, 1971).
Holladay, A. J., and Poole, J. F. C., 'Thucydides and the Plague of Athens', *Classical Quarterly* 29 (1979), pp. 282–300.
Hornblower, Simon, *A Commentary on Thucydides*, vol. 1 (Oxford: Clarendon Press, 1991).
Jouanna, Jacques, 'Air, Miasma, Contagion in the Time of Hippocrates and the Survival of Miasmas in Post-Hippocratic Medicine (Rufus of Ephesus, Galen and Palladius)', in *Greek Medicine from Hippocrates to Galen. Selected Papers*, ed. by Jacques Jouanna (Leiden: Brill, 2012), pp. 121–37.
Lichtenthaeler, Charles, *Thucydide et Hippocrate vus par un historien-medecin* (Droz: Geneve, 1965)
Lloyd, Geoffrey Ernest Richard, *In the Grip of Disease. Studies in Greek Imagination* (Oxford: Oxford University Press, 2003).
Loraux, Nicole, 'Thucydide et la sédition dans les mots', in Ead., *La tragédie d'Athènes. La politique entre l'ombre et l'utopie* (Paris: Seuil, 2005), pp. 84–87.
MacLeod, Colin, 'Thucydides on Faction', *Proceedings of the Cambridge Philological Society*, 205 (1979), pp. 52–68.
Mittelstadt, Michael, 'The Thucydidean Tragic View: The Moral Implications', *Ramus*, 14 (1985), pp. 59–73.
Morgan, Thomas E., 'Plague or Poetry? Thucydides on the Epidemic at Athens', *Transactions of the American Philological Association*, 124 (1994), pp. 197–209.
Orwin, Clifford, '*Stasis* and Plague: Thucydides on the Dissolution of Society', *Journal of Politics*, 50 (1988), pp. 831–47.
Paci, Enzo, *Storia del pensiero presocratico* (Rome: ERI, 1957).
Page, Denys Lionel, 'Thucydides' Description of the Great Plague at Athens', *Classical Quarterly*, 47 (1953), pp. 97–119.
Parry, Adam, 'The Language of Thucydides' Description of the Plague', *Bulletin of the Institute of Classical Studies*, 16 (1969), pp. 106–18.
Ponchon, Pierre, *La rationalité tragique. Essai sur la constitution d'une forme de pensée d'Héraclite à Thucidyde et sur sa critique platonicienne*, Ph.D. thesis, Clermont-Ferrand.
Price, Jonathan J., *Thucydides and Internal War* (Cambridge: Cambridge University Press, 2001).
Rawlings, Hunter R., *A Semantic Study of* prophasis *to 400 B.C.* (Wiesbaden: Hermes, 1975).
Rechenhauer, Georg, *Thukydides und die hippokratische Medizin* (Hildesheim: Olms, 1991)
Thomas, Rosalind, 'Thucydides Intellectual Milieu and the Plague', in *Brill's Companion to Thucydides*, ed. by Antonios Rengakos and Antonis Tsamakis (Leiden: Brill, 2006), pp. 87–108.
Visvardi, Eirene, *Emotion in Action. Thucydides and the Tragic Chorus* (Leiden: Brill, 2015).

MARCO DI BRANCO

2. Between Religion and Science

The Debate on the Concept of Contagion in the Medieval Islamic World and its Western Parallels

▼ **ABSTRACT** The notion of contagion was looked upon with suspicion in the Arabic medical tradition. Medieval Islamic theologians generally ascribed epidemics to the will of God, denied contagion, and believed that an epidemic disease was to be accepted as a fatality, or even a blessing for the believer, as dying of plague could be regarded as a form of martyrdom that granted direct access to paradise. By contrast, in the works of two fourteenth-century Arab Andalusian intellectuals, Ibn Ḫātima, d. 1369 *c.*, and Ibn al-Ḫaṭīb, 1313–1374, we find clear clinical evidence of the contagious nature of the fourteenth-century plague outbreak. The paper explores the contribution Ibn Ḫātima and Ibn al-Ḫaṭīb gave to the concept of contagion, understood as disease transmission through direct contact or by proximity.

As is known, one of the first detailed descriptions of an epidemic which has come down to us is that of the so-called 'plague of Athens' (*c.* 429–426 BCE) by the Greek historian Thucydides (d. 399/398 BCE), a section of which is dedicated to the problem of contagion:

> The plague (ἡ νόσος) is said to have come first of all from Ethiopia beyond Egypt and from there it fell on Egypt and Libya and on much of the [other] lands. It struck the city of Athens suddenly. People in the Piraeus caught it first, and so, since there were not yet any fountains there, they actually alleged that the Peloponnesians had put poison in the wells. Afterwards, it arrived in the upper city too, and then deaths started to occur on a much larger scale. Everyone, whether doctor or layman, may say from his own experience what the origin of it is likely to have been, and what causes he thinks had the power to bring about so great a change. I shall give a statement of what it was like, which people can study in case it should ever attack again, to equip themselves with foreknowledge so that they shall not fail to recognize it. I can give this account because I both suffered the disease myself and saw other victims of it [...]. The nature of the disease was

Epidemics and Pandemics, ed. by Michele Nicoletti and Alessandro Palazzo (Turnhout: Brepols, 2024), pp. 37–52
BREPOLS PUBLISHERS 10.1484/M.STPH-EB.5.136406

> beyond description, and the sufferings that it brought to each victim were greater than human nature can bear. There is one particular point in which it showed that it was unlike the usual run of illnesses: the birds and animals which feed on human flesh either kept away from the bodies, although there were many unburied, or if they did taste them, it proved fatal. To confirm this, there was an evident shortage of birds of that kind, which were not to be seen either near the victims or anywhere else. What happened was particularly noticeable in the case of dogs, since they live with human beings. Apart from the various unusual features in the different effects which it had on different people, that was the general nature of the disease. None of the other common afflictions occurred at that time; or any that did end in this. Some victims were neglected and died; others died despite a great deal of care. There was not a single remedy, you might say, which ought to be applied to give relief, for what helped one sufferer harmed another. No kind of constitution, whether strong or weak, proved sufficient against the plague, but it killed off all, whatever regime was used to care for them. The most terrifying aspect of the whole affliction was the despair which resulted when someone realized that he had the disease: people immediately lost hope, and so through their attitude of mind were much more likely to let themselves go and not hold out. In addition, one person caught the disease through caring for another, and so they died like sheep: this was the greatest cause of loss of life. If people were afraid and unwilling to go near to others, they died in isolation, and many houses lost all their occupants through the lack of anyone to care for them. Those who did go near to others died, especially those with any claim to virtue, who from a sense of honor did not spare themselves in going to visit their friends, persisting when in the end even the members of the family were overcome by the scale of the disaster and gave up their dirges for the dead.[1]

The plague of Athens is treated by Thucydides with careful attention to the recording of empirical detail without suggesting any reasons for the epidemic. His purpose is entirely instructive in the hope that future generations would be able to learn from the lessons of the past. In this sense, the consideration that persons caught the disease through caring for others, and that people were afraid and unwilling to go near others, since those who did died, especially those who did not spare themselves in going to visit their friends, is particularly interesting. These reflections of Thucydides suggest an awareness of the fact that contact with the sick could expose

---

1 Thucydides, *History of the Peloponnesian War*, 2. 7. 3–54, ed. and trans. by Martin Hammond and Peter John Rhodes (Oxford: Oxford University Press, 2009) pp. 112–16. On this famous description see A. James Holladay and J.C.F. Poole, 'Thucydides and the Plague of Athens', *Classical Quarterly*, 29 (1979), pp. 282–300; Clifford Orwin, 'Thucydides on the Dissolution of Society', *Journal of Politics*, 50 (1988), pp. 831–47; Thomas E. Morgan, 'Plague or Poetry? Thucydides on the Epidemic at Athens', *Transactions of the American Philological Association*, 124 (1994), pp. 197–209; Donald A. Nielsen, 'Pericles and the Plague: Civil Religion, Anomie, and Injustice in Thucydides', *Sociology of Religion*, 57 (1996), pp. 397–407; Elizabeth M. Craik, 'Thucydides on the Plague: Physiology of Flux and Fixation', *Classical Quarterly*, 51 (2001), pp. 102–08.

First of all, Muslim intellectuals devoted themselves to organizing the vast body of knowledge they had acquired. The theoretical discourse on the causes and symptoms of diseases was enriched, taking as a model the methods of Greek medicine, without any consideration for the medical treatises of the Byzantine era. One of the greatest scholars of medieval Arabic medicine was Abū Bakr Muḥammad b. Zakariyyā al-Rāzī (*c.* 865–925 CE). In his opinion, neither Plato nor Aristotle nor Hippocrates nor Galen could be overcome, but he does not hesitate to modify their philosophical conclusions and to add to the mass of medical knowledge derived from the Greco-Roman tradition the results of of his own research and observations. For example, whenever he deals with a particular disease, he begins by summarizing the set of data that could be found on the subject in the Greek or Indian sources available in Arabic translation and in the works of the Islamic physicians of his time, before always adding his own opinion or personal judgment.[15] Rāzī was a doctor at the Samanid court of Bukhara and directed the hospitals of Rayy and Baghdad. His most famous work is the treatise *Kitāb fī 'l-ǧadarī wa-'l-ḥaṣba* (*On Smallpox and Measles*), a topic that had already been addressed in a little known treatise by Tābit b. Qurrà (d. 901 CE). Rāzī's text clearly shows his interest in therapeutics and this contrasts strongly with the silence on the subject that characterizes the Greek and Byzantine treatises that have come down to us. In general, Rāzī's works contain numerous extracts from ancient authors concerning diseases and therapeutics, to which he adds the description of the clinical cases he himself deals with. However, he seems to be disinterested in the classification of symptoms: his respect for Galen is not enough to prevent him from correcting the theories of the great Greek physician and his criticisms mainly concern questions of logic and clinical application. For example, he states that in his hospital experiences of Rayy and Baghdad he had had many clinical cases that, in their evolution, had not followed the descriptions of the diseases by Galen. And yet, Rāzī does not dispute the foundations of Galen's medical theory and indeed considers it substantially correct and reliable. As a result, Rāzī's work completely lacks reflection on the concept of contagion.[16]

The best-known figure in the field of medieval Arabic medicine is undoubtedly Abū 'Alī al-Ḥusayn b. 'Abdallāh b. Sīnā, latinized as Avicenna (980–1037 CE). Born in a small village near Bukhara, after studying philosophy and medicine, he traveled through the territories of the Middle East, serving as a minister to the Buyid dynasty of Persia. He was an extremely prolific author and composed treatises on sexual hygiene, cardiology, respiratory diagnostics, phlebotomy, dietetics, and various works dedicated to the treatment of colic, intermittent fevers, and diabetes. The great work of Ibn Sīnā, for which he is famous in the West, is the *Kitāb al qānūn fī 'l-ṭibb* (*Canon of Medicine*). It was composed over a long period of time: it was begun in Gurgān, in northern Persia, continued in Rayy, and completed in Hamadān. This great encyclopedia replaced all the other circulating medical treatises. Ibn Sīnā, who, unlike Rāzī,

15 See, e.g., Richard Walzer, *Greek into Arabic: Essays on Islamic Philosophy* (Oxford: Bruno Cassirer, 1962), pp. 14–16.

16 Savage-Smith, 'Médecine', pp. 166–72.

never cites his sources, divides his treatise into five books. The first book consists of four parts: 1) the elements, the humours, the anatomy of the homogeneous parts (muscles, bones, nerves, arteries, and veins), and the three faculties; 2) the general symptoms of diseases and diagnostics; 3) hygiene and dietetics, the medical problems of childhood, adulthood, and old age, the effects of climate change, and medical advice to travelers; and 4) general methods of treatment, surgical interventions, and pain relief. The second book of the *Qānūn* concerns medicinal products (*materia medica*), classified in alphabetical order; the third book deals with the diseases typical of certain parts of the body presented in an order that goes from head to toe; the causes, symptoms, and treatments of these diseases are extensively examined; the fourth book deals with diseases not specific to a single part and is divided into four sections: 1) fevers; 2) pustules, abscesses, ulcers, swellings, leprosy, smallpox, wounds, fractures, and dislocations; 3) infections, insect bites, and animal bites; and 4) cosmetics, obesity and thinness, hair, skin, nail care, and unpleasant odors.[17] In the work by Ibn Sīnā, the Greek, Byzantine, and Syriac medical traditions are enriched by the personal observations of the author and this produces a coherent and organized medical system. This system, essentially Galenic in nature, but very modified and extremely elaborate, actually became the real canon of Islamic medicine, although it was sometimes criticized for its excessive difficulty and for its 'philosophical' character. In any case, the concept of contagion is once again absent from the methodological horizon of Ibn Sīnā: according to him, for example, a sure sign of an approaching plague epidemic was that rats and subterranean animals flee to the surface of the earth, and behave as if they were intoxicated before dying. Although this is an exact description of the effects of a plague epizootic, it was believed at that time that animals perceived the evil miasma before men. Thus, Ibn Sīnā considered the rats only a forewarning of the plague, not its cause and his analysis of the disease is strongly influenced by the *De differentiis febrium* by Galen, which had been translated into Arabic by Qusṭā ibn Lūqā (d. *c.* 912 CE).

When confronted with the phenomenon of the epidemics, Muslims generally ascribed its ultimate cause to the will of God. As Michael Walters Dols has written, 'the majority of the Muslim legal scholars who wrote plague treatises were more interested in the theological explanation of the disease than in physical causation; the latter was of greater concern to the physicians, various naturalistic interpretations are usually found randomly lumped together with religious explanations, differing only in degrees of emphasis according to an individual author's point of view'.[18] Consequently, the Muslim authors at the time of the Black Death adopted the 'miasmatic' theory of epidemics from Hippocrates and Galen, either directly or indirectly through the commentaries of Muslim doctors, especially Ibn Sīnā. In fact, the study of Hippocrates and Galen was the mainstay of the general medical education in the

17 For an introduction to the work by Ibn Sīnā, see, e.g., Lenn E. Goodman, *Avicenna* (London–New York: Routledge, 1992) and Olga Lizzini, *Avicenna* (Roma: Carocci, 2012).

18 Michael Walters Dols, *The Black Death in the Middle East* (Princeton: Princeton University Press, 1977), p. 85.

medieval period.[19] For example, in his monograph *Kitāb fī 'l-ʿidā* (*Book of Transmission [of Diseases]*), Qusṭā ibn Lūqā explains the phenomenon in the following way: penetrating into the organism of other individuals, the air infected by the patient first damages their vital pneuma, then the blood, and finally the organs, exactly as it happens in the patient, and consequently the symptoms presented by the various patients are the same. This author reactualizes the tradition of the already mentioned *problemata physica,* in which some immaterial forms of contagion by 'sympathy' were described, which were believed to pass, for example, through a smile or yawn. In this way, however, the medical concept of contagion ran the risk of remaining confined to the field of magic, which was very widespread in popular beliefs but condemned by Islamic religious authorities. The Prophet had in fact forbidden magic and divination as part of those pagan customs fought by Islām. Moreover, since in a saying attributed to the Prophet (*ḥadīṯ*) on the ineffectiveness of the various divinatory practices there was the mention of the term *ʿidā* ('transmission'), here understood in a magical sense, and since the same term was used by doctors to designate the transmission of a disease, theologians deduced that contagion as such did not exist and that the fact of contracting a disease during an epidemic was to be accepted as inevitable. Other sayings of the Prophet then affirmed the prohibition on entering a region infested by the plague and leaving it to escape the disease. The plague was declared a blessing for the believer: death as a result of the disease was considered a form of martyrdom and as such would ensure direct access to paradise.[20] In the manuals and practical compendiums, the sentence of theologians relating to contagion had not yet found any echo, and this was also because the concrete opportunity to experience the phenomenon had been missed. Their authors merely supplemented the Galenic list of contagious diseases, adding some of them, such as diaphragmitis, smallpox, and leprosy. Only the plague of the fourteenth century, a highly infectious disease, with its sudden onset and ability to affect a large part of the population,[21] provided the opportunity to study more closely the contagion and its mechanism. In this field, a fundamental role was played by two Andalusian intellectuals: Ibn Ḫātima (d. 770/1369 *c.*) and Ibn al-Ḫaṭīb (1313–1374).[22] Alongside terrestrial and

19 On the idea of epidemics in the Early Islamic world, see Lawrence I. Conrad, 'Tāʿūn and Wabāʾ Conceptions of Plague and Pestilence in Early Islam', *Journal of the Economic and Social History of the Orient*, 25 (1982), pp. 268–307. Cf. also Giovanni Filoramo and Rosa Maria Parriniello, *Guarire dal contagio. Riti e parole delle grandi religioni* (Milano: Jaca Book, 2020), pp. 99-116.

20 On this topic, see for example Ursula Weisser, *Zeugung, Vererbung und pränatale Entwicklung in der Medizin des arabisch-islamischen Mittelalters* (Erlangen: Lüling, 1983), passim.

21 On the subject, see in general Anna Montgomery Campbell, *The Black Death and Men of Learning* (New York: Coloumbia University Press, 1931); *Pandemic Disease in the Medieval World: Rethinking the Black Death*, ed. by Monica H. Green (Kalamazoo–Bradford: ARC Medieval Press, 2015); John Aberth, *Doctoring the Black Death: Medieval Europe's Medical Response to Plague* (Lanham–Boulder–New York–London: Roman and Littlefield, 2021).

22 On these two scholars and their works, see in particular Dols, *The Black Death*, pp. 92–94; Ernst Seidel, 'Die Lehre von der Kontagion bei den Arabern', *Archiv für Geschichte der Medizin*, 6 (1912), pp. 81–93; Russell Hopley, 'Contagion In Islamic Lands: Responses from Medieval Andalusia and North Africa', *Journal for Early Modern Cultural Studies*, 10 (2010), pp. 45–64; William B. Ober and Nabil Alloush, 'The

celestial explanations for the causation of the pestilential miasma, an immediate cause was believed to be contagion: in fact, in the treatises of the Andalusian physicians there is clear clinical evidence of the contagious nature of the pandemic. Like in the Boccaccio's description of the plague, contamination of the air may arise from the sick and their clothing, bedding, and utensils.

Ibn Ḫātima described the spread of the plague in his hometown in southern Spain, Almería, and gave an exact picture of its symptoms, already distinguishing between bubonic plague and pneumonic plague and describing the primary pneumonic plague, of which he emphasized its highly infectious character. In an interesting illustration of the concept of contagion, the author observed that among the inhabitants of the Sūq al-Ḫalq in Almería, where the flea-laden clothes and bedding of the sick were sold, almost everyone perished. Furthermore, Ibn Ḫātima shed light on the fact that contact with individuals suffering from the disease caused the appearance of the disease in the same form, either bubonic or pulmonary:

> I have noticed, after long efforts, that when a man touches a sick person, he is seized by the same disease and the signs of this appear on him: if the blood drips from the sick, it also drips from the other; if a tumor appears in the first, it also appears in the second in the same place, and if abscesses are formed in the first and pus drips from him, the same thing happens to the other. Identical is the way of propagation from the second sick person to the third.[23]

In order not to conflict with religion, he rejected the magical interpretation of the contagion spread among the Bedouins and traced the phenomenon back to a law of nature established by God. The miasmas coming from the breath and exhalations of the sick were not only transmitted through the air, but also infected the objects with which they had come into contact; this would have explained the high mortality among the rags of the bazaar, where the clothes and beds belonging to the victims of the plague were sold.

In his treatise *Muqniʿat al-sā'il ʿan al-marad al-hā'il* (*A very useful inquiry into the horrible sickness*), Ibn al-Ḫaṭīb, an historian and physician who served as vizier at the Nasrid court in Granada, explained in detail the different forms of the course of the plague on the basis of the doctrines of Galen; he also analysed the modalities of the transmission of the disease that could occur indirectly through the clothes or jewelry. In order to show that the spread of the plague occurred through contagion, he made a series of epidemiological observations, such as the concomitance between the arrival of an individual from an infected region and the manifestation of the epidemic, the spread of individual outbreaks, as well as several cases in which groups of people kept in strict isolation in an environment where the disease was raging remained immune from contagion:

Plague at Granada, 1348–1349: Ibn al-Khatib and Ideas of Contagion', *Bulletin of the New York Academy of Medicine*, 58 (1982), pp. 418–24, and *Ibn al-Jaṭīb y su tiempo*, ed. by Celia del Moral and Fernando Velásquez Basanta (Granada: Editorial Universidad de Granada, 2012).

23 Cited in Djebbar, *Storia della scienza araba*, p. 293.

> It becomes clear to anyone who has diagnosed or treated the disease that most of the individuals who have had contact with a plague victim will die, whereas the man who has had no exposure will remain healthy. A garment or vessel may carry infection into a house; even an earring can prove fatal to the man who has put it in his ear. The disease can make its first appearance in a single house of a given town, then spread from that focus to other persons — neighbors, relatives, visitors. The disease can break out in a coastal town that had been free of the disease until a plague victim landed there, coming across the sea from a town where plague is raging. The date at which plague appears in the town coincides with [i.e. occurs a few days after] the debarkation of this carrier. Many people remained in good health who kept themselves in isolation from the outside world, for example the pious Ibn Abī-Madyān in Salé. He believed in contagion; therefor he laid by a store of provisions and bricked up his house, sequestering his large family. The town was severely stricken, but no one in his household took ill. There are many accounts of communities remote from highways and commerce that remained unscathed. There is also the remarkable example of the prisoners in the Arsenal at Seville who were unaffected even though the city itself was hard hit. Other reports tell us that itinerant nomads who live in tents in North Africa remained free of disease because the air is not shut in, and the corruption from it is only mildly infectious.[24]

Unlike Ibn Ḫātima, Ibn al-Ḫaṭīb directly attacked theologians, accusing them of having caused the death of countless people. This was because they had denied contagion, despite overwhelming evidence to the contrary, prohibiting in their legal opinions the escape from infected places:

> And amidst the horrible afflictions that the plague has imposed upon the people, God has afflicted the people with some learned religious scholars who issue *fatwās* [against fleeing the plague], so that the quills with which the scholars wrote these *fatwās* were like swords upon which the Muslims died [...]. Although the intent of the divine law is innocent of harm, when a prophetic statement is contradicted by the senses and observation, it is incumbent upon us to interpret it in a way so that the *ḥadīṯ* fits reality, even if we claim to subscribe to the literal meaning of the *ḥadīṯ* and, lest we forget, to the fundamentals of the divine law that everybody knows about. And the truth of this matter is that it should be interpreted in accordance with those who affirm the theory of contagion. Moreover, there are in the divine law many indications that support the theory of contagion, such as the statement of Muḥammad: 'A disease should not visit a healthy man', or the statement that: 'One escapes the fate of God to meet the fate of God'. But this is not the place to go on at length concerning this matter, because the discussion about whether the divine law agrees or disagrees with the contagion theory is not the business of the medical art, but is incidental to it. And

24 Ibn al-Ḫaṭīb, *Muqni'at al-sā'il 'an al-marad al-hā'il*, cited in Ober and Alloush, 'The Plague at Granada, 1348–1349', p. 422.

> in conclusion, to ignore the proofs for plague contagion is an indecency and an affront to God and holds cheap the lives of Muslims. And some of the learned holy men have retracted their *fatwās* for fear of helping people to their deaths. May God keep us from committing error in word and deed![25]

According to Ibn al-Ḫaṭīb, therefore, it would have been necessary to try to harmonize the tradition with direct experience or rather to follow the *ḥadīṯ* of the Prophet favourable to the hypothesis of the contagious character of the disease.

Although Ibn al-Ḫaṭīb was not yet able to provide a theory of contagion, as Girolamo Fracastoro did in his famous treatise *De Contagione* (1546),[26] his clear statement in favour of the pre-eminence of direct experience rather than religious tradition is particularly noteworthy; in fact, he did observe contagion-infection empirically. Unlike all other Muslim scholars, and possibly as a rebuttal to Ibn Ḫātima's maintenance of orthodoxy specifically, Ibn al-Ḫaṭīb denied the legal statements of the Islamic jurisconsults against the theory of contagion, and stated: 'The existence of the contagion is well-established through experience, research, sense perception, autopsy and authenticated information, and this material is the proof'.[27]

As Dols has rightly underlined, 'it should be borne in mind that Ibn al-Ḫaṭīb's treatise was conceived within the framework of the miasmic theory, which differs radically from the modern germ theory of disease. In any case, the human transmission of the plague as interpreted by Ibn al-Ḫaṭīb was unacceptable to the orthodox Muslim view of a divine act. The studies of this author are a clear example of innovation at a time of crisis, within a traditional and authoritative body of thought'.

The conflict between Ibn al-Ḫaṭīb and the Islamic jurisconsults should not, however, be interpreted in modernist terms as a clash between religion and science: in fact, the debate takes place within the Islamic worldview, and, ultimately, concerns the correct interpretation of the Prophet's statements.

This brief history of the concept of contagion highlights on the one hand the very long persistence of the Hippocratic-Galenic model, which remained for centuries at the base of Western and Islamic medicine, on the other the limits of the attempt to apply the experimental method within a framework dominated by religion. In this sense, Ibn al-Ḫaṭīb has much in common with Galileo Galilei.

---

25 Ibn al-Ḫaṭīb, *Muqniʿat al-sāʾil ʿan al-maraḍ al-hāʾil*, cited in John Aberth, *The Black Death. The Great Mortality of 1348–1350: A Brief History with Documents* (New York: Palgrave Macmillan, 2005), pp. 115–16.

26 See, e.g., Vivian Nutton, 'The Seeds of Disease: An Explanation of Contagion and Infection from the Greeks to the Renaissance', *Medical History*, 27 (1983), pp. 1–34 as well as chapters 5 and 6 of this volume.

27 Cited in Dols, *The Black Death*, p. 93.

Bibliography

Boccaccio, Giovanni, *Il Decameron*, ed. by Carlo Salinari (Roma-Bari: Laterza, 1986).

Ibn Qayyim al-Jawziyya, *La Médecine du Prophète Muḥammad* (Paris: Les Éditions Albouraq, 2021).

Procopius, *The History of the Wars, Books 1 and 2*, trans. by Henry Bronson Dewing (London–New York: William Heinemman–The Macmillan Co., 1914).

Thucydides, *History of the Peloponnesian War*, ed. and trans. by Martin Hammond and Peter John Rhodes (Oxford: Oxford University Press, 2009).

***

Aberth, John, *The Black Death. The Great Mortality of 1348–1350: A Brief History with Documents* (New York: Palgrave Macmillan, 2005).

———, *Doctoring the Black Death: Medieval Europe's Medical Response to Plague* (Lanham–Boulder–New York–London: Roman and Littlefield, 2021).

Allen, Pauline, '*The "Justinianic" Plague*', *Byzantion*, 49 (1979), pp. 5–20.

Boudon-Millot, Véronique, *Galeno di Pergamo. Un medico greco a Roma*, trans. by Maria Luisa Garofalo (Roma: Carocci, 2020) (orig. ed. *Galien de Pergame, un médicin grec à Rome* [Paris: Les Belles Lettres, 2012]).

Campbell, Anna Montgomery, *The Black Death and Men of Learning* (New York: Columbia University Press, 1931).

Conrad, Lawrence I., 'Ṭāʿūn and Wabāʾ Conceptions of Plague and Pestilence in Early Islam', *Journal of the Economic and Social History of the Orient*, 25 (1982), pp. 268–307.

Craik, Elizabeth M., 'Thucydides on the Plague: Physiology of Flux and Fixation', *Classical Quarterly*, 51 (2001), pp. 102–8.

———, *The 'Hippocratic' Corpus. Content and Context* (London: Routledge, 2014).

D'Ancona, Cristina, *La casa della sapienza. La trasmissione della metafisica greca e la formazione della filosofia araba* (Bologna: Guerini e associati, 2005).

del Moral, Celia, and Velásquez Basanta, Fernando, *Ibn al-Jaṭīb y su tiempo* (Granada: Editorial Universidad de Granada, 2012).

Djebbar, Ahmed, *Storia della scienza araba. Il patrimonio intellettuale dell'Islam*, trans. by Massimo Campanini (Milano: Raffaello Cortina, 2002) (orig. ed. *Une histoire de la science arabe : Introduction à la connaissance du patrimoine scientifique des pays d'Islam*. Entretiens avec Jean Rosmorduc [Paris: Le Seuil, 2001]).

Dols, Michael Walters, *The Black Death in the Middle East* (Princeton: Princeton University Press, 1977).

Endress, Gerhard, 'Die wissenschaftliche Literatur', in *Grundriß der arabischen Philologie*. Vol. 2: *Literaturwissenschaft*, ed. by Helmut Gätje (Wiesbaden: Ludwig Reichert, 1987), pp. 400–506.

———, 'Die wissenschaftliche Literatur', in *Grundriß der arabischen Philologie*. Vol. 3: *Supplement*, ed. by Wolfdietrich Fischer (Wiesbaden: Ludwig Reichert, 1992), pp. 3–152.

Filoramo, Giovanni and Rosa Maria Parriniello, *Guarire dal contagio. Riti e parole delle grandi religioni* (Milano: Jaca Book, 2020).

Goodman, Lenn E., *Avicenna* (London–New York: Routledge, 1992).
Green, Monica H. (ed.), *Pandemic Disease in the Medieval World: Rethinking the Black Death* (Kalamazoo–Bradford: ARC Medieval Press, 2015).
Gutas, Dimitri, *Greek Thought, Arabic Culture: The Graeco-Arabic Translation Movement in Baghdad and Early Abbasid Society (2nd-4th/8th-10th Centuries)* (London–New York: Routledge, 1998).
Holladay, A. James, and Poole, J.C.F., 'Thucydides and the Plague of Athens', *Classical Quarterly*, 29 (1979), pp. 282–300.
Hopley, Russell, 'Contagion In Islamic Lands: Responses from Medieval Andalusia and North Africa', *Journal for Early Modern Cultural Studies*, 10 (2010), pp. 45–64.
Little, Lester K. (ed.), *Plague and the End of Antiquity: The Pandemic of 541–750* (Cambridge, Cambridge University Press, 2006).
Lizzini, Olga, *Avicenna* (Roma: Carocci, 2012).
Marafioti, Martin, 'Post-*Decameron* Plague Treatises and the Boccacian Innovation of Narrative Prophylaxis', *Annali d'Italianistica* 23, *Literature & Science*, (2005), pp. 69–87.
Morgan, Thomas E., 'Plague or Poetry? Thucydides on the Epidemic at Athens', *Transactions of the American Philological Association*, 124 (1994), pp. 197–209.
Nielsen, Donald A., 'Pericles and the Plague: Civil Religion, Anomie, and Injustice in Thucydides', *Sociology of Religion*, 57 (1996), pp. 397–407.
Nutton, Vivian, 'The Seeds of Disease: An Explanation of Contagion and Infection from the Greeks to the Renaissance', *Medical History*, 27 (1983), pp. 1–34.
Ober, William B., and Alloush, Nabil, 'The Plague at Granada, 1348–1349: Ibn al-Khatib and Ideas of Contagion', *Bulletin of the New York Academy of Medicine*, 58 (1982), pp. 418–24.
Oikonomopoulou, Katerina, 'The *Problemata*'s Medical Books: Structural and Methodological Aspects', in *The Aristotelian* Problemata Physica*: Philosophical and Scientific Investigations*, ed. by Robert Mayhew, (Leiden: Brill, 2015), pp. 61–78.
Orwin, Clifford, 'Thucydides on the Dissolution of Society', *Journal of Politics*, 50 (1988), pp. 831–47.
Savage-Smith, Emilie, 'Médecine', in *Histoire des sciences arabes, 3. Technologie, alchimie et sciences de la vie*, ed. by Roshdi Rashed (Paris: Éditions du Seuil, 1997) pp. 155–212.
Seidel, Ernst, 'Die Lehre von der Kontagion bei den Arabern', *Archiv für Geschichte der Medizin*, 6 (1912), pp. 81–93.
Testa, Giuseppe, *La peste antonina. Storia della prima pandemia dalla Cina alla Roma imperiale* (Roma: Salerno Editrice, 2021).
Walzer, Richard, *Greek into Arabic: Essays on Islamic Philosophy* (Oxford: Bruno Cassirer, 1962).
Weisser, Ursula, *Zeugung, Vererbung und pränatale Entwicklung in der Medizin des arabisch-islamischen Mittelalters* (Erlangen: Lüling, 1983).

ALESSANDRO PALAZZO

3. Pestilences and Contagious Diseases in the Middle Ages

Albert the Great and the Fourteenth-Century Plague Treatises[*]

▼ **ABSTRACT** This paper explores Albert the Great's views on pestilences and contagious diseases. Albert did not dedicate a specific work or part of a work to these topics, but upon thorough inspection it is evident that pestilences were given careful attention within his corpus. Despite objective historical limitations (he did not experience any plague outbreaks during his lifetime and in his works the terms *pestis* and *pestilentia* are vague, covering a large variety of different sicknesses), Albert's investigation of the causes of pestilential and contagious diseases is worthy of consideration. My first claim is that he explained these phenomena in scientific terms and not as a result of God's will, which in the Middle Ages was often invoked as the cause of natural calamities. My second thesis is that Albert's explanatory models provided the basis for the late-medieval discourse on plague. In his works, the fourteenth-century treatises on plague, the so-called *Pestschriften*, found some of the conceptual tools they used to construct the etiological and nosological identity of this devastating disease.

1. Introduction

In the Middle Ages, people were familiar with a whole range of catastrophic events (earthquakes, floods, fires, famines, and wars). Among such calamities, pestilences had particularly devastating and lasting effects, and left deep traces in medieval societies: the undoing of family ties, the undermining of social structures, the impair-

* This publication is part of the research project *Itineraries of Philosophy and Science from Baghdad to Florence: Albert the Great, his Sources and his Legacies* (2023-2025), funded by the Italian Ministry of University and Reserach (PRIN 2022, 20225LFCMZ).

Epidemics and Pandemics, ed. by Michele Nicoletti and Alessandro Palazzo (Turnhout: Brepols, 2024), pp. 53–104
BREPOLS PUBLISHERS 10.1484/M.STPH-EB.5.136407

ment of political institutions, the collapse of economic life, and a sharp demographic decline.

Two plague pandemics hit the medieval world: the Justinianic plague — after the name of the Emperor Justinian, a sufferer himself — and the mid-fourteenth-century pandemic, the so-called Black Death. A large body of contemporary sources inform us about the dire consequences of medieval plague outbreaks, especially of the Black Death. The disaster was not only chronicled by historians, but also elicited philosophical and medical explanations, invited theological reflections, and provided a subject for literary reworking. Moreover, plague figured as a key element in private correspondences, account books, charters, and political documents of different kinds and origin.[1] The medieval understanding of plague, being mostly based on the description of symptoms, was far from the modern-day laboratory perception.[2] This

1 On the 1347–50 plague pandemic, see, e.g, Philip Ziegler, *The Black Death* (London: Collins, 1969); Jean-Noel Biraben, *Les hommes et la peste en France dans les pays européens et méditerranéens*, 2 vols (Paris-La Haye: Mouton, 1975–76); *La peste nera: dati di una realtà ed elementi di una interpretazione*. Atti del XXX Convegno storico internazionale, Todi, 10–13 ottobre 1993 (Spoleto: Centro italiano di studi sull'Alto Medioevo, 1994); Klaus Bergdolt, *Der Schwarze Tod in Europa. Die Große Peste und das Ende des Mittelalters* (München: Beck, 1994); *The Regulation of Evil. Social and Cultural Attitudes to Epidemics in the Late Middle Ages*, ed. by Agostino Paravicini Bagliani and Francesco Santi (Firenze: Sismel-Edizioni del Galluzzo, 1998); William Naphy and Andrew Spicer, *Plague. Black Death and Pestilence in Europe* (Stroud: Tempus Publishing Limited, 2004); Ole J. Benedictow, *The Black Death 1346–1353. The complete history* (Woodbridge: Boydell Press, 2004); Joseph P. Byrne, *Encyclopedia of the Black Death* (Santa Barbara, California-Denver, Colorado-Oxford: ABC-CLIO, 2012); Kay Peter Jankrift, *Im Angesicht der 'Pestilenz'. Seuchen in westfälischen und rheinischen Städten (1349–1600)* (Stuttgart: Steiner Verlag, 2020); Alberto Luongo, *La peste nera. Contagio, crisi e nuovi equilibri nell'Italia del Trecento* (Roma: Carocci, 2022). For an up to date account of plague in general, see at least Dominique Buchillet, 'Epidemic Diseases in the Past: History, Philosophy, and Religious Thought', in *Encyclopedia of Infectious Diseases: Modern Methodologies*, ed. by Michel Tibayrenc (Hoboken: John Wiley and Sons, 2007), pp. 517–24; Frank M. Snowden, *Epidemics and Society: From the Black Death to the Present* (New Haven: Yale University Press, 2019).

2 See Andrew Cunningham, 'Transforming Plague: The Laboratory and the Identity of Infectious Disease', in *The Laboratory Revolution in Medicine*, ed. by Andrew Cunningham and Perry Williams (Cambridge: Cambridge University Press, 1992), pp. 209–44. Towards the end of the nineteenth century, Alexandre Yersin discovered the bacillus causing the plague disease (*Yersinia pestis*). Usually present in rats and wild rodents, this bacterium is transferred to humans through the bite of fleas (of rodents or humans), giving rise to the infection, which may be bubonic, pneumonic, or septicemic. In the pneumonic form, it is transmitted from person to person by coughing, sneezing, spitting, or even speaking. Recent studies, benefitting from the growing use of the resources of modern sciences (paleogenetics, archeobiology, microbiology, immunology, etc.), have started to question the identification of the 14th-century plague pandemic with the contagious disease caused by *Yersinia pestis*. On the new genetic and biological approach to medieval plague, see, e.g., Graham Twigg, *The Black Death: a biological reappraisal* (London: Batsford, 1984); Susan Scott and Christopher Duncan, *Biology of Plagues. Evidence from Historical Population* (Cambridge: Cambridge University Press, 2001); Susan Scott and Christopher Duncan, *Return of the Black Death: the world's greatest serial killer* (Chichester: Wiley, 2004); Vivian Nutton (ed.), *Pestilential complexities: understanding medieval plague, Medical History. Supplement*, 27 (London: Wellcome Trust Centre for the History of Medicine at UCL, 2008), in particular Vivian Nutton's introduction and the papers by Lars Walløe, Samuel K John Jr., Daniel Antoine, and Elisabeth Carniel; Lester K. Little, 'Plague Historians in Lab Coats', *Past and Present*, 213 (November 2011), pp. 267–90; *Pandemic Disease in the Medieval World: Rethinking the Black Death*, ed. by Monica H. Green (Kalamazoo–Bradford: ARC Medieval Press, 2015); George Dameron, 'Identificazione di un killer. Recenti scoperte scientifiche e storiche sulla natura della peste nera', in *Boccaccio 1313–2013*, ed. by Francesco Ciabattoni, Elsa Filosa, and Kristina Marie

medieval approach explains why the words *pestis* and *pestilentia* had a broad meaning, covering a wide range of different epidemic and contagious diseases having more or less similar symptoms.

This paper focuses on Albert the Great's views on pestilences and contagious diseases. As is well known, Albert the Great (1200–80) was a key figure in the intellectual life of the Middle Ages. A Dominican friar, a master regent in theology at the University of Paris and the Dominican *studium generale* at Cologne, he was a systematic commentator of the *Corpus Aristotelicum* and thus an attentive scholar of natural processes, including biological and medical phenomena.[3] His scientific interests spanned from human physiology, psychology and embryology to the theory of the elements, from cosmology to zoology and botany. He was already called *doctor universalis* in his lifetime due to his encyclopedic scientific knowledge.

Even though he has not left us a specific work specifically dedicated to pestilences and contagious diseases, we find his views on these subjects scattered throughout his works. As we will see, Albert explained pestilences in strictly naturalistic terms, relying on some of the most prominent sources on natural philosophy, medicine, and astrology at his disposal (above all, Aristotle, Galen, Avicenna, and Albumasar), on the Bible, on his personal 'experience', and on secondhand observations. Albert took the same approach to pestilences and contagious diseases as he did to other natural and human-related catastrophes (deluges, fires, floodings, earthquakes, wars, and famines).[4]

Olson (Ravenna: Longo, 2015), pp. 57–70; Pierre Toubert, 'La Peste Noire (1348), entre histoire et biologie moléculaire', *Journal des Savants*, 1 (2016), pp. 17–31. On a paleogenetic and phylogenetic basis, Monica H. Green, 'The Four Black Deaths', *American Historical Review*, 125 (2020), pp. 1601–31, has recently laid out a scenario in which the *Yersinia pestis*, present in a latent form throughout Asia as early as the thirteenth century due to the Mongol conquests, became visible in Asia, the Black Sea, and the Mediterranean with its devastating effects only between the 1330s and 1340s.

3 On Albert's medical expertise and theories, see at least Nancy Siraisi, 'The Medical Learning of Albertus Magnus', in *Albertus Magnus and the Sciences. Commemorative Essays 1980*, ed. by James Weisheipl (Toronto: Pontifical Institute of Medieval Studies, 1980), pp. 379–404; Heinrich Shipperges, 'Das medizinische Denken bei Albertus Magnus', in *Albertus Magnus. Doctor Universalis 1280/1980*, ed. by Gerbert Meyer and Albert Zimmermann (Mainz: Matthias-Grünewald-Verlag, 1980), pp. 279–94; Miguel de Asúa, 'War and Peace: Medicine and Natural Philosophy in Albert the Great', in *A Companion to Albert the Great. Theology, Philosophy, and the Sciences*, ed. by Irven M. Resnick (Leiden-Boston: Brill, 2013), pp. 269–97; Katja Krause, 'Grenzen der Philosophie. Albert der Großen Kommentar zu De animalibus und die Medizin', *Documenti e Studi sulla Tradizione Filosofica Medievale*, 30 (2019), pp. 265–93; Amalia Cerrito, *Albert the Great (c. 1193-1280) and the Configuration of the Embryo: Virtus Formativa* (London: Palgrave Macmillan, 2023).

4 The scholarly debate on the definition of natural catastrophes and their difference from human-induced calamities cannot be gone into here. For different positions on these issues, see, e.g., Jacques Berlioz, *Catastrophes naturelles et calamités au Moyen Age* (Firenze: Sismel-Edizioni del Galluzzo, 1998), pp. 20–25, (p. 24); Michael Matheus, 'L'uomo di fronte alle calamità ambientali', in *Le calamità ambientali nel Tardo Medioevo europeo: realtà, percezioni, reazioni*. Atti del XII convegno del Centro di Studi sulla civiltà del tardo Medioevo S. Miniato, 31 maggio — 2 giugno 2008, ed. by Michael Matheus and others (Firenze: Firenze University Press, 2010), pp. 1–20. Gian Maria Varanini, 'Presentazione', in *Le calamità ambientali nel Tardo Medioevo europeo*, proposes the concept of 'environmental calamities' ('calamità ambientali'), which expands the usual notion of catastrophe to also include human agency and society's perception of, and reaction to, catastrophic events.

In what follows, after briefly providing basic historical information on the two medieval plague pandemics, I intend first to thoroughly comment on the several passages wherein Albert analyses pestilences. I will then explore the reception of Albert's views in the plague literature originated with the great pandemic of the mid-fourteenth-century. In the attempt to understand the etiology of the pestilence and the mechanisms of contagion, describe the symptoms, work out prophylactic countermeasures, and devise a therapy, physicians and natural philosophers of the fourteenth century often used Albert's ideas as a framework for a rational approach to the pandemic.

2. The Medieval Plague Pandemics: the Justinianic Plague and the Black Death

We know about the beginnings of the sixth-century Justinianic pandemic from the historian Procopius of Caesarea who, being at the court of Justinian in the early 540s, was an eyewitness to the dramatic beginnings of the plague.[5] From 543 onward, the pestilence hit vast areas in Western Europe, striking several regions of Europe on a recurrent basis during the sixth century (543–47, 571, 582–84, 588, 591–94), and returning in frequent waves at least until the eight century.

Gregory of Tours (538/39–594) was the most renowned and authoritative among the Western chroniclers of the Justinianic plague. He viewed the pestilence as the fundamental event of his lifetime. His works accurately describe several waves of the disease. He interpreted the plague from a theological point of view as a manifestation of God's anger at human wrongdoing and viewed it as a tragic event in the history of salvation. In the pages he devotes to the plague we read that the catastrophe was heralded by prodigies (comets, eclipses, floods, etc.). Gregory also describes the liturgical measures (processions, vigils, fasting, prayers, pilgrimages, and sessions of collective confession and penitence) that were taken to counter the disease and seek the intercession of angels and bishop saints.[6]

A similar interpretive pattern is adopted by Paul the Deacon (Paulus Diaconus) in the *Historia Langobardorum*. An historian from the eighth century, Paul described supernatural events that were taking place in 680 when the epidemic was ravaging

---

5 On the Justinianic plague, see *Plague and the End of Antiquity. The Pandemic of 541–750*, ed. by Lester K. Little (Cambridge: Cambridge University Press, 2007); Merle Eisenberg and Lee Mordechai, 'The Justinianic Plague and Global Pandemics: The Making of the Plague Concept', *American Historical Review*, 125 (2020), pp. 1632–67. For an analysis of the two medieval plague pandemics, see Gundolf Keil, 'Seuchenzüge des Mittelalters', in *Mensch und Umwelt im Mittelalter*, ed. by Bernd Herrmann (Stuttgart: Deutsche Verlags-Anstalt, 1986), pp. 109–28.

6 On Gregory's views on plague, see Michael McCormick, 'Gregory of Tours on Sixth-Century Plague and Other Epidemics', *Speculum*, 96/1 (2021), pp. 38–96. The theurgic conception characteristic of the High-Medieval battle against pestilences underlies the liturgical measures described by Gregory: see Mirko D. Grmek, 'Le concept d'infection dans l'Antiquité et au Moyen Age, les anciennes mesures sociales contre les maladies contagieuses et la fondation de la première quarantaine à Dubrovnik (1377)', *Rad Jugoslavenske Akademije Znanosti i Umjetnosti*, 384 (1980), pp. 9–55 (p. 24).

Rome. Almost simultaneous lunar and solar eclipses prefigured the calamity. Paul writes that at that time many people saw an evil angel holding a hunting-spear in his hand and being ordered by a good angel to bang with it on the doors of the houses of the people doomed to die. Someone had the revelation that the plague would stop if an altar dedicated to the martyr Saint Sebastian were installed in the basilica of St Peter's 'ad Vincula'. Once this was done, the epidemic ceased to sweep across the city.[7]

The second medieval plague pandemic, known today as the Black Death, but named differently by the medieval people (*mortalitas, epidemia, pestilentia*), was a fundamental event in the later Middle Ages, marking a turning point in the European history according to many historians.[8] After first appearing in Central or Eastern Asia, plague struck the region around the Caspian Sea around 1345, moved from the Eastern to the Mediterranean ports along the trade routes in 1347, expanded inland, and swept across Europe until around 1352.[9] There were several pandemic resurgences in the second half of the fourteenth century and epidemic outbreaks continued to strike in localized areas in Europe until the eighteenth century.

The plague also drew a wide range of reactions from all components of medieval society.[10] Like the Justinianic plague, the Black Death was considered from a supernatural perspective as a collective punishment inflicted by God for human crimes.[11] This idea led to public rites of repentance and to invocations of the saints, the angels,

---

7 Paulus Diaconus, *Historia Langobardorum*, ed. Georg Waitz (Monumenta Germaniae Historica. Scriptores rerum Langobardicarum et Italicarum sec. VI–IX) (Hannover: Hahn, 1988; repr. of ed. Hannoverae, impensis bibliopolii Hahniani 1878), VI. 5, p. 166, 20–34.

8 The scale of the demographic collapse that followed the Black Death outbreak is often adduced as a proof of its being a watershed in history. On the demographic aspect, see Rinaldo Comba, 'Il rilevamento demografico: prima e dopo la peste nera', in *La peste nera: dati di una realtà ed elementi di una interpretazione*, pp. 155–73.

9 The traditional view that the early spread of the pandemic was due to the Tartars besieging the Crimean city of Caffa in 1346 and throwing plague-infected cadavers over the walls of the city has recently been rejected: see Hannah Barker, 'Laying the Corpses to Rest: Grain, Embargoes, and *Yersinia pestis* in the Black Sea, 1346–48', *Speculum*, 91/1 (2021), pp. 97–126. Interestingly, the episode, narrated in Gabriele de Mussis' *Historia de morbo*, has been interpreted by several scholars as an early example of bacteriological warfare: see, e.g., Vincent J. Derbes, 'De Mussis and the Great Plague of 1348. A Forgotten Episode of Bacteriological Warfare', *Journal of the American Medical Association*, 196. 1 (1996), pp. 59–62; Mark Wheelis, 'Biological Warfare at the 1346 Siege of Caffa', *Emerging Infectious Diseases*, 8 (2002), pp. 971–75.

10 See e.g., *The Black Death*, trans. and ed. by Rosemary Horrox (Manchester-New York: Manchester University Press, 1994); John Aberth, *The Black Death. The Great Mortality of 1348–1350. A Brief History with Documents* (New York: Palgrave Macmillan, 2005).

11 This notion, which we often find linked to what can be called a pastoral of fear, was widespread in the fourteenth century among authors with different backgrounds: see, e.g., Gabriele de Mussis, *Historia de morbo*, ed. by August Wilhelm Henschel, 'Document zur Geschichte des schwarzen Todes', *Archives für die gesammte Medicin*, 2 (1842), pp. 45–59 (pp. 45–46); Boccaccio, *Decameron*, ed. Vittore Branca, vols 2 (Torino: Einaudi, 2014^4), vol. 1, Intr. p. 15, § 8, p. 21, § 25; Iohannes de Rupescissa, *De consideratione quintae essentiae* (Basel: 1561), p. 163; Giovanni Villani, *Nuova Cronaca*, ed. Giuseppe Porta (Milano-Parma: Fonazione Pietro Bembo-Ugo Guanda, 1991), vol. 3, XIII. 84, pp. 485–86; Matteo Villani, *Cronica con la continuazione di Filippo Villani*, ed. Giuseppe Porta (Milano-Parma: Fondazione Pietro Bembo-Ugo Guanda, 1995), vol. 1, I. 1–2, pp. 5, 1–9, 20; Francesco Petrarca, *Prose*, ed. P. G. Ricci, E. Carrara, and E. Bianchi (Milano-Napoli: Ricciardi, 1955), p. 1122.

and the Virgin Mary. The need for self-mortification reached shocking peaks with the bands of flagellants wandering through German lands and performing violent penitential rites by scourging themselves.[12] The plague outbreaks and the wondrous events foreshadowing or surrounding it (earthquakes, eclipses, fires, hail, rains of toads and snakes, etc.) were interpreted in eschatological terms as harbingers of the nearness of the apocalypse.[13] The sense of a looming catastrophe led many to perceive no moral limitations and forget human dignity. These people exceeded in merrymaking and indulged in debauchery, as though they were living their last hours.[14] The need to find a cause for the pandemic facilitated the dissemination of conspiracy theories that considered the plague to be man-made. Several human groups (lepers, foreigners, the wealthy, and Jews) were scapegoated. In particular, the Jews were accused of poisoning wells and spreading the plague, an accusation that led to massacres of innocent people.[15]

After the first onslaught of the plague outbreak, public authorities responded by issuing ordinances concerning quarantine, isolation of the plague-affected, and sanitation. All these measures suggest that there was awareness that interhuman contagion was the reason for the spread of the disease.[16]

Physicians, however, were unable to understand the speedy propagation of the disease within the traditional nosological Hippocratic-Galenic framework, and could

---

12 See, e.g., Henricus de Hervordia, *Liber de rebus memorabilioribus sive Chronicon*, ed. August Potthast (Gottingae: Sumptibus Dieterichianis, 1959), pp. 280–81. On the flagellants, see F. Graus, *Pest — Geissler — Judenmorde. Das 14. Jahrhundert als Krisenzeit* (Göttingen: Vandenhoeck & Ruprecht, 1987; 2. durchges. Aufl.), pp. 38–59.

13 Robert E. Lerner, 'The Black Death and Western European Eschatological Mentalities', *The American Historical Review*, 86 (1981), pp. 533–52; Laura A. Smoller, 'Of Earthquakes, Hail, Frogs, and Geography: Plague and the Investigation of the Apocalypse in the Later Middle Ages', in *Last Things. Death and the Apocalypse in the Middle Ages*, ed. by Caroline Walker Bynum and Paul Freedman (Philadelphia: University of Pennsylvania Press, 2000), pp. 156–87, pp. 316–37, claims that the hallmark of the fourteenth-century discussion on plague was the interweaving of apocalyptic explanations with naturalistic analyses. On the medieval apocalyptic interpretation of catastrophes, see the recent Robert E. Bjork, *Catastrophes and the Apocalyptic in the Middle Ages and the Renaissance* (Turnhout: Brepols, 2019). Useful remarks can also be found in John Aberth, *From the Brink of the Apocalypse: Confronting Famine, War, Plague, and Death in the Later Middle Ages* (New York-London: Routledge, 2001).

14 Boccaccio, *Decameron*, vol. 1, Intr. pp. 19–20, § 21–22, p. 27, § 44; Matteo Villani, *Cronica*, I. 6, pp. 16, 10–17, 29. David Herlihy, *The Black Death and the Transformation of the West*, ed. and introd. by Samuel K. Cohn, Jr. (Cambridge, Mass.-London: Harvard University Press, 1997), pp. 63–65, regards this behaviour as 'revulsion toward death' or a 'victory, however temporary, over death'. For further links between pandemics and conspiracy theories, see section 4 of chapter 10 of this volume.

15 Graus, *Pest — Geissler — Judenmorde*, pp. 155–389; Samuel K. Cohn Jr., 'The Black Death and the Burning of the Jews', *Past and Present*, 196 (2007), pp. 3–36; Jan Philipp Weber, *Die Jugendpogrome zur Zeit des Schwarzen Todes 1348–1350. Was waren die Ursachen?* (München: Grin Verlag, 2019).

16 Paul Slack, 'Responses to Plague in Early Modern Europe: The Implications of Public Health', *Social Research*, 55 (1988), pp. 433–53, makes interesting remarks on the responses of medieval political authorities. For political reactions in later centuries, see Carlo Maria Cipolla, *Miasmi e umori* (Bologna: Il Mulino, 1989), Id., *Il pestifero e contagioso morbo. Combattere la peste nell'Italia del Seicento* (Bologna: Il Mulino, 2012). One should not forget that some of the treatises on the plague were commissioned by town governments, city leaders, or sovereigns. Therefore, a sharp distinction between the public health policies enacted by political authorities and the remedies suggested by medical treatises seems to be untenable.

only devise preventive remedies and curative measures with a limited impact on the plague's spread. The recourse to alchemical therapies and magical amulets is a clear sign of the inadequacy of the usual humoral medical approaches.[17]

3. Albert the Great on Pestilences

3.1. A Philosophical Approach

Since he died in 1280, Albert did not experience the ravages of the Black Death. By the words *pestis* and *pestilentia*, he did not refer to proper plague, caused by the bacterium *Yersinia pestis*, but to unspecified epidemics, contagious diseases, leprosy, miasmatic contamination, or malaria-like sickness due to an unhealthy environment.[18]

He accounted for this large body of pestilences and contagious diseases in different ways, but all of his explanations had a scientific basis. This is one of the reasons why Albert's analyses were so successful among fourteenth-century authors.

A crucial passage from Albert's commentary on the *De causis proprietatum elementorum* (= *DCPE*) helps us clarify his attitude towards pestilences. Even though here Albert deals with deluges, his words describe a scientific approach to be applied to catastrophes of any kind, including pestilences.

> Sunt autem quidam qui omnia haec divinae dispositioni tantum attribuunt et aiunt non debere nos de huiusmodi rebus quaerere aliam causam nisi voluntatem dei. Quibus nos in parte consentimus, quia dicimus haec nutu dei mundum gubernantis fieri ad vindictam maleficii hominum. Sed tamen dicimus haec deum facere propter causam naturalem, cuius primus motor est ipse qui cuncta dat moveri. Causas autem suae voluntatis non quaerimus nos, sed quaerimus causas naturales, quae sunt sicut instrumenta quaedam per quae sua voluntas in talibus producitur ad effectum.[19] (There are some who ascribe everything to the divine disposition, saying that we ought to seek no other cause of such things than God's will. We agree with them partly because we maintain that these events happen by the will of God, Who governs the world, as a punishment for men's misdeeds; yet,

17 Chiara Crisciani and Michela Pereira, 'Black Death and Golden Remedies. Some Remarks on Alchemy and the Plague', in *The Regulation of Evil*, pp. 7–39; Byrne, *Encyclopedia of the Black Death*, pp. 9–10. According to Nicolas Weill-Parot, 'La rationalité médicale à l'épreuve de la peste: médecine, astrologie et magie (1348–1500)', *Médiévales*, 46 printemps (2004), pp. 73–88, available at https://journals.openedition.org/medievales/884 (last accessed 01.02.2022), the recourse to seals against plague must be linked to the rational framework of scholastic medicine.

18 On the fluctuation of the meaning of the terms 'pestilence' and 'epidemics' in the thirteenth and fourteenth centuries, see Joël Chandelier, 'Définition et terminologie des épidémies dans la médicine latine de la fin du Moyen Âge', in *Épidémies, épizooties. Des représentations anciennes aux approches nouvelles*, ed. by François Clément (Rennes: Presses universitaires de Rennes, 2017), pp. 29–42 (pp. 30–35).

19 Albertus, *De causis proprietatum elementorum*, ed. by Paul Hossfeld (Alberti Magni Opera omnia, 5. 2) (Münster i.W.: Aschendorff, 1980), I. 2. 9. pp. 76, 75–77, 2. The work has been translated into English: Albert the Great, *On the Causes of the Properties of the Elements (Liber de causis proprietatum elementorum)*, trans. with introduction and notes by Irven M. Resnick (Milwaukee: Marquette University Press, 2010).

we state that God does these things by means of a natural cause, of which the first mover is He himself that sets everything in motion. However, we do not search for the causes of His will, but search for the natural causes, which are like instruments by which His will is put into effect in such events).

He did not exclude the possibility of a divine punishment of human misdeeds. Such an explanation, however, had no scientific value in the context of the commentary on the *DCPE* because it did not identify the secondary causes used by God as a means by which He accomplished His will. Albert's scientific stance vis-à-vis cataclysms is condensed in the words 'However, we do not search for the causes of His will, but search for the natural causes', which constitute a programmatic principle opposed to the fideistic attitude of those who believe that all depends on divine disposition.

Our extension of Albert's explanatory model of deluges to his study of pestilences is not only conceptually pertinent, but also justified on a historical basis, because the aforementioned passage was to be quoted by some fourteenth century scholars dealing with the plague (in particular, Conrad of Megenberg and Henry of Herford).

3.2. Physical Causes

All the theories put forward by Albert relate pestilences to the corruption of the air. Already documented in the *Corpus Hippocraticum* (*Nat. hom.* 9), the idea that epidemics were airborne diseases, caused by corrupt air or noxious exhalations, was the backbone of medieval etiological analyses. Moreover, according to the Galenic conception of the six non-natural things, air was the thing that acted more effectively on human beings than any other, including food and drink (*De regimine sanitatis* I. 1).[20] Further, the aerist theory was endorsed by Avicenna[21] and remained dominant in the fourteenth-century *Pesttraktate.*[22]

In a passage from his commentary on the *DCPE*, Albert mentions both a physical and an astrological origin of air corruption. The air is either corrupted by an inferior poisoning and corrupting cause ('ex inferiori invenenante et corrumpente'), namely

---

20 See also Galenus, *De febrium differentiis*, I. 6, where several causes for the corrupt air are put forward.

21 See Avicenna, *Liber canonis*, IV. fen i. tract. 4. cap. 1. (Venetiis: 1507; repr. Hildesheim: Georg Olms Verlag, 2003) f. 416ra-b.

22 The literature on medieval conceptions of contagion is extensive and cannot be summarized here. See at least Grmek, 'Le concept d'infection dans l'Antiquité et au Moyen Age', pp. 9–55; Vivian Nutton, 'The Seeds of Disease: An Explanation of Contagion and Infection from the Greeks to the Renaissance', *Medical History*, 27 (1983), pp. 1–34; *Contagion. Perspectives from Pre-Modern Societies*, ed. by Lawrence I. Conrad and Dominik Wujastyk (London-New York: Routledge, 2000); Saul Jarcho, *The Concept of Contagion in Medicine, Literature and Religion* (Malabar: Krieger Publishing Company, 2000); *Air, miasmes et contagion. Les épidémies dans l'Antiquité et au Moyen Âge*, ed. by Sylvie Bazin-Tacchella and others (Langres: Dominique Guéniot, 2001); Aurélien Robert, 'Contagion morale et transmission des maladies: histoire d'un chiasme [XIIIe-XIXe siècle]', *Tracés. Revue de Sciences humaines*, 21 (*Contagions*) (2011), pp. 41–60. On the ancient roots of the concept of contagion, see Fabio Stok, 'Il lessico del contagio', in *Atti del Seminario Internazionale di Studi 'Letteratura scientifica e tecnica greca e latina'* (Messina 29–31 ottobre 1997), ed. by Paola Radici Colace and Antonino Zumbo (Messina: Edizioni Dr Antonino Sfameni, 2000), pp. 55–89.

the breath of poisonous animals ('ex spiritu animalium venenosorum'), a corruption similar to that arising from a poisonous vapour, a corpse, a swamp, or whatever else has decomposed ('ex vapore venenoso, ex cadavere vel palude vel aliquo alio resoluto'), or by the influence of a superior celestial body ('ex superiori corpore aliquo caelesti').[23]

Albert goes into detail about each of the specific cases of physical corruption. With regard to animals' corruptive breath, he refers to the two great *dracones* mentioned in the *DCPE*. In his commentary on the text, Albert clarifies that *draco* was the name of a species of a cubit-long snake whose bite was venomous and deadly.[24] According to the *DCPE*, in Philip of Macedon's time there was a valley between two mountains in *Armenia Minor* infested by a poisonous air killing whoever crossed it. Socrates was asked to find the reason for the contamination. He ordered to construct a structure as high as the mountains and to set a flat, clean, and polished mirror on top of it. In this way, he was able to see reflected in the mirror two snakes, one on each of the two mountains. The vapour released from their stomachs and expelled through their mouths was infecting the air.[25] Once he had learned the cause of the poisoning, the king commanded the snakes to be slain by someone who had covered his mouth, nostrils, and all the body's pores through which the contaminated air could have penetrated into his body ('tecto ore et naribus et omnibus poris, per quae poterat attrahi aër infectus [...]').

In itself, the episode narrated by the *DCPE* is significant because it gives Albert authoritative support for his view that the air is tainted by the vapour let out by some animals ('Corruptio autem illa aeris fuit ex vapore resoluto ex draconibus [...]') and indicates that his knowledge about contamination and pestilences is often derived from previous sources.

---

23 *DCPE*, II. 2. 1. p. 95, 14–20: 'Corrumpitur autem aer dupliciter, aliquando videlicet ex inferiori invenenante et corrumpente, aliquando autem ex superiori corpore aliquo caelesti corrumpente ipsum; ex inferiori quidem sicut ex spiritu animalium venenosorum, cui corruptioni similis est, quae est ex vapore venenoso, ex cadavere vel palude vel aliquo alio resoluto [...]'. On Albert's views, see also the analysis contained in Alessandro Palazzo, 'Forms and Models of Contagion According to Albert the Great. Pestilence, Leprosy, the Basilisk, the Menstruating Woman, and Fascination', *Quaestio*, 23 (2023), pp. 221–51.

24 *DCPE*, II. 2. 1. p. 95, 43–44: '[...] est enim serpens cubitalis, qui draco vocatur et habet morsum et venenum mortiferum'. On the *dracones*, see Albertus, *De animalibus libri XXVI nach der Cölner Urschrift*, ed. by Hermann Stadler, 2 vols (Münster i.W.: Aschendorff, 1916–1920), vol. 2, XXV. 2. nn. 25–29. pp. 1565, 18–1567, 26. These *magni dracones* have nothing to do with the Biblical 'draco magnus' (see *Revelation* 12. 3 and *Psalms* 73. 13–14). For the recourse to the Biblical terminology of *dracones* in relation to natural calamities, see Isabelle Draelants, 'Phénomènes célestes et tremblements de terre au Moyen Âge: enquête sur l'historiographie médiévale dans les limites de la Belgique actuelle (600–1200)', in *Les catastrophes naturelles dans l'Europe médiévale et moderne*, ed. by Bartolomé Bennassar (Toulouse: Presses universitaires du Midi, 1996), pp. 187–222 (pp. 208–10); for the pestilential dragon in early-medieval hagiographic contexts, see Peregrine Horden, 'Disease, dragons and saints: the management of epidemics in the Dark Ages', in *Epidemic and ideas. Essays on the historical perception of pestilence*, ed. by Terence Ranger and Paul Slack (Cambridge: Cambridge University Press, 1992), pp. 45–76.

25 *DCPE*, II. 2. 1. p. 95, 21–59 (p. 95, 47–50.53–54): 'Hi autem dracones *aperuerunt ora* contra se invicem et infecerunt *aërem* in medio ex *vapore* ventris sui, qui *egrediebatur ex orificiis eorum* [...] infectio causabatur ex *vapore* resoluto *de ventribus draconum*'.

It is interesting to note that in this particular case Albert does not explicitly mention the concept of pestilence; rather he describes the infection of air due to the breath of the *dracones* as a form of poisoning ('ex veneno diffuso in aërem'). However, the distinction between pestilences and poisoning is not always clear-cut. As we shall see, some of the fourteenth-century treatises on plague were to refer to poison both to explain the cause of the pestilence and to explain how the disease works within the human body.[26] According to Albert, the *dracones* are not the only animals able to emit poison. Elsewhere, he claims that the basilisk snake spreads poison by breathing or by looking.[27] It should be stressed that Albert does not explicitly associate the basilisk with pestilences, even though it cannot be denied that the basilisk's property of infecting the air through the spirit issuing from its eyes makes this animal a fitting explanatory model for air corruption — the same holds true for the menstruating woman, whose eyes release a spirit able to infect the air and cloud the surface of a polished and a clean mirror.[28] Unsurprisingly, therefore, the basilisk will feature as one of the possible causes of air infection in a few fourteenth-century plague tractates.

Water is also subject to be infected, as Albert shows by describing the poisoning effects of the *iusquiamus* (its scientific name is *Hyoscyamus niger*), a toxic herb[29] that can cause the death of fish. Yet, being warm, the air is contaminated more intensively than water, which, due to its coldness, does not putrefy (*putrescere*) as fast and strongly as the air. The poisoning of water also has destructive effects on reason and memory and causes suffocation.[30]

---

26 On this point, see Frederick W. Gibbs, *Poison, Medicine, and Disease in Late Medieval and Early Modern Europe* (London-New York: Routledge, 2019), chapter 4, who claims that these treatises understood plague epidemic as a form of poisoning, identifying poison as the cause and the agent of the disease and not merely using it as a metaphor of the epidemic. The 'poison thesis' has been thoroughly illustrated by John Aberth, *Doctoring the Black Death: Medieval Europe's Medical Response to Plague.* (Lanham-Boulder-New York-London: Roman and Littlefield, 2021), Intr. and Chap. 1, pp. 48–148. For a more nuanced position on the role of poison, see Danielle Jacquart: 'Les multiples facettes des relations entre empoisonnement et peste dans les explications médicales de la fin du Moyen Âge', in *Poison. Knowledge, Uses, Practices*, ed. by Caterina Mordeglia and Agostino Paravicini Bagliani (Firenze: Sismel-Edizioni del Galluzzo, 2022), pp. 223–48. On the medieval writings on poisons and venoms, see Franck Collard, *Les écrits sur les poisons* (Turnhout: Brepols, 2016).

27 Albertus, *De animalibus*, vol. 1, VII. 2. 5. p. 553, 18–23; Id., *De anima*, ed. by Clemens Stroick (Alberti Magni Opera omnia, 7. 1) (Münster i.W.: Aschendorff, 1968), II. 3, 1. p. 97, 84–85. On the medieval tradition on basilisk and its ancient roots, see Robert McNeill Alexander, 'The Evolution of the Basilisk', *Greece and Rome*, 10 (1963), pp. 170–81. Albert claims that the hiss of the basilisk can also infect the surrounding air: see Albertus, *De animalibus*, vol. 2, XXV. 2. p. 1555, 32–35, p. 1561, 27–31.

28 See Albertus, *De anima*, II. 3. 1. p. 97, 82–83. Similarly, the eyes of a wolf can poison the surrounding air and, through the air, the eyes of human beings: see Albertus, *Quaestiones super De animalibus*, ed. Ephrem Filthaut (Alberti Magni Opera omnia, 12) (Münster i.W.: Aschendorff, 1955), VIII. 34, p. 199, 71–78. On 'visual contagion', see Justin K. Stearns, *Infectious Ideas. Contagion in Premodern Islamic and Christian Thought in the Western Mediterranean* (Baltimore: The Johns Hopkins University, 2011), pp. 91–105.

29 Albertus, *De vegetabilibus libri VII*, ed. by Ernst Heinrich Friedrich Meyer and Karl Friedrich Wilhelm Jessen (Berlin: Typis et impensis Georgii Reimeri, 1867), VI. 2. 10, pp. 526–27. This herb is also used by necromancers to invoke demons (p. 527).

30 *DCPE*, II. 2. 1. pp. 95, 61–96, 20.

Albert makes it clear that air corruption spreads much farther than the released vapour. This is due to the fact that a vapour can only rarefy to a limited extent, while the bad smell and the ensuing contamination can spread far through the air.

> Et oportet scire, quod haec corruptio aëris multo longius dispergitur, quam possit extendi vapor resolutus; vapor enim resolutus non extenditur multum, eo quod fumus non potest tantum rarificari. Sed odor et corruptio cum odore ad longinquas partes inficit aerem[31] (It must be known that this corruption of the air spreads much further than the exhaled vapour can; indeed, the exhaled vapour does not expand very far because the smoke cannot rarefy very much. Yet, the stench and corruption caused by it corrupts the air to far-off regions).

In other words, stinking things can act both through their smoke-like and vaporous substance ('ex substantia vaporativa et fumosa') or through the quality of being reeky ('ex foetore qualitativo'): in the former case, they contaminate from nearby and by a strong infection, whereas in the latter they contaminate faraway locations only through a qualitative alteration, locations where nothing of the vapour released by their substances ever arrived.[32]

The idea of corruption 'ex foetore' is behind the popular practice of disseminating pleasant scents through the air to counter the spread of pestilences, which will be one of the most common remedies prescribed in the fourteenth-century plague tractates.[33]

To clarify the difference between noxious vapours and corruptive smells, Albert uses a zoological example. Vultures are believed to sense the smell of the air polluted by a mass of cadavers of men and horses lying on a battleground at a distance of five hundred leagues. No smoke-like evaporation ('nulla fumalis evaporatio') can spread to such a distance, not even if it becomes as thin as fire.[34] In this case too, Albert

31 *DCPE*, II. 2. 1. p. 96, 21–26.

32 *DCPE*, II. 2. 1. p. 96, 38–45: 'Sed oportet scire, quod odorifera et foetida dupliciter inficiunt, scilicet ex substantia vaporativa et fumosa et ex foetore qualitativo. Et primo quidem modo inficiunt de prope et forte infectione, secundo autem modo inficiunt alterando solum et longe multum in locis, ubi numquam aliquid fuit de fumali evaporatione ipsorum'. The distinction between a qualitative alteration of the air linked to seasonal changes and a substantial change such as putrefaction of the air we find in some fourteenth-century plague treatises does not seem to be patterned after Albert's distinction: see John Arrizabalaga, 'Facing the Black Death: perceptions and reactions of university medical practitioners', in *Practical Medicine from Salerno to the Black Death*, ed. by Luis García-Ballester and others (Cambridge: Cambridge University Press, 1994), pp. 237–88 (pp. 246–47). This view is entertained, among others, by Jacme d'Agramont: *Regiment de preservació de pestilència* (Lleida, 1348), intr. by Jon Arrizabalaga, Luis García Ballester, and Joan Veny, ed. by Joan Veny (Barcelona: Enciclopèdia Catalana, 1998), Intr. Chap. 1 and Art. V, Chap. 1, pp. 53b, 22–55a, 19. For an English translation of the text, see 'Regimen of Protection Against Epidemics or Pestilences and Mortality', trans. by María Luisa Duran-Reynals and Charles-Edward A. Winslow, *Bulletin of the History of Medicine*, 23 (1949), pp. 57–89.

33 John M. Riddle, 'Pomum ambrae: Amber and Ambergris in Plague Remedies', in *Sudhoffs Archiv für Geschichte der Medizin und der Naturwissenschaften*, 48 (1964), pp. 111–22.

34 *DCPE*, II. 2. 1. p. 96, 30–38: '[…] vultures enim corruptionis, quae de cadaveribus resolvitur, foetorem coniciuntur aliquando per quingentas leucas sensisse et illuc advenisse, ubi infra quingentarum leucarum spatium ante numquam visi sunt, propter multitudinem cadaverum, quae in terra illa post caedem quandam ciderunt ex hominibus et equis, ad quod spatium nulla fumalis evaporatio posset extendi,

is not relying on experience-based information, but is quoting a well-known passage, widespread across the works of Arab and Latin authors.[35]

The physical corruption of the air (*ex inferiori*) can be also explained on a geographic basis. In this regard, Albert maintains that the tainted air disperses through vaster spaces and is especially abundant in Africa.[36] In his *De natura loci* (= *DNL*), he adds that Africa was not a pleasant place to live in both because of its deserts and because of its poisonous and monstrous animals infecting the air and making the region uninhabitable.[37] Here too, Albert is relying on a written source, the *Cosmographia* by Aethicus Ister.[38]

In *DNL*, Albert explores the climatic and environmental factors producing miasmatic contamination in temperate locations on the seacoast. These areas are made warm and humid by the corruptive action of an overabundant liquid (*superfluo umore*). Heat cannot consume the liquid (*umor*) in excess; on the contrary, it multiplies and corrupts the liquid. As a consequence, these areas are full of pestilential vapours and there are thunder and lightning. All of this results in high mortality of human beings and other animals, because the humid and poisonous air penetrates the inner parts of vital organs, leading to immediate death. Here Albert gives a slight hint at the biological side of the process of infection ('aër umidus corrumpitur et efficitur venenosus et penetrat indigestus ad interiora vitalium et perimit subito'). Moreover, he adds that these pestilential locations are often swampy and the water on the ground contaminates habitations. Therefore, the products of farming are often contaminated in accordance with the ontological principle that a place (*locus*) is connatural with what is located in it (*locatum*). Hence, Albert urges to flee regions

etiam si ad ignis raritatem, ut diximus, perveniret'. The fact that a smell is different from the smoke-like evaporation of an odorous thing is demonstrated by Albert in the *De anima* within the discussion of the physiology of smell: see Albertus, *De anima*, II. 3. 25. p. 135, 12–51, where he also quotes the passage on the vultures.

35 See Eckhart, *Expositio s. evangelii secundum Iohannem*, ed. by Karl Christ and others (*Die lateinischen Werke*, Bd. 3), (Stuttgart-Berlin-Köln: Kohlhammer, 1994), n. 700, pp. 614–15 and n. ad loc.

36 *DCPE*, II. 2. 1. p. 96, 49–52: 'Haec autem corruptio in aëre longius spargitur et abundat praecipue in Africa, sicut diximus in libro de natura locorum. Ex his igitur et similibus sunt corruptiones aeris causatae ex inferiori'.

37 Albertus, *De natura loci*, ed. by Paul Hossfeld (Alberti Magni Opera omnia, 5. 2) (Münster i.W.: Aschendorff, 1980), 3. 5, p. 38, 40–44: '([…] habeat [*scil.* Africa] nec delectabilem habitationem propter eremos multas et venenata et monstruosa animalia, quibus est plena, quae aërem inficientia non permittunt homines habitare in ea'.

38 Aethicus Ister, *Cosmographia*, ed. by Michael W. Herren (Publications of the Journal of Medieval Latin, 8) (Turnhout: Brepols, 2011), § 110, p. 212, 4–6: 'Plures itaque gentes uultu horribile et nonnulla monstruosa; serpentium et ferarum multitudinem, rinocerotas, camilopardus, basiliscus et dracones inmensus […]'. It should however be noticed that the passage referred to is an implicit quotation from Isidore's *Etymologiarum sive originum libri XX*, ed. Wallace Martin Lindsay, (Oxford: Clarendon, 1911) XIV, 5, 14–15: 'Aethiopia dicta a colore populorum […] plurimas habens gentes, diverso vultu et monstruosa specie horribiles. Ferarum quoque et serpentium referta est multitudine. Illic quippe rhinoceros bestia et camelopardus, basiliscus, dracones ingentes, ex quorum cerebro gemmae extrahuntur'.

of this kind, a warning that will be often repeated by the fourteenth-century plague tractates as an effective way to avoid the pestilential disease.[39]

In another passage, Albert insists that an excess in humidity is a factor in corruption. A place is infected by nearby ponds (*stagnis*), swamps (*paludibus*), and mud (*lutis*), and is affected by thick humidity (*grossa umiditate*). Sometimes, a pestilence is said to break out as a consequence of the corruption caused by mud and marshes. Even though it is unclear what the vague term *pestilentia* refers to, one can safely guess that in both abovementioned passages Albert has in mind endemic malaria-like diseases.[40]

Forests are also unwholesome, because since their soil (*fundus*) is filled with vapour that is trapped (*conclusus*) under the branches of trees, they contain clouds and whirlwinds ('nebulas et turbines') of a thick suffocating air. Among trees, some are especially harmful (e.g., the walnut and the oak), for they either corrupt the air with their pungency (*amaritudine*) or, since they are tall, they contain the air, without allowing it to be ventilated and purified.[41]

In the *Meteora* (= *Met.*), Albert identifies earthquakes as another physical cause of aerial contamination. As is well-known, this work is concerned with those phenomena that occur near stars (the Milky Way, comets, etc.) or in the air (rainbows, vapours, etc.), or that arise from vapours trapped in water or the earth (wind and earthquakes). Based on Aristotle's *Meteora*, Albert argues that when the sun acts on the earth made humid by rain, two vapours, moist and dry, rise up. Sometimes the vapour arises from the depths of the earth ('extrahitur de profundo terrae'), where it is coerced into subterranean cavities. When it is compressed underground, the vapour is shaken in the bowels of the earth and its agitation impacts on what ecloses it, causing an earthquake.[42]

Frequently an earthquake is followed by a pestilence because after being trapped in the earth and deprived of light and air, the vapour somehow has the nature of poison. For several days before its complete eruption during the earthquake, the

39 *DNL*, 1. 13. pp. 21, 85–22, 10: 'Loca autem, quae sunt remotiora a meridie et accedunt ad climata frigidiora et temperatiora, sita super mare aliquod, efficiuntur calida et umida superfluo umore et corrumpente; locus enim talis plus habet umidi, quam calor consumere possit, et ideo calor multiplicat ipsum et corrumpit, et ideo talia loca frequenter sunt vaporosa et pestifera habitantibus ea, et in locis illis fuerunt multa tonitrua et coruscationes. Corrumpentur et inficientur multum, ita quod inducunt gravem mortalitatem in homines et animalia alia, quia aër umidus corrumpitur et efficitur venenosus et penetrat indigestus ad interiora vitalium et perimit subito. Talia autem loca etiam paludosa sunt frequenter ex umore diffuso in terram et corrumpente habitationem; quandocumque enim calidum non est nisi corrumpens umidum et non vincens ipsum, inducit pestiferas corruptiones, et ideo talia loca fugienda sunt, quia etiam ea quae cultura nascuntur in talibus locis, frequenter corrumpunt, quia, sicut diximus superius, locus et locatum connaturalitatem multam habent'.

40 *DNL*, 1. 13. p. 22, 88–96.

41 *DNL*, 1. 13. pp. 22, 97–23, 7.

42 Albertus, *Meteora*, ed. by Paul Hossfeld (Alberti Magni Opera omnia, 6. 1) (Münster i.W.: Aschendorff, 2004), III. 2. 6, pp. 133, 42–134, 2, p. 134, 46–48.

corrupt vapour leaks gradually out through the pores of the earth, killing animals (e.g., sheep) that take their nourishment from the soil and thus absorb the poison.[43]

Albert also affirms that he was once an eyewitness to the poisoning effect of the vapour arising from below the surface of the earth.

> Ego autem vidi in Paduana civitate Lombardiae quod puteus ab antiquo tempore clausus inventus fuit, qui cum aperiretur et quidam intraret ad purgandum puteum, mortuus fuit ex vapore cavernae illius. Et similiter mortuus est secundus, et tertius voluit scire, quare duo moras agerent, inclinatus in puteum adeo debilitatus est quod spatio duorum dierum vix rediit ad seipsum. Cum autem exspirasset vapor putrefactus in puteo, factus est bonus et potabilis.[44] (In Padua, a city of Lombardy, I saw that a well that had long been closed was found. After the well was opened, someone got in to purge it, but died from the vapour coming out of that cave. The same happened to a second person. Since he wanted to know why the two were delaying, a third man leant into the well, but was so weakened that only after two days he could barely come back to himself. Only after the putrefied vapour had exhaled, did [the water in] the well become good and drinkable).

The episode shows that here Albert understands *pestilentia* as a form of poisoning due to inhalation of toxic vapours.

3.3. *Astrological Causes*

Let us now return to the initial passage from Albert's commentary on the *DCPE* and examine the second type of causes of air contamination evoked there, namely, celestial bodies. In particular, Albert refers to the doctrine of planetary conjunctions, i.e., the theory relating natural catastrophes and momentous historical events to the alignments of the planets moving along the ecliptic. One of the forms of the so-called universal astrology, this theory had been advanced by the Arab astrologer Albumasar in his renowned work *On the great conjunctions* (*Book of Religions and Dynasties*), written in Arabic towards the end of the ninth century and translated into Latin in the twelfth century by John of Seville, then revised in Toledo later in the twelfth century. Conjunctionist astrology enjoyed great success in the Latin Middle Ages and Early Modern Times, Albert being one of the Western scholars most fascinated with it.[45]

---

43 *Met.*, III. 2. 12. p. 141, 30–58, esp. p. 141, 48–58: 'Scias etiam quod frequenter pestilentia et praecipue omnem sequitur terraemotum. *Vapor* enim inclusus et privatus sic luce et aëre libero grossus est habens quasi veneni naturam. Et ideo animalia interficit, praecipue quae terrae quasi semper proximum os tenent sicut oves. Quia antequam totus erumpat vapor, per plures dies semper aliquid eius paulatim per poros terrae evadit et laedit animalia pastum in loco terraemotus accipientia et continue os iuxta terram habentia, quia ex hoc quasi continue hauriunt vaporem venenosum'.

44 *Met.*, III. 2. 12. p. 141, 30–72.

45 Alessandro Palazzo, 'Astrology and Politics: the Theory of Great Conjunctions in Albert the Great', in *Stars, Kingdoms, Beliefs, and Masses. Political Astrology in the Mediterrenean Area from the Middle Ages to the Renaissance*, ed. by Marienza Benedetto and others, *Quaestio*, 19 (2019), pp. 173–203, with extensive bibliography on the medieval discussion on great conjunctions.

The theory of great conjunctions was a very effective scientific tool, which enabled Albert to explain natural phenomena and human affairs taking place on the whole Earth, in a specific region, or in a city in terms of celestial causality. Since planetary conjunctions were seen as causes — and thus signs — of events to come, this astrological doctrine was believed to also provide information about the future. Although the periodic alignments of Saturn and Jupiter ('great conjunctions') constituted the core of conjunctionism,[46] Mars too played a crucial role and, by coming into conjunction with other planets, had a major impact on the sublunar world.

In his commentary on the *DCPE*, Albert ascribes several types of calamities — including pestilences — to the conjunctions of the planets.

> Coniunctio enim duarum praecipue stellarum, quae sunt Iuppiter et Mars, cum aliis coadiuvantibus in signo Geminorum, quod est triplicitatis aëreae, faciunt ventos pestilentes et aëres corruptos, qui subito necant multitudinem hominum et animalium, sicut ventus fuit, qui in Adremoth interfecit exercitum unum subito; Iuppiter enim, cum calidus et umidus in natura, habet elevare ventos et vapores et praecipue in signo Geminorum, quod signum est calidum et umidum in ultimo statu naturae aëris. Mars autem, cum sit intemperate calidus et siccus, ignit vapores elevatos, et ideo incipiunt per aërem multiplicari fulgura et scintillationes et pestiferi vapores et ignes et veneno peracuto et ideo inducunt frequenter pestilentias[47] (The conjunction of Jupiter and Mars, aided by other celestial bodies in the sign of Gemini, a sign belonging to the airy triplicity, brings about pestilential winds and contaminates the air, which kills multitudes of men and animals, as did the wind that in Adremoth instantaneously destroyed an entire army. Being naturally warm and humid, Jupiter must raise winds and vapours, mainly in the sign of Gemini, which is a warm and humid sign in the extreme condition of the airy nature. By contrast, Mars, being excessively warm and dry, inflames the risen vapours. Hence, the air gets filled with bolts of lightning and sparkles, and pestilential vapours and flames poison the air and thus cause frequent pestilences).

While the reference to the wind of Adramoth is already in the *DCPE*, Albert himself provides the scientific explanation of how the conjunction of Jupiter and Mars causes the air to be poisoned and pestilences to take place. In the *DCPE*, Albert also finds a mention of a wind that was produced by the conjunction of some planets in the sign of Virgo and that brought about a pestilence in Iamen, a region of India.[48]

Albert also relates the pestilential air to the joint effects of Mars and Jupiter in the section of the *Met.* dealing with thunders.[49]

---

46 *DCPE*, I. 2. 2. pp. 64, 82–65, 17.

47 *DCPE*, II. 2. 1. p. 96, 53–68.

48 Ps.-Aristoteles, *De causis proprietatum elementorum*, ed. by. Paul Hossfeld, in Albertus, *De causis proprietatum elementorum*, p. 62, 72–74. See *DCPE*, I. 2. 2. p. 64, 10–17.

49 *Met.*, III. 3. 22. p. 173, 36–47: '[...] tonare attribuunt, cuius nulla alia causa est, nisi quia Iuppiter habet in proprietate elevare ventorum fortium et siccorum materiam, ut supra diximus, praecipue quando fuerit coniunctus in virtute aliqua cum Marte tempore aestivo in signis aquilonaribus; quia tunc certissime potest

3.4. Medical Explanations

In the texts we are analysing, Albert does not deal with curative measures to be taken against pestilences. In a few passages, however, in addition to the causes and the process of air corruption, he also examines the impact of contaminated air on the human body and the development of the disease. In the commentary on the *DCPE*, he argues that excessive dryness of the air excites (*acuit*) the humors produced by the human body, giving rise to serious illnesses (*aegritudines pravae*) and lethal pestilences. Wise physicians, Albert continues, state that corrupted air contaminates even more than food and drink, because it reaches, unaltered, the lung, the heart, and, through hidden pores, the whole body, while food and drink reach the inner vital organs only after being cooked and digested.[50]

Albert also takes a medical approach in the *quaestio de animalibus* no. 32 ('Utrum morbus pestilentialis proveniat ex infectione aëris') of Book 7.

> Ad istud dicendum, quod morbus pestilentialis maxime provenit ex infectione aëris, quia cum aër infectus inspiratur, inficit pulmonem, quia rarae compositionis est, et pulmone infecto inficitur cor, et ideo respirantibus et inspirantibus accidit talis morbus.[51] (It must be replied to this that a pestilential disease to a largest extent arises from the corruption of the air, because once the corrupted air has been inspired, it infects the lung, which is composed of a thin substance, and after the lung the heart gets infected; therefore, this disease affects those who breathe in and breathe out).

In the same *quaestio*, once again Albert mentions carcasses and other rotten beings as causes of aerial contamination, adding that since cadavers and putrid things are more numerous (*magis abundant*) on the surface of earth than in the upper part of the air, birds are less affected than ground-bound animals by the abovementioned disease.[52]

Moreover, domestic animals tend to die more than wild animals for several reasons:[53] first, since they are more numerous and live in a smaller spaces, the mingling

---

praedici quod multae scintillationes et tonitrua fient in aëre, ita ut etiam periculum sit futurum hominibus propter aëris pestilentiam ex nimia corruptione futura propter vapores incensos pestiferos immixtos aëri; quia Iuppiter cum sole elevat eos et Mars incendendo corrumpit eosdem; et ita fit aër venenosus'.

50 *DCPE*, II. 2. 1. p. 96, 69–78: 'Aliis etiam de causis similibus accidit *aëri superflua siccitas*, quae acuit umores generatos in hominibus, et ideo *habitatoribus* illius aëris *accidunt aegritudines pravae et pestilentiae mortiferae*; plus enim inficit aër corruptus quam corruptus cibus vet potus, sicut dicunt Sapientes Medicorum, eo quod aër corruptus non alteratus transit ad pulmonem et ad cor et per poros occultos in corpus totum. Cibus autem et potus ad interiora vitalia non pertingunt nisi alterata per decoctiones et digestiones'. From a parallel passage in the *De animalibus* we learn that Albert was certainly referring to Galen (*De regimine sanitatis*, I. 1): see Albertus, *De animalibus*, vol. 1, VII. 3. 5. p. 569, 10–13. The passage is also quoted by Henry of Herford (*Catena aurea entium*, V. 2. 7; VIII. 6. 17), who mentions Galen explicitly.

51 Albertus, *Quaestiones super De animalibus*, VII. 32. p. 186, 27–32.

52 Id., *Quaestiones*, ed. Ephrem Filthaut, VII. 32. p. 186, 42–45: 'Praeterea, aër inficitur ex cadaveribus mortuorum animalium et aliis putrefactis, quae magis abundant in superficie terrae quam in superiore parte aëris, et ideo iste morbus minus accidit avibus quam gressibilibus'.

53 Id., *Quaestiones*, ed. Ephrem Filthaut, VII. 32. p. 186, 47–59.

of their breaths makes air more infectious ('ex multiplicatione sui anhelitus magis inficitur aër');[54] second, domestic animals are more humid than wild animals, because they are fatter, and humidity is the principal agent of corruption and putrefaction;[55] especially sheep and oxen die of this disease ('ex tali morbo'), the former feeding on the products of farming (*ex terraenascentibus*) and being unable to distinguish what is toxic from what is innocuous, the latter having a lung of thin substance (*rarae compositionis*), which means their heart and breath (*spiritus*) get more easily infected when they inspire polluted air.

In the *Met.*, Albert once again has recourse to conjunctionism. He describes the different types of fires that are formed in the cold region of the air by drawing on Seneca's *Naturales Quaestiones*. When all these different kinds of flames are under the influence of Mars, especially in the years of its conjunction with Jupiter, they foreshadow storms, outbreaks of anger in human beings, and pestilences. In particular, flames (*scintillationes*) spread through the air, corrupting and poisoning it. The poisoned air causes abscesses and pustules ('ad apostemata generanda et variolas').[56]

In the texts examined so far, the term 'pestilence' is used to designate a wide range of epidemic, endemic, and contagious diseases, whose exact identity, however, is often difficult to pinpoint.

3.5. *Leprosy*

Leprosy is a contagious disease whose specific nature Albert seems to be aware of. One of the main sources for the medieval discussion on leprosy is the Bible, which Albert also cites in this regard several times. The biblical background explains a distinctive trait of the medieval discourse on leprosy, namely, the interplay between the spiritual (leprosy as a disease of the soul, which is a consequence and a manifestation of sin) and the physical level (leprosy as a disease affecting the body).[57] In the

---

54 The trasmission of the disease through contaminated breath foreshadows the concept of contagion through contiguity, an idea which Albert does not further elaborate upon.

55 See Galenus, *In Hippocr. Epidem.*, III. 1, Kühn XVII, 651. Humidity [*humidum*] is the subject of putrefaction: see *Met.*, IV, 1, 8, p. 220, 1–30. On the process of putrefaction in general, see *Met.* IV. 1. 5–11, pp. 216, 21–224, 65.

56 *Met.*, I. 4. 9. p. 39, 58–66: 'Significationes omnium istorum sunt secundum effectum Martis, et praecipue quando fiunt in anno, quando Mars et Iuppiter sunt coniuncti. Tunc enim in aëre signant huiusmodi ignes tempestates et in hominibus iras et pestilentias ex aëreo veneno, quia scintillationes huiusmodi saepius discurrentes per aërea, cum sit vapor frigidus et siccus combustus, corrumpunt aërem et faciunt venenosum, praecipue ad apostemata generanda et variolas et huiusmodi'. See also *Met.*, I. 4. 9. p. 40, 6–9: 'Vult autem Albumasar quod etiam ista aliquando mortes regum et principum significent propter dominium Martis, praecipue quando fiunt in forma inconsueta et saepius solito'.

57 Saul Nathaniel Brody, *The Disease of the Soul. Leprosy in Medieval Literature* (Ithaca-London: Cornell University Press, 1974); Grmek, 'Le concept d'infection dans l'Antiquité et au Moyen Age', pp. 18–23; Stearns, *Infectious Ideas*, pp. 37–66. Scholarship on medieval conceptions of leprosy is extensive and ever growing: see, e.g., Richard Palmer, 'The Church, Leprosy and Plague in Medieval and Early Modern Europe', in *The Church and Healing*. Papers Read at the Twentieth Summer Meeting and the Twenty-First Winter Meeting of the Ecclesiastical History Society, ed. William J. Sheils (Oxford: Basil Blackwell, 1982), pp. 79–99; François-Olivier Touati, 'Contagion and Leprosy: Myth, Ideas and Evolution in Medieval

Commentary on the *Gospel of Luke*, Albert addresses a difficulty arising from the apparent contrast between the Biblical passages (*Leviticus* 14 and 2 *Kings* 5) forbidding contacts with lepers and the episode of Christ touching the lepers. The inconsistency is avoided by arguing that since leprosy is a contagious disease, the prohibition was imposed to avoid disseminating it. Since, in the case of Christ, touching does not propagate the infection, but is aimed at curing the disease, the law is not abolished, but rather it is respected according to the intention of the lawgiver ('non solvitur lex, sed impletur secundum legislatoris intentionem').[58]

The religious characterization of leprosy is also behind Albert's reflection on its contagiousness. In Book 4 of the *Sentences* commentary, Albert reflects on the phrase 'mentis contagione ac cecitate', used in Peter Lombard's *Liber Sententiarum* to qualify sin, and contrasts contagion with sin.[59] What is important for us in this passage is not the denial of the ability of sin 'to produce a contagion' ('contagionem faciens'), a point Albert will refute in his reply to this argument, but the notion of contagion as a disease originating from contact, a definition which is reminiscent of Isidore of Seville's *Etymologiae*.[60]

> Contagio enim est morbus proveniens ex simili contactu: sicut dicitur morbus contagiosus, qui ex convictu et contactu quodam conversationis et communicationis quae in conversatione est, contrahitur: non autem omne peccatum est tale: ergo non omne peccatum est contagionem faciens[61] (Indeed, contagion is a disease arising from a similar contact, just as a contagious disease is called that which is contracted from both living together and some contact caused by being associated and mutually interacting. But not every sin is such; therefore, not every sin produces a contagion).

The text affirms that contagion is not the process of transmission of the sickness, but the sickness itself. This point is reiterated in Albert's reply to the argument, where he clarifies that every sin causes contagion. He also adds that contagion is the corruption produced by the influence of a noxious cause.

Minds and Societies', in *Contagion. Perspectives from Pre-Modern Societies*, pp. 179–201; Luke Demaitre, *Leprosy in Pre-Modern Societies. A Malady of the Whole Body* (Baltimore: Johns Hopkins University Press, 2007), and bibliography quoted in both contributions.

58 Albertus, *Enarrationes in primam partem Evangelii Lucae (I–IX)*, ed. by Auguste Borgnet (Alberti Magni Opera omnia, 22) (Paris: Vivès, 1894), 5. 13, p. 374b: 'Videtur autem contra legem facere, Levit. XIV, 1 et seq., ubi dicitur, quod qui tangit leprosum immundus erit. Adhuc, IV Reg. V, 10, Eliseus non tetigit leprosum, sed verbo curavit. Sed ad hoc dicendum, sicut diximus in Matthaeo, quod lex non tangendi leprosum ideo data est, quia lepra morbus contagiosus est: et ideo praecipiuntur non tangi, ne leprosi per factum multiplicentur. Ubi ergo per tactum non fit infectio, sed leprae curatio, ibi non solvitur lex, sed impletur secundum legislatoris intentionem. Et hoc modo secundum Chrysostomum, ostendit se Christus non contrarium legi, sed super legem ut legis Dominum'.

59 Petrus Lombardus, *Sententiae in IV libris distinctae*. T. II, *Liber III et IV*, Editiones Collegii S. Bonaventurae Ad Claras Aquas (Grottaferrata: 1981), IV. 18. 4. p. 357, 8–9.

60 Isidorus, *Etymologiarum libri*, IV. 6: 'Idem et contagium a contingendo, quia quemquem tetigerit, polluit'.

61 Albertus, *Commentarii in IV Sententiarum (dist. I–XXII)*, ed. by Auguste Borgnet (Alberti Magni Opera omnia, 29) (Paris: Vivès, 1894), IV. 18. 8, p. 778a.

> [...] dicendum quod omne peccatum contagionem imprimit: dicitur enim hic contagio, non quae serpit tantum ab uno in alium, sed etiam corruptio contracta ex impressione foedantis et putrefacientis[62] ([...] it must be said that every sin causes a contagion. Indeed, we call contagion not only that which creeps from one to another, but also the corruption caused by what pollutes and putrefies).

In other works,[63] Albert draws on the explanatory model of leprosy set forth by Avicenna in the *Canon*,[64] according to which leprosy is an illness whose origin lies in the mental representations of lepers.[65]

This conception is closely related to Avicenna's understanding of the connection between soul and body, as set out in the psychological section of his major encyclopedic work, *Kitāb al-Šifā'*. Here, Avicenna depicts the body-mind relationship in terms of the soul being superior to and independent of the body. This fact is evident in the soul's ability to modify the body without physical intermediation, only through mental representations (emotions, images, and so on). For instance, when a sick man is truly convinced that he will recover and the form of this conviction becomes firmly rooted in his mind, this form affects his body and he becomes well; the opposite happens when a healthy man believes he is ill. The action of the form conceived of by the man is more effective than any medical treatment involving the use of material instruments and media.[66]

Whether leprosy originates from physical contact between bodies or is due to the influence of the soul on the body, the etiologies proposed by Albert make leprosy a natural event which does not involve supernatural causes, notwithstanding the aforementioned intermingling of two levels (spiritual and physical) in the analysis of the disease.

Albert's strictly scientific approach to pestilences and infectious diseases becomes even more evident when it comes to commenting on the famous apocalyptic verses of the *Gospel of Luke* mentioning earthquakes, famine, pestilences, and great signs from the sky.

> Tunc dicebat illis: Surget gens contra gentem, et regnum adversus regnum; et terrae motus magni et per loca fames et pestilentiae erunt, terroresque et de

62 Albertus, *Sent.*, IV 18. 8. p. 780a.

63 See Albertus, *De fato*, ed. by Paul Simon (Alberti Magni Opera omnia, 17. 1) (Münster i.W.: Aschendorff, 1975), 2. p. 70, 15–18 with references to other passages in Albert's corpus.

64 Robert, 'Contagion morale et transmission des maladies'.

65 Albertus, *De causis et processu universitatis a prima causa*, ed. by Winfried Fauser (Alberti Magni Opera omnia, 17. 2) (Münster i.W.: Aschendorff, 1993), II. 2. 21, p. 115, 70–79: 'Propter quod dicit Avicenna, quod omnis materia subiecta motori alicui, statim ut concipit formam motoris, appetit eam et movetur ad ipsam induendam. Sicut videmus, quod concipiente anima aliquod delectabile, quod dum corpori immittitur per spiritum, statim appetit illud corpus et movetur ad iuduendum ipsum. Propter quod medicus cognoscit accidentia animae inter alias causas aegritudinum. Iam enim quidam, ut dicit Avicenna, ex cogitatione et timore lepre leprosi facti sunt'. See Avicenna, *Liber canonis*, IV. fen 3. tr. 3. cap. 1, f. 442vb-443ra; see also I. fen 1. doctr. 4. c. 2., f. 6vb.

66 Avicenna, *Liber de anima seu Sextus de naturalibus IV–V*, ed. by Simone Van Riet (Louvain-Leiden: Éditions Orientalistes-Brill, 1968), IV. 4. p. 64, 20–24.

caelo signa magna erunt (Then he said to them: Nation will rise against nation, and kingdom against kingdom. There will be powerful earthquakes, famines, and plagues from place to place; and awesome sights and mighty signs will come from the sky; *Luke* 21. 10–11).

In this case, Albert applies aerial etiology to supernaturally induced pestilences, figuring out the chain of natural processes eventually leading to them. God's anger ('igne furoris Domini') is seen as the first origin of the calamity, which is however the product of a series of natural processes. As in *DNL*, Albert claims that the air is corrupted by thunder and lightning produced by a burning and poisonous vapour. As a consequence, dew and rain infect the earth and poison what is born from it, the products of farming become contaminated, and the underground vapours are shaken, causing earthquakes.[67] By explaining the pestilences and catastrophes in natural terms (*naturaliter*), Albert deprives Luke's verses and other apocalyptic Biblical passages (e.g., *Revelation* 8,5) of their eschatological value. This philosophical exegesis is in line with Albert's general uneasiness with prophetic eschatologism.[68]

4. The Aftermath of Albert's Discussion of Pestilences

According to John Arrizabalaga, the reactions of the mid-fourteenth-century plague treatises to the Black Death 'are the first attempts in late medieval Europe to construct it [scil., plague] as a disease-entity'.[69] In his fundamental article, Arrizabalaga

67 Albertus, *Enarrationes in secundam partem Evangelii Lucae (X–XXIV)*, ed. Auguste Borgnet (Alberti Magni Opera omnia, 23) (Paris: Vivès, 1894), p. 635a: '"Et pestilentiae". Secundum signum quod est ab aere. Aere enim corrupto cadit ros corruptus, et guttae pluviarum corruptae super terrae nascentia, et faciunt ea venenosa, et pestem sive mortalitatem inducentia. Unde pestilentia, ut dicit Isidorus, dicitur quasi pastulentia: quia pestis illa a pastu venenatorum causatur. Ezechiel. V, 17: *Pestilentia et sanguis transibunt per te*. Jerem. XXI, 6: *Percutiam habitatores civitatis hujus*, scilicet Jerusalem: *homines et bestiae pestilentia magna morientur.* De utroque istorum simul dicitur, Apocal. VIII, 5: *Accepit Angelus thuribulum, et implevit illud de igne altaris, et misit in terram: et facta sunt tonitrua, et voces, et fulgura, et terrae motus magnus.* Angelus autem est Christus Dominus, qui thuribulum cordis sui implevit igne furoris Domini in Judaeos, et effudit in terram Judaeam. Et facta sunt tonitrua et coruscationes, quae naturaliter ex vapore ignito venenoso et corrumpunt aerem, et pastum qui de terra nascitur: et commovendo vapores subterraneos faciunt terrae motum. Haec autem plaga spiritualiter ab eis procuratur, qui mala dant exempla: pastu enim illorum alii corrumpuntur'.

68 Albertus, *Commentarii in IV Sententiarum dist. XXIII–L*, ed. Auguste Borgnet (Alberti Magni Opera omnia, 30) (Paris: Vivès, 1894), IV. 43. 7, pp. 516–18, "An scibile sit tempus adventus Domini ad judicium".

69 John Arrizabalaga, 'Facing the Black Death', pp. 238, 286–87. On the numerous plague treatises related to the Black Death, see Dorothea Waley Singer, 'Some Plague Tractates (Fourtheenth and Fifteenth Centuries)', *Proceedings of the Royal Society of Medicine*. Section of the History of Medicine, 9 (1916), pp. 159–212; Anna Montgomery Campbell, *The Black Death and Men of Learning* (New York: Coloumbia University Press, 1931); Dominick Palazzotto, *The Black Death and medicine: a report and analysis of the tractates written between 1348 and 1350* (PhD dissertation, University of Kansas, 1973); Robert S. Gottfried, *The Black Death. Natural and Human Disaster in Medieval Europe* (New York-London-Toronto-Sydney: The Free Press, 1983), pp. 92–111; Irma Naso, 'Individuazione diagnostica della "Peste nera". Cultura medica e aspetti clinici', in *La peste nera: dati di una realtà*, pp. 351–81; Weill-Parot, 'La rationalité médicale', 73–88; Danielle Jacquart, 'La perception par les contemporains de la peste de 1348', in *L'homme*

has thoroughly explored some of the most authoritative plague treatises with specific regard to the arguments they put forward, the issues they address, and the sources they use. Yet, despite the accuracy and depth of his reconstruction, Arrizabalaga has failed to grasp the crucial role played by Albert's works in this plague literature. It is important to note that behind several of the theses and explanations advanced there were Albert's views on pestilences, and in particular on their etiology. The use of Albert's works is sometimes explicit, mostly silent, and in any case massive, so that it can legitimately be argued that Albert had already initiated the conceptual construction of plague as a 'disease-entity' about a century before the great plague pandemic broke out in Europe in 1347–48.

The recourse to Albert's interpretive categories is also a consequence of the initial widespread perception that the Black Death was not a new type of disease, but only one of the many pestilences occurred in the past, the only difference being its extreme severity and contagiousness.[70] The difficulty to conceptualize the specific character of this disease is also mirrored in the use of a rather traditional and unspecific nosographic vocabulary.[71] The situation changed some time after 1350, when physicians gained awareness of the peculiar features of the plague outbreak compared to past epidemics.[72] John of Burgundy, the author of an important work on plague, affirmed that modern physicians had become much more knowledgeable about the nature of the plague thanks to a long-lasting practice of cures — the statement is found in a tractate written in 1365, i.e., some eighteen years after the plague outbreak had first hit Europe. He also added that their competence in pestilential diseases was incomparably superior to that of medical practitioners and authors of the past because they, with the exception of Hippocrates, had not experienced such a general and enduring epidemic in their life.[73]

Before examining some of the fourteenth-century plague treatises individually, it is worth briefly summarizing some of the main ideas these treatises share with Albert.

---

face aux calamités naturelles dans l'Antiquité et au Moyen Âge. Actes du 16ème colloque de la Villa Kérylos à Beaulieu-sur-Mer les 14 & 15 octobre 2005 (Paris: Académie des Inscriptions et Belles-Lettres, 2006), pp. 237–47; John Aberth, *Doctoring the Black Death*.

70 Arrizabalaga, 'Facing the Black Death', pp. 247–48, claims that only Gentile da Foligno changed his view expressed in his earliest and major *consilium*, by acknowledging the unprecedented nature of the 1348 pestilence in two subsequent *consilia*. On the persuasion of a continuity with previous pestilences, see Sabine Krüger, 'Krise der Zeit als Ursache der Pest? Der Traktat De mortalitate in Alamannia des Konrad von Megenberg', in *Festschrift für Hermann Heimpel zum 70. Geburtstag am 19. September 1971*, 2 Bd., ed. by Mitarbeitern des Max-Planck-Instituts für Geschichte (Göttingen: Vandenhoeck & Ruprecht, 1972), pp. 839–83 (p. 839, n. 2).

71 Naso, 'Individuazione diagnostica', pp. 357–61, pp. 372–73.

72 Melissa P. Chase, 'Fevers, Poisons and Apostemes: Authority and Experience in Montpellier Plague Treatises', *Annals of the New York Academy of Sciences*, 441 (1985), pp. 153–69, argues that from 1360 onward Montepellier physicians felt the need for an accurate taxonomy of epidemic diseases and were concerned with fitting plague within an appropriate category. In other words, their clinical experience and the requests of public authorities led this generation of doctors to re-categorize plague and outline its nosographic contours more clearly.

73 Karl Sudhoff, 'Pestschriften aus den ersten 150 Jahren nach der Epidemie des "schwarzen Todes" 1348. III', *Archiv für Geschichte der Medizin*, 5 (1912), pp. 62–69.

As a preliminary remark, it is important to stress that the Aristotelian *Meteora* and the Pseudo-Aristotelian *DCPE*, along with Albert's commentaries on the two works, were given primary importance among the many philosophical and medical works the fourteenth-century literature on plague drew upon and quoted from.[74]

The plague tracts generally agreed with Albert on the theorization of two levels of causes for epidemics — remote and astrological causes, on the one hand, close and physical causes, on the other. Arrizabalaga traces this distinction back to Avicenna, who had differentiated the forms of the heavens from the near causes of pestilential fevers.[75] However, several plague tractates had a more markedly astrological understanding of the remote causes than Avicenna. By celestial and universal causes these treatises usually meant planetary conjunctions, in particular that of Saturn, Jupiter, and Mars in Aquarius which occurred in 1345.[76] Arrizabalaga mentions a few works referring to this famous conjunction (Augustine of Trento's tractate, the *Compendium* of the masters of the Paris medical Faculty, the tractate of the anonymous practitioner of Montpellier),[77] but there were many more.[78] Almost all of them were indebted,

74 Albert's commentary on the *DCPE* is quoted not only by the works we examine below, but also by other plague treatises, for instance by Petrus de Amousis' *Tractatus de epydimia*: see Jacquart, 'La perception par les contemporains', 240. On this work, see Alfred Coville, 'Écrits contemporains sur la peste de 1348 à 1350', in *Histoire littéraire de la France*, t. 37 (Paris: Imprimerie Nationale, 1938), pp. 325–90 (pp. 327–359).

75 Arrizabalaga, 'Facing the Black Death', pp. 251–52. For the general Avicennian scheme, see Avicenna, *Liber canonis*, IV. fen i. tract. 4. cap. 1. f. 416ra.

76 According to Bernard R. Goldstein and David Pingree, 'Levi ben Gerson's Prognostication for the Conjunction of 1345', *Transactions of the American Philosophical Society*, 80. 6, (1990) pp. 1–60 (p. 52), the triple conjunction was in fact not a single conjunction of the three planets but a series of three conjunctions, of Mars with Jupiter (1st of March), Mars with Saturn (4th of March), and Jupiter with Saturn (21st of March).

77 Arrizabalaga, 'Facing the Black Death', pp. 252–54. Apart from the reference to the 1345 conjunction of the three major planets, Augustine's treatise stands out for the prominent place it gives to astrological factors for the understanding of pestilences. On Augustine's work, see Lynn Thorndike, 'A pest tractate before the black death', *Sudhoffs Archiv für Geschichte der Medizin*, 23 (1930), pp. 346–56 (repr. with additions as 'Augustine of Trent; a pest tractate before the black death', in Lynn Thorndike, *A History of Magic and Experimental Science*, vol. 3 [New York: Columbia University Press, 1934], pp. 224–32); Domenico Gobbi, *Agostino da Trento. Astrologia e medicina* (Trento: Civis, 2009); Francesca Bonini, 'Forms of Pronosticatio in the Plague Tractate by Augustine of Trento', in *Prophecy and Prophets in the Middle Ages*, ed. by Alessandro Palazzo and Anna Rodolfi (Firenze: Sismel-Edizioni il Galluzzo, 2020), pp. 215–34; Ead., 'The Plague Tractate by Augustine of Trento', *Studi Filosofici*, 43 (2020), pp. 53–74; Ead., 'Plague and Astrology in the Fourteenth Century: The Plague Tractate by Augustine of Trento', *Bulletin de Philosophie Médiévale*, 63 (2022), pp. 383–472.

78 See Campbell, *The Black Death and Men of Learning*, pp. 37–44; Coville, 'Écrits contemporains sur la peste de 1348 à 1350', pp. 363–65, pp. 372–82, with specific regard to the *Causa epidemiae et preservatio eiusdem* and Simon de Couvin's allegorical poem *De judicio Solis in conviviis Saturni*; Palazzotto, *The Black Death and medicine*, pp. 64–72. See, e.g., Symon de Covino, *De judicio Solis in conviviis Saturni*, ed. by Emile Littré, 'Opuscule relatif à la peste de 1348, composé par un contemporain', *Bibliothèque de l'école des chartes*, 2 (1841), pp. 206–43; Raimundus Chalmelli de Vivario, *De peste*, ed. by Robert Hoeniger, in Id., *Der schwarze Tod in Deutschland: ein Beitrag zur Geschichte des vierzehnten Jahrhunderts* (Berlin: Grosse, 1882), pp. 159–77 (p. 161); *Causa epidemiae et preservatio eiusdem*, ed. by Karl Sudhoff, *Archiv für Geschichte der Medizin*, 5, 1/2 (1911), no. 23, pp. 41–46 (p. 42); *Quaestiones*, ed. Karl Sudhoff, *Archiv für Geschichte der Medizin*, 11, 1/2 (1918), no. 107, pp. 52–55 (p. 53). The importance of the conjunction of

either explicitly or implicitly, to Albert on this point. In fewer cases, eclipses were also included among celestial causes of the plague.

The view that pestilence was caused by air corruption was predominant in the fourteenth-century plague treatises, whether or not they attributed this corruption to celestial causes.[79] Some tractates went as far as identifying plague with pestilential air *tout court*.[80] As said above, 'aerist' theory was a widespread etiological model of epidemics in Antiquity and the Middle Ages; therefore, it is difficult to regard Albert as the only source on this point.

However, more specific ideas put forward by some treatises might be traced back to Albert as a main source. Plague tractates shared Albert's conviction about the link between stench and pestilential air,[81] and thus his advice to avoid places contaminated by the presence of stagnant waters or corpses. A few animals — especially the basilisk — were viewed as a cause of poisonous vapours, just as Albert had held the *dracones* responsible for poisoning the air. Albert's view that often a pestilence followed an earthquake was a common conception among fourteenth-century authors.[82] Some of them saw this theory confirmed by the devastating earthquake that struck Carinthia and other areas of Austria, Southern Germany, and Friuli in 1348.

A few treatises explained the pestilence on the basis of the Avicennian soul-body doctrine, urging people not to entertain negative thoughts about or have fear of the plague, because mental images were thought to cause the sickness.[83] As said above,

---

the three superior planets also emerges in the vernacular adaptations of some of the Latin treatises: see, e.g., one of the vernacular versions of the Parisian *Compendium* and Guy de Chauliac's *La grande Chirurgie* in *Sylvie Bazin-Tacchella*, 'Rupture et continuité du discours médical à travers les écrits sur la peste de 1348: Le *Compendium de epidemia* (1348) et ses adaptations françaises. La relation de peste contenue dans la *Chirurgia Magna* de Guy de Chauliac (1363)', in *Air, miasmes et contagion*, pp. 105–56 (pp. 133–34 [Albert is quoted], p. 155).

Petrus de Amousis also refers to the 1345 conjuntion and uses astral configurations to explain the selectivity of contagion, human bodies being more or less subject to contamination depending on astral influences. For this reason, the fate of people living in the same climate may be different, with some dying and some surviving: see Jacquart, 'La perception par les contemporains', pp. 244–45. The selectivity of contagion is also explained on an astrological basis by Michele Savonarola and Antonio Guaineri, two fifteenth-century physicians: see Danielle Jacquart, 'Theory, Everyday Practice and Three Fifteenth-Century Physicians', *Osiris*, 6 (1990), pp. 140–60 (p. 146).

79 See Campbell, *The Black Death and Men of Learning*, pp. 48–56; Palazzotto, *The Black Death and medicine*, pp. 72–84.

80 See Arrizabalaga, 'Facing the Black Death', pp. 245–46.

81 Arrizabalaga, 'Facing the Black Death', 275–77, 285, mentions the Parisian *Compendium*, Gentile da Foligno, and Jacme d'Agramont. See also Palazzotto, *The Black Death and medicine*, pp. 165–91.

82 Besides the treatises examined below, see, e.g., *Epistola et regimen Alphontii Cordubensis, de pestilentia*, ed. by Karl Sudhoff, *Archiv für Geschichte der Medizin*, 3, 3 (1909), pp. 223–26 (p. 224); Karl Sudhoff, 'Pestschriften aus den ersten 150 Jahren nach der Epidemie des "schwarzen Todes" 1348. XI Ausarbeitungen über die Pest vor der Mitte des 15. Jahrhunderts entstanden im niederen Deutschland', *Archiv für Geschichte der Medizin*, 11, 1/2 (1918), no. 108, p. 56 (this is however a late treatise dating to the fifteenth century).

83 The idea is advanced not only by Jacme d'Agramont (Art. V, Part 2, Chap. 6), but also by several other treatises: see, e.g., *Ad preseruandum a pestilencia regimen bonum*, ed. by Karl Sudhoff, *Archiv für Geschichte der Medizin*, 11, 1/2 (1918), no. 113, p. 72.

the process whereby bodily transformations are induced by mental representations had been used by Albert to explain the genesis of leprosy.[84]

4.1. *Jacme d'Agramont*, Regiment de preservació de pestilència

A physician working at the medical *Studium* of Lérida, Jacme d'Agramont wrote a tractate on the plague titled *Regiment de preservació de pestilència* (= *Regiment*). The work is noteworthy for several reasons. First of all, since it dates to 24 April 1348, it is likely to be the first treatise to have been written after the outbreak of the Black Death in Europe. Furthermore, since Jacme intended to lay down a regimen of prevention for the benefit of ordinary people, he addressed his work not to professional physicians, but to the noble men and councillors of the town of Lérida in Catalonia. Moreover, due to its very purpose and addressees, the tractate was written in the Catalan vernacular.[85]

Albert's influence is more significant in the etiological section of this work. Jacme makes his debt clear through two explicit Albert quotes. Their importance cannot be underestimated, because apart from the often-quoted Sacred Scriptures there are only few *auctoritates* (Aristotle, Avicenna, Galen, Rhazes) cited by name in the *Regiment*. Jacme therefore contributed to the dissemination of some of Albert's natural-philosophical ideas about pestilences among a wider non-Latin readership.

But what notions does Jacme owe to Albert? Among the causes of a universal pestilence, Jacme includes planetary conjunctions, quoting the passage in Albert's commentary on the *DCPE* (I, 2, 2) dealing with the great conjunctions between Saturn and Jupiter as causes of mortality and depopulation. Jacme finds the deadly influence of the conjunction difficult to understand, because the qualities of Jupiter are opposed to those of Saturn and should prevent its negative action.[86] Albert is quoted once again as saying that the influence is due to an occult property without a proper name, just like the properties causing the purgative action of rhubarb or the attraction exerted by the magnet.[87]

Besides these explicit citations of Albert's work, in the *Regiment* we find some of his most important ideas. For instance, Jacme shares the view that a pestilence may be brought about by an infection of the air caused by unburied remains of men and horses lying on a battleground.[88] Moreover, he also agrees with the claim

---

84 On this, see also *Pesttraktat*, ed. by Karl Sudhoff, *Archiv für Geschichte der Medizin*, 11, 1/2 (1918), nos 114–15, p. 92 (dating to the fifteenth century).

85 On Jacme's *Regiment*, see Charles-Edward A. Winslow and María Luisa Duran-Reynals, 'Jacme d'Agramont and the first of the plague tractates', *Bulletin of the History of Medicine*, 22 (1948), pp. 747–65; Francisco José Cremades Rodríguez, *Traducció al castellà del* Regiment de preservació a epidèmia o pestilència e mortaldats *de Jacme d'Agramont* (Tesi doctoral, Universitat d'Alacant, 2009); Id., *El Regiment de preservació de pestilència (1348) de Jacme d'Agramont. Història del manuscrit guardat a Verdú, context i versió en català actual* (Tàrrega-Lleida: Museu Comarcal de l'Urgell-Tàrrega, 2016).

86 Jacme d'Agramont, *Regiment*, ed. Veny, Article II, Part 1, Ch. 2. p. 56b, 33–41.

87 *Regiment*, Article II. Part 1, Ch. 2. p. 56b, 42–46. I was not able to trace this passage in Albert's works.

88 *Regiment*, Article II. Part 1, Ch. 2. pp. 56b, 53–57a, 4.

that vapours formed inside the earth could sometimes cause earthquakes and, once emitted, mixed with the air, corrupting and thickening it.[89] Among the causes of a particular pestilence taking place in a specific city, Jacme also mentions high trees which impede ventilation and thus corrupt the air, but while Albert had referred specifically to walnut and oak trees, he mentions poplars, walnut trees, and fig trees — these differences probably depended on the different natural environments the two authors lived in.[90] Among the signs announcing the coming of a plague, the *Regiment* mentions the appearance in the sky of a fiery body called *drach*, which seems to be the same as the flying dragon mentioned by Albert and, in his wake, by the Parisian physicians in their *Compendium*.[91]

There is, however, a major difference between the *Regiment* and Albert's analyses. The *Regiment* contains frequent biblical references and often advances the view that the plague was a divine punishment for human iniquities. As said, Albert did not accept this theological explanation in a philosophical context. In the last article of the *Regiment*, Jacme goes even so far as to endorse the view that there was a moral plague parallel to the natural pestilence he had examined in the previous parts of the tractate.[92]

4.2. Compendium de epidimia per collegium facultatis medicorum Parisius ordinatum

Albeit not the first plague tractate from a chronological point of view — it dates to October of 1348 — the *Compendium de epidimia per collegium facultatis medicorum Parisius ordinatum* (= *Compendium*)[93] was highly influential due to its origin and official nature. It was a document written by the doctors of the medical faculty at the University of Paris upon request of the king Philipp VI of France and soon became a reference point for many other tractates on plague.[94]

89 *Regiment*, Article II. Part 1, Ch. 2. p. 57a, 26–33.

90 *Regiment*, Article II. Part 2, Ch. 1. p. 57b, 51–55.

91 *Regiment*, Article III. Ch. 1. p. 59a, 7–9.

92 *Regiment*, Article VI. pp. 65b, 25–66b, 47.

93 On the 'opinion' of the medical faculty of the University of Paris and its vernacular versions (contained respectively in the manuscripts Paris, Bibliothèque nationale de France, fr. 2001 and fr. 12323), see Hippolyte Émile Rébouis, *Étude historique et critique sur la peste* (Paris: Alphonse Picard–Croville-Morant & Foucart, 1888), pp. 34–46; Karl Sudhoff, 'Pestschriften aus den ersten 150 Jahren nach der Epidemie des "schwarzen Todes" 1348. XVIII. Pestschriften aus Frankreich, Spanien und England', *Archiv für Geschichte der Medizin*, 17, 1/3 (1925), pp. 12–139 (pp. 65–76); Coville, 'Écrits contemporains sur la peste de 1348 à 1350', pp. 336–59. Rudolf Sies, *Das 'Pariser Pestgutachten' von 1348 in altfranzösischer Fassung* (Würzburger medizinhistorische Forschungen, 7) (Hannover: Pattensen, 1977), has prepared the critical edition of the vernacular version in Paris, Bibliothèque nationale de France, fr. 12323. Bazin-Tacchella, 'Rupture et continuité du discours médical', pp. 105–31, carries out a comparative analysis of the two vernacular versions of the *Compendium* and Guy of Chauliac's *La Grande Chirurgie*.

94 Campbell, *The Black Death and Men of Learning*, p. 16; Naso, 'Individuazione diagnostica', p. 361; Smoller, 'Earthquakes, Hail, Frogs, and Geography', pp. 172–74, defines the document as the 'best-known scientific discussion of plague from the mid-fourteenth century' (p. 172), while Bazin-Tacchella, 'Rupture et continuité du discours médical', 128, qualifies it as 'un text de référence'.

At the outset of the *Compendium*, the Parisian doctors affirm that they will rely on the statements of ancient renowned philosophers as well as modern wise men, both astrologers and physicians. Albert too must be counted among these sources.[95]

First of all, his influence can be discerned in the idea that the epidemic (*epidimia*) — this is one of the names used by the Parisian masters to refer to the plague — is brought about by both a superior and celestial cause and an inferior and earthly one.[96]

The *Compendium* regards a celestial constellation as the remote and first cause of the 1347–48 pestilence.[97] In particular, the plague pandemic is ascribed to the 'greatest' conjunction of the three major planets (Saturn, Jupiter, and Mars) in Aquarius on 20 March 1345, at one o'clock in the afternoon. This conjunction, aided by other conjunctions and eclipses, corrupted the air surrounding the physicians (*nos*) and heralded both death and famine.[98]

This explanation is bolstered with a quote from the Pseudo-Aristotelian *DCPE* alluding to the great conjunctions of Saturn and Jupiter, occurring every 240 years at every shift of triplicity and producing devastating effects.[99] Albert's influence is explicit because a quote from his commentary on the *DCPE* follows immediately (II, 2, 1). In this passage, which I have already analysed above, Albert depicts the conjunction of Mars and Jupiter as the origin of a pestilential air.[100] It is important

95 *Compendium de epidimia per collegium Facultatis medicorum Parisius ordinatum*, ed. by H. Émile Rébouis, in Id., *Étude historique et critique sur la peste*, pp. 70–145 (p. 72): 'clarissimorum philosophorum antiquorum dictis, ac etiam modernorum sapientium, tam astronomorum quam medicorum'. Other, full or partial, editions of the text are in Justus Friedrich Karl Hecker, 'The Black Death in the fourteenth century', *Wissenschaftliche Annalen der gesammten Heilkunde*, 29 (1834), pp. 219–39; L.-A. Joseph Michon, *Documents inédits sur la grande peste de 1348 (Consultation de la Faculte de Paris, consultation d'un praticien de Montpellier, description de Guillaume de Machaut)* (Paris: J.-B. Baillière et fils, 1860), pp. 49–70; Hoeniger, *Der schwarze Tod in Deutschland*, pp. 152–56.

96 *Compendium*, p. 74.

97 *Compendium*, p. 76: 'Dicamus igitur quod remota causa et primeria istius pestilentie fuit et est aliqua constellatio celestis'.

98 *Compendium*, p. 76: 'Anno namque domini MCCCXLV fuit maxima conjunctio trium planetarum superiorum, scilicet XX[a] die mensis martii, in aquario, prima hora post meridiem: que quidem conjunctio, cum aliquibus conjunctionibus et eclipsibus prioris corruptionis pernecabilis ipsius aeris nos cicumdantis causa existens, mortalitatem et famem nec non et alia multa signat [...]'.

99 *Compendium*, p. 76: '[...] testatur Aristoteles, libro suo de causis proprietatum elementorum, circa medium, dicens quod: mortalitas gentium et regna vacua fiunt apud conjunctionem stellarum duarum, Saturni scilicet et Jovis; propter permutationem duarum ipsarum de triplicitate ad triplicitatem, accidunt accidentia magna; et hoc est inventum apud antiquos philosophos''. See Ps.-Aristoteles, *De causis proprietatum elementorum*, pp. 63, 80–82.

100 *Compendium*, p. 78: 'Et Albertus de Colonia, libro suo de causis proprietatis elementorum, tractatu 2°, cap. 1, dicit quod conjunctio duarum stellarum, scilicet Martis et Jovis, inducunt magnam pestilentiam in aere [...]'. See *DCPE*, II. 2. 1. p. 96, 53–68. The same combination of the two passages, that on the great conjunctions of Saturn and Jupiter from Ps.-Aristotle's *De causis proprietatum elementorum* and that on the conjunction of Jupiter and Mars from Albert's commentary on the *DCPE*, are also quoted in Raimundus Chalmelli de Vinario, *De peste*, ed. Robert Hoeniger, in, Id., *Der schwarze Tod in Deutschland*, p. 164. The quote from Albert's commentary on the *DCPE* is present not only in *Pesttraktate*, but also in astrological literature, for instance the *Summa iudicialis de accidentibus mundi* by John of Eschenden, a specialist in conjunctionist astrology: see Thorndike, *A History of magic and experimental science*, vol. 3, pp. 332–33, pp. 718–19.

to understand that Albert's description of the conjunction of Mars and Jupiter was designed to explain the genesis of the deadly wind that killed an army in Adremoth — a past event recounted by the *DCPE*. On the contrary, the *Compendium* analyses the recent astrological configuration of the two planets and remarks that, from the sixth day of October of 1347 to the end of May of the present year (1348), Mars was in Leo together with the Head of the Dragon, was retrograde, and was in an unfavourable aspect — the fourth — to Jupiter. This astrological configuration is said to be the cause of toxic vapours arising from the earth and infecting the air.[101]

The *Compendium* adds another quotation from Albert's *Met.* explaining the power of Jupiter to raise strong winds.[102] Once again, the *Compendium* adapts the Albert quotation to different geographical and astrological conditions: while Albert asserts that the power of Jupiter depended on the conjunction with Mars taking place in summer in the Northern signs, the *Consilium* speaks of southern winds and the region around Paris ('in nostra regione').

> Jupiter habet a proprietate sua elevare materiam ventorum fortium qui, ut plurimum meridionales existentes, caliditatem et humiditatem superfluas in istis inferioribus induxerunt. Humiditas tamen in nostra regione caliditatem superavit[103] (Jupiter has the property of rising the matter of strong winds, which, being mostly southern winds, produced excessive heat and humidity in these inferior regions. Yet in our region dampness outweighed heat).

In light of the aforesaid, it is clear that the doctors of the Parisian medical Faculty entirely depend on Albert as regards the universal and remote cause of the plague. To describe the 1345 conjunction of three superior planets, they adopt the theory of the great conjunctions, which they significantly do not read in the standard source on this topic — Albumasar's Book on *Great conjunctions* — but in a more concise version provided by the *DCPE*. In so doing, they are strongly influenced by Albert's commentary on the *DCPE*, which contains an exhaustive and technical account of the theory of conjunctions. Moreover, they understand the noxious interaction of Mars and Jupiter on the basis of the two above-mentioned passages in Albert's commentaries on the *DCPE* and the *Met.*

The *Compendium* points to air corruption as the particular and immediate cause of the epidemic,[104] adhering to Albert's views. Apart from this general agreement,

---

101 *Compendium*, p. 78.

102 *Compendium*, pp. 78–80: 'Exinde generati sunt venti validi, quia, secundum Albertum, libro quarto metereorum, Jupiter habet a proprietate sua elevare materiam ventorum fortium [...]'; see *Met.* III. 2. 22. p. 173, 36–47.

103 *Compendium*, pp. 78, 80.

104 *Compendium*, pp. 80–84. Joëlle Ducos, 'L'air corrompu dans les traités de peste', in *Air, miasmes et contagion*, pp. 87–104 (pp. 94–98), problematizes the concept of air corruption by arguing that the *Compendium* interweaves a meteorological perspective with medical discourse. As a consequence, she singles out four different meanings of air (the location of atmospheric phenomena, matter endowed with qualities and subject to be corrupted, air surrounding physical places and affecting physical states, and matter penetrating into the human body) in the text, remarking that many ambiguities arise concerning the concepts of air corruption, vapours, exhalations, etc.

we also find several tacit textual parallels: the Paris doctors implicitly refer to the passage of Albert's commentary on the *DCPE* (II, 2, 1) stating that contaminated air is more noxious than food and drink because it quickly penetrates into the heart and lung with its evil;[105] moreover, the *Consilium* shares Albert's view that putrid vapours can arise from swamps, ponds, deep valleys (*DNL*, 1, 13), and unburied corpses;[106] furthermore, the Parisian doctors accept the notion that the pestilence may be caused by the putrid vapours that give rise to earthquakes;[107] finally, we find that both Albert's *Met.* (I, 4, 8) and the Parisian physicians refer to that fiery body in the sky known as 'draco'.[108] In sum, the Parisian doctors give voice to some of Albert's most characteristic views on pestilences. Given the authoritativeness of the *Compendium*, these views became part of the fundamental concepts expounded by the plague treatises written during or after the Black Death. Whether or not Albert's name is mentioned, his ideas started enjoying wide currency.

Yet there were differences, too, between the *Compendium* and Albert's theories. Given the urgency of the health crisis and the need to counter the spread of the disease, the Parisian doctors do not limit themselves to the study of the etiology of the plague, but also devote a long section of their *Compendium* to prevention and therapy, aspects mostly neglected by Albert. Furthermore, in contrast with Albert's prominently scientific attitude, the *Compendium* urges the readers to turn to God with humility when the epidemic is caused by divine will. Nevertheless, not even in this case must physicians' advice be overlooked.[109]

4.3. Quidam tractatus de epidemia compositus a quodam practico de Montepessulano

A treatise written by an anonymous practitioner from Montepellier (= Practicus de Montepessulano) in 1349 offers us an example of what can be defined as Albert's conceptual influence.[110] From its beginning, the text shows an evident dependence on the *Compendium* of the Parisian physicians on a few specific points. In particular, in their wake it emphasizes the crucial role of the celestial causes by asserting that

---

105 *Compendium*, p. 80: 'aer enim malus nocibilior est cibis et potibus, eo quod velociter penetret ad cor et pulmonem cum sui malitia'.

106 *Compendium*, p. 82: 'ut puta a palludibus, lacubus, profundis vallibus, nec non et mortuis corporibus non sepultis nec combustis'.

107 *Compendium*, p. 82, p. 84: 'propter putrefactiones in interioribus coartatas que quando motum terre inducunt, et de facto nuper induxerunt; et sic nocere faciunt et fecerunt, aerem et aquam putrefaciendo'.

108 *Compendium*, p. 88.

109 *Compendium*, p. 92: 'Amplius pretermittere nolumus, quod quando epidimia a voluntate divina procedit, in quo casu non est aliud consilium nisi quod ad ipsum humiliter recurratur, consilium tamen medici non deserendo. Altissimus enim de terra creavit medicinam; unde sanat solus langores Deus qui de fragilitatis solo producit in largitate sua medicinam. Benedictus Deus, gloriosus et excelsus qui, auxiliari non desinens, certam curandi doctrinam timentibus explicavit'.

110 Text published in Michon, *Documents inédits sur la grande peste de 1348*, pp. 71–81. On the text, see Coville, 'Écrits contemporains sur la peste de 1348 à 1350', pp. 359–62. Another edition is Hecker, 'The Black Death in the fourteenth century', pp. 240–48.

the epidemic is identical with air corruption, and all air corruptions can be traced back to celestial causes.[111] The practitioner of Montepellier considers the planetary constellation of the three superior planets taking place in 1345 to be the cause of the plague outbreak. In this regard, he quotes the *Compendium*'s aforementioned passages concerning planetary conjunctions.[112] Since, as we know, the Parisian doctors had drawn their ideas on planetary conjunctions from Albert's views, the practitioner of Montepellier can be seen as being indirectly influenced by Albert via the *Compendium* of the Parisian doctors.

The most original trait of the Montepellier practitioner's treatise resides in its explanation of plague as a contagion due to an aerial spirit going out of the eyes of the sick person and striking the eyes of a healthy person standing nearby and looking at the sick person.[113] 'Visual contagion' gives the epidemic a greater strength and causes instantaneous death. Far from being regarded as miraculous, this form of contagion is considered to be a natural process similar to the phenomenon of burning mirrors described in the Euclidean *Catoptrica*[114]. The Montpellier practitioner describes the genesis of the infectious spirit issuing forth from the eyes in specific medical terms. As the brain expels the 'windy' and poisonous material through the concave optical nerves toward the eyes, the sick person is agonizing and his or her eyes are immobilized and thus unable to move from place to place. The first ventosity (*prima ventositas*), which is still and steady, continually produces a toxic spirit that seeks accommodation in some nature ('quaerit habitaculum in aliqua natura') into which it can enter and be at rest. If a healthy person gazes at this visible spirit (*spiritum visibilem*), he or she is contaminated by the pestilential disease. To clarify this process, the Montepellier physician adduces the example of the basilisk. As soon as this mythical animal firmly looks at a healthy person who observes it in turn, the venomous aerial spirit issuing forth from its eyes impacts the eyes of the person, poisoning him or her. And the basilisk's sight is by nature attracted by clearer body parts (*membra clariora*), like the eyes.[115]

111 Practicus de Montepessulano, p. 72: 'omnes enim corruptiones aeris reducuntur in causas coelestes'.

112 Practicus de Montepessulano, p. 72, p. 74.

113 Practicus de Montepessulano, pp. 72–73: 'sed major fortitudo hujus epidemiae, et quasi subito interficiens, est quando spiritus aerius egrediens ab oculis aegroti repercusserit ad oculum sani hominis circumstantis, et ipsum aegrum respicientis'. On this theory, see Stearns, *Infectious Ideas*, pp. 95–96. The idea of contagion through sight is also advanced by Guido de Cauliaco, *Chirurgia Magna*, II, doctr. 2, 5. (see Aberth, *The Black Death*, pp. 63–66: p. 64). Sound remarks on the concept of contagion in the plague tractates here examined are found in Palazzotto, *The Black Death and medicine*, pp. 93–99.

114 Practicus de Montepessulano, p. 73.

115 Practicus de Montepessulano, pp. 75–76: '[...] et aliquando cerebrum expellit hanc ventosam et venenosam materiam, per nervos opticos, concavos ad oculos, et tunc aeger est in agone, tenens oculos quasi non possent moveri de loco ad locum, et ibi prima ventositas recipit proprietatem mirabilem, quae, sic stans et permanens, continuo fit spiritus ille toxicus, et quaerit habitaculum in aliqua natura in quam possit intrare, et quiescere. Et quem spiritum visibilem si quis sanus aspexerit, suscipit impressionem morbi pestilentialis, et intoxicatur [...] Exemplum de basilisco, qui quando respexerit fortiter aliquem sanum, ipsum respicientem, statim spiritus visibilis et aereus, et venenosus, egrediens ab oculis basilisci, transiens in objecto, scilicet in oculo respicientis basiliscum, statim et subito intoxicat praedictum hominem; vel alias mutatum sit, quod ipsum mori oportet, et de proprietate ejus est semper respicere membra clariora,

As we have seen above, the poisoned spirit issuing from the eyes of a basilisk has parallels in Albert's works. It would probably be going too far to affirm that the physician of Montpellier depended on Albert as his only and immediate source on this point; it is certain, however, that Albert was one of the most authoritative medieval proponents of the view that the basilisk infects by sight and that he influenced all those who in the late Middle Ages evoked this extraordinary property of the basilisk, including the practitioner of Montpellier.

4.4. Tractatus de mortalitate in Alamannia (De epidimia magna)

Scholarly accounts of Conrad of Megenberg's scientific career have already demonstrated that Albert the Great was a fundamental source for his works.[116] Even though Conrad was not properly a physician, but a master of natural philosophy, he deserves our attention as the author of a tractate in the form of a *quaestio* devoted to the plague, entitled *Tractatus de mortalitate in Alamannia* (*Treatise on the Mortality in Germany*).

It must first be mentioned that before writing the Latin *Tractatus de mortalitate*, dating to 1350, Conrad had addressed the issue of plague in Book 2, Chapter 33 of the *Buch von der natürlichen Dingen* (1348–50), a vernacular encyclopaedia.[117] In contrast to previous scholarship, Dagmar Gottschall has emphasized that in the *Buch* Conrad has the attitude of a scientist concerned with understanding plague as a natural phenomenon of the physical world.[118]

Conrad adopts an identical scientific approach and puts forth the same views on plague in the *Tractatus de mortalitate*.[119] In this work, he singles out four possible causes of the plague: the Jews poisoning sources of drinking water; the celestial

---

scilicet oculos'. On this, see Arrizabalaga pp. 263–64. The vapour released from the menstruating woman's eyes too acts on clear bodies — mirrors and eyes: see Albertus, *De anima*, II. 3. 1. p. 97, 82–83, p. 98, 27–33.

116 See in particular Dagmar Gottschall, *Konrad von Megenbergs* Buch von den natürlichen Dingen*: ein Dokument deutschsprachiger Albertus Magnus-Rezeption im 14. Jahrhundert* (Leiden-Boston: Brill, 2004), esp. pp. 25–131.

117 Dagmar Gottschall, 'Scienza in volgare: Corrado di Megenberg e la peste del 1348', in *Filosofia in volgare nel medioevo*. Atti del convegno della Società italiana per lo studio del pensiero medievale (S.I.S.P.M.). Lecce, 27–29 settembre 2002, ed. by Nadia Bray and Loris Sturlese (Louvain-la-Neuve: FIDEM, 2003), pp. 107–31. As for Conrad's view on the earthquake as the cause of the plague in his vernacular work, his sources — among them Albert the Great — and the contemporary debates on this topic, see pp. 110–22.

118 Gottschall, 'Scienza in volgare', p. 113.

119 See Dagmar Gottschall, 'Conrad of Megenberg and the Causes of the Plague: a Latin Treatise on the Black Death Composed *c.* 1350 for the Papal Court in Avignon', in *La vie culturelle, intellectuelle et scientifique à la cours des papes d'Avignon*, ed. by Jacqueline Hamesse (Turnhout: Brepols, 2006), pp. 319–32 and the bibliography quoted therein. For the opposite interpretation of the treatise as the moral response of a theologian to the general crisis of his time, see Krüger, 'Krise der Zeit als Ursache der Pest?', pp. 839–62. On the tractate, see also Jens Pfeiffer, 'Macht der Sterne oder Miasmen der Erde: Heinrich von Mügeln und Konrad von Megenberg über die Pest von 1348', in Artes *im Mittelalter*, ed. by Ursula Schaefer (Berlin: Akademie Verlag, 1999), pp. 110–23. An abbreviation of Konrad's treatise, titled *Utrum mortalitas, que fuit hijs annis, fit ab ultione divina propter iniquitates hominum vel a cursu quodam naturali*, has been critically edited by Karl Sudhoff, 'Pestschriften aus den ersten 150 Jahren nach der Epidemie des "schwarzen

virtue due to specific planetary conjunctions; God punishing mankind's iniquities; and corrupted and venomous vapours released by the earth.

What about the presence of Albert in Conrad's *De mortalitate*? As in his other works, Conrad takes Albert's views as an unavoidable reference point, but he does not hesitate to take distance, wherever he finds them incorrect.

After easily rejecting the human agency theory,[120] Conrad examines the astrological explanation at some length. This theory is excluded for several reasons. First, since Saturn completes its orbit around the zodiac sphere in thirty years, mortality would happen every thirty years, but this is not the case. Nor could the conjunctions of Saturn with other planets cause mortality, for no conjunction would last as long as the pestilence, which at the time Conrad was writing the treatise had already been on the rampage for five or six years. Furthermore, whereas what is immediately caused in the sublunary realm by a conjunction occurs according to an orderly process, the pestilence was spreading randomly across regions without following any pattern.[121] For all of these reasons, Conrad concludes that the mortality does not seem to derive from the stars immediately, but in a mediated and very remote way.

Conrad subsequently cites Albert who, along with other natural philosophers, said that, when all planets are aligned in Aquarius, a universal deluge of water occurs by nature, while when they are all in Leo there is a universal deluge of fire. Conrad disagrees with Albert, even though Avicenna entertained the same idea regarding natural deluges.[122]

From another work by Conrad, his commentary on Tempier's *Syllabus* written around 1354, we learn the reason of this disagreement. With regard to article no. 182 of the Piché edition ('Quod possibile est quod fiat naturaliter universale diluvium ignis'), Conrad maintains that if a universal deluge took place naturally, all humankind and all perfect animals could be destroyed in a natural way and afterwards regenerated naturally without sexual reproduction ('naturaliter sine seminum propagacione'). In other words, a universal deluge caused by nature would imply spontaneous generation as the only way to repopulate the world in a natural way. This is an error, Conrad adds, into which Albert fell by following Avicenna's natural

---

Todes" 1348. XI. Ausarbeitungen über die Pest vor der Mitte des 15. Jahrhunders entstanden im niederen Deutschland', *Archiv für Geschichte der Medizin*, 11, 1/2 (1918), no. 106, pp. 44–92 (pp. 44–51).

120 Konrad von Megenberg, *Tractatus de mortalitate in Alamannia (De epidimia magna)*, ed. by Sabine Krüger, in Ead., 'Krise der Zeit als Ursache der Pest?', pp. 866–68.

121 Konrad von Megenberg, *Tractatus de mortalitate*, pp. 868–70. The same argument was advanced by *Die Pestschrift des Blasius Brascinonensis*, ed. Karl Sudhoff, *Archiv für Geschichte der Medizin*, 17, 1/3 (1925), no. 273, p. 117, where it is argued that, since the epidemic had lasted 57 years — the treatise dated to 1406 — it could not have arisen from any planet or conjunction of two planets, because these celestial periodicities (planetary orbits or conjunctions) were of different length.

122 Konrad von Megenberg, *Tractatus de mortalitate*, p. 870: 'Propter hec et similia non apparet michi hanc mortalitatem immediate fore ab astris, sed pocius mediate ac multum remote. Cuius exemplum pono. Aliqui etenim naturalium opinantur, sicut Albertus super De proprietatibus elementorum, quod omnibus planetis simul dyametraliter existentibus in Aquario fiat diluvium universale aque a natura, et eisdem dyametraliter stantibus in Leone fiat diluvium universale ignis, quod si verum esset, quamvis non credam illud, licet Avicenna fuerit hoc idem opinatus de diluvio naturali [...]'.

explanation of the universal deluges of water and fire.[123] Moreover, Conrad makes clear his rejection of spontaneous generation with regard to Tempier's article no. 188 (the Piché edition).[124]

If Conrad's attitude toward Albert's astrological explanation of universal deluges is negative, why does he quote the passage from Albert's commentary on the *DCPE* in the *De mortalitate*? Even though Conrad contests Albert's theory because it implies spontaneous reproduction of human beings, nevertheless he cites the very same theory as a confirmation that the death of living beings by water or fire would not be immediately produced by the stars, but by the elements. By the same token, Conrad imagines (*imaginor*) that the epidemic of the air ('epidimiam aeris') is caused by a corporeal essence existing in the air.[125] As we shall see, he will reveal the nature and origin of the epidemic of the air further in the text. Conrad's interpretive move is rather interesting: he makes his point that the stars are only remote causes of the pestilence by referring to Albert's very theory that he criticizes for its implication of spontaneous generation.

More relevant are the last two opinions. Conrad believes absolutely true ('veram esse omnino') the opinion — the third — that the epidemic is God taking vengeance

123 Konrad von Megenberg, *Werke. Ökonomik (Buch III)*, ed. by Sabine Krüger (Monumenta Germaniae Historica. Staatsschriften des späteren Mittelalters III, 5. 3) (Stuttgart: Anton Hiersemann, 1984), III. 1, cap. 14, pars 8, p. 155, 12–20: 'Quintus articulus est, quod possibile est, ut naturaliter fiat diluvium universale. Error est, quia tunc secundum viam nature possent omnes homines atque omnia animalia perfecta destrui et naturaliter sine seminum propagacione regenerari, quod est prius reprobatum. In hoc errore dominus Albertus olim nostre Ratisponensis ecclesie episcopus imitatus est Avicennam, sicut patet in commento suo De proprietatibus elementorum, ubi dicit, quod, cum omnes planete dyametraliter fuerint in Aquario, erit diluvium universale aque, sed cum omnes dyametraliter fuerint in Leone, fiet diluvium universale ignis'. Significantly, Conrad drops the mention of 'fire' ('fiat diluvium universale'), thus interpreting Tempier's article 182 as referring to a deluge of water too. On Conrad's understanding of Albert's theory of the deluge, I allow myself to refer to Alessandro Palazzo, 'Deluges, the Great Year, and Great Conjunctions in Albert the Great's Aristotelian Paraphrases', *Giornale critico della filosofia italiana*, s. VII, vol. XVII, a. C (CII), fasc. 3 (2021), pp. 495–520.

124 Konrad von Megenberg, *Werke. Ökonomik (Buch III)*, III. 1, cap. 14, pars 7, pp. 152, 14–153, 5. See David Piché, *La condamnation Parisienne* (Paris: Vrin, 1999) p. 136, no.188(82): 'Quod si in aliquo humore virtute stellarum deveniretur ad talem proportionem cuiusmodi proportio est in seminibus parentum, ex illo humore posset generari homo; et quod homo posset sufficienter generari ex putrefactione'. On the connection between the two articles in Conrad's commentary: see Roland Hissette, '*Le Symbolum Parisinum*: approche de trois commentaires médiévaux et évocation de doctrines significatives d'Albert le Grand', in *Il commento filosofico nell'Occidente latino (secoli XIII–XV)*, ed. by Gianfranco Fioravanti and others (Turnhout: Brepols, 2002), pp. 469–98 (pp. 482–83).

125 Konrad von Megenberg, *Tractatus de mortalitate*, p. 870: '[...] tunc absque dubio mortalitas, qua suffocarentur animata in aqua vel igne, non diceretur immediate fieri astris, sed pocius ab elementis, sicut ymaginor epidimiam aeris, id est interfectionem ipsius, a quodam corporeo esse in illo existente'. Ann G. Carmichael, 'Universal and Particular: The Language of Plague, 1348–1500', in *Pestilential complexities: understanding medieval plague*, pp. 17–52, calls attention to the problematic character of the universal language applied to plague; in this regard, she also refers to the comparison between the allegedly universal plague and the Universal Flood found in Matteo Villani (*Cronica*, I. 1, pp. 5, 1–7, 33) and Conrad of Megenberg (pp. 25–26). Gottschall claims that, according to Conrad, plague, unlike the Universal Flood, is a localized, however widespread, natural event and thus does not affect the whole world: Gottschall, 'Scienza in volgare', pp. 125–26.

on human beings for their wickedness.[126] However, it remains unclear how exactly divine omnipotence puts the punishment into effect. Conrad hesitates between two possible solutions: either God inflicts His punishment by spreading a deadly matter throughout the air and affecting human beings (*inflictive*) or He allows nature to have its course and lets the plague work its evil to punish human iniquity although He could have spared humans from the plague by acting against nature (*permissive*). What is important to note here is that even though both solutions fall into the third opinion as two species within the same genus, the latter (God's punishment *permissive*) leaves room for a natural explanation of the plague epidemic based on the analysis of its proximate causes.

This analysis is the fourth opinion, Conrad's own theory, according to which the immediate and independent cause of the epidemic is a corrupted and poisonous exhalation from the earth ('exalacio terrestris corrupta et venenosa'). For several pages (877–83) Conrad engages in a demonstration of the validity of this conception and the rejection of several counterarguments.[127] Tacitly quoting from Albert's *Met.*, Conrad explains aerial contamination as due to a vapour which, long trapped in the bowels and caves of the earth, is made poisonous. He also mentions the example of the well, for in Conrad's lifetime something similar happened in Regensburg.[128]

126 Konrad von Megenberg, *Tractatus de mortalitate*, p. 877: 'Sic ergo tot et tantis talibus(que) viciis mundo depravato irascitur deus et homines peccatores per diversa mundi climata stravit. [...] Quam opinionem credo veram esse omnino, quia vel permissive aut inflictive de sua omnipotentia magistravit corpora hominum infirmari et sanguinem in ipsis corrumpi'. For several pages he depicts the cultural and philosophical decline of his time leading to the pestilence: Konrad von Megenberg, *Tractatus de mortalitate*, pp. 871–77. On the cultural crisis portayed by Conrad, see Krüger, 'Krise der Zeit als Ursache der Pest?', pp. 844–57.

127 It should be noticed that Conrad initially introduces this thesis conditionally and hypothetically. Only at the end of the treatise the question addressed at the beginning (whether the great epidemic of those years was brought about by God's revenge or by the course of nature) will be answered definitely: see Konrad von Megenberg, *Tractatus de mortalitate*, p. 877: '(Q)uapropter hanc quartam pono opinionem in sensu condicionis et locucionis ypotetice [...]'. By contrast, the theory that plague is caused by corrupt vapours coming out of the earth (fourth opinion) is deemed as the most likely by the abbreviation published by Sudhoff: see *Utrum mortalitas, que fuit hijs annis* [...], ed. by Sudhoff, pp. 47, 131–32: 'Qua propter quarta opinio, quam probabiliorem alijs credo [...]'.

128 Konrad von Megenberg, *Tractatus de mortalitate*, pp. 877–78: '[...] aer vaporosus et plenus fumo terrestri diu clausus et incarceratus in aliquo mansorio terre adeo corrumpitur, ut venenum efficacissimum efficiatur humane nature et precipue in cavernis et ventribus terre, ubi per novum et recentem aerem adventari non poterit. Illud probatur experienciis quam plurimis sumptis a puteis longo tempore desertis et superius obstructis per plurimos annos. Nam quando tales putei aperiuntur et purgari debent, accidit nonnumquam, quod primus qui ingreditur, statim suffocatur et quandoque plures sibi mutuo succedentes. Sic accidit olim in Veneciis, ut recitat Albertus, in quodam puteo longis annis obstructo, in quo duo homines velociter moriebantur et tercius volebat videre, cur primi duo tantum moritentur et quid facerent, et accedens puteum respexit deorsum, qui statim cecidit et iacuit per triduum non loquens neque compos sui. Simile huic accidit temporibus nostris in Ratispona civitate Bawarie, ubi in apercione cuiusdam putei longis annis deserti tres ingredientes in illum mortui sunt, et vulgares causam ignorantes basiliscum putabant intus latitare et iterato eundem puteum obstruxerunt et obruerunt'. See, p. 881: '[...] videtur michi aer infectus et venenatus per vapores corruptos et exalaciones venenosas in terre motibus exalantes et egredientes causa esse et fuisse sepedicte mortalitatis'.

Conrad is not the only one to describe a contemporary event similar to the one experienced by Albert in Padua — Henry of Herford does the same. Therefore, it is reasonable to suppose that in the fourteenth century Albert's anecdote became a narrative frame for recasting accounts of real events. Conrad also evokes the belief that a basilisk lurking in a well was the cause of poisonous vapours, but disqualifies it as a belief held by 'commoners' (*vulgares*). On this point, one should notice that Henry of Herford has a different position, since he adduces the basilisk theory as a possible explanation for toxic exhalations. In general, by considering the basilisk explanation irrational, Conrad runs counter to Albert's theory that the breathing of some animals is one of the causes of air corruption.

In sum, Conrad advocates the specific version of the 'aerist' theory predicated on Aristotle's and Albert's natural-philosophical explanation of the earthquake as the effect of fumes enclosed in the bowels of the earth.[129]

This etiological explanation of the plague outbreak seems to be confirmed by the famous earthquake which in 1348 took place in Carinthia and nearby areas of Austria, southern Germany, and Friuli and released noxious vapours, killing human beings in several regions of the world.[130] In other words, to Conrad's mind a real contemporary catastrophe corroborates Albert's explanation of pestilences as a consequence of an earthquake.[131] Albert is also cited as the source of one of the arguments adduced in support of this theory. According to this passage, during some earthquakes human beings are transmuted into rocks, particularly salt rocks, due to the strong mineral virtue of earthly vapours.[132]

4.5. *Henry of Herford's* **Chronicon** *and* **Catena aurea entium**

Henry of Herford was a German Dominican friar of the fourteenth century (*c.* 1300–1377). The scanty information about his life and career has already been investigated,

---

129 Konrad von Megenberg, *Tractatus de mortalitate*, p. 878: 'Secundum fundamentum est, quod motus terre causatur ab exalacione terrestri seu fumo clauso in visceribus terre, qui quando pulsat cum impetu ad latera terre et exire non potest, terram quassat et movet illam. Ista causa de motu terre ab omnibus philosophis sciencie naturalis est approbata, nec oportet hic raciones philosophorum ad hoc inducere'.

130 Konrad von Megenberg, *Tractatus de mortalitate*, pp. 878–79. Conrad dates the earthquake to 1347.

131 Arno Borst, 'Das Erdbeben von 1348. Ein historischer Beitrag zur Katastrophenforschung', *Historische Zeitschrift*, 233 (1981), pp. 529–69 (pp. 542–45) on Conrad of Megenberg's reactions. On the earthquake, see Christa Hammerl, *Das Erdbeben vom 25. Jänner 1348 — Rekonstruktion des Naturereignisses* (Phd diss.: University of Vienna, 1992); Christian Rohr, 'Man and Natural Disaster in the Late Middle Ages: The Earthquake in Carinthia and Northen Italy on 25 January 1348 and its Perception', *Environment and History*, 9 (2003), pp. 127–49, who adopts a bound-mentality approach.

132 Konrad von Megenberg, *Tractatus de mortalitate*, p. 880: 'Octava racio est, quia visum est, ut recitant experti philosophi Avicenna et Albertus, quod in aliquibus terre motibus homines in lapides sunt transubstanciati et precipue in lapides salis propter fortem virtutem mineralem in vaporibus terrestribus existentem'. See Albertus, *De mineralibus*, ed. Auguste Borgnet (Alberti Magni Opera omnia, 5), (Paris: Vivès, 1890), I. 2. 8, p. 21b. The story of the transformation of people into salt rocks (salt pillars in the *Buch von der natürlichen Dingen*) became widespread in Early Modern Times: see Rohr, 'Man and Natural Disaster', p. 142, n. 42.

so there is no need here to insist on it.[133] His literary production was astonishingly vast and diversified, embracing several areas of study. His two main works are relevant for our analysis because they also address, among other issues, epidemics and the plague outbreak of the mid-fourteenth century. They are the *Chronicon*, a universal chronicle spanning all of human history, from the beginning of the world to Henry's lifetime,[134] and the *Catena aurea entium*, a large encyclopedia addressing in ten books all aspects of reality, from God to the elements, from the realms of minerals, plants, and animals to human beings.[135]

Henry's *Chronicon* is one of the richest historical sources on the Black Death in the German lands. The text, completed in 1355 — which is when Henry stops his historical account — recounts the tragic effects of the pestilence.[136] Henry provides us with first-hand information on the flagellants and the attacks on Jews, accused of propagating the epidemic by poisoning water sources.[137]

Yet Henry is far from giving us a merely fact-based account of the events. Not only because he reshapes contemporary facts through the Ovidian account of the plague on the island Oenopia in the time of king Aeacus,[138] but also because the pages he devotes to the plague are an astonishing interweaving of wondrous events,

---

133 See Klaus Peter Schumann, 'Wundergeschichten des Mindener Dominikaners Heinrich von Herford', *Mitteilungen des Mindener Geschichtsvereins*, 55 (1983), pp. 87–102; Id., *Heinrich von Herford. Enzyklopädische Gelehrsamkeit und universalhistorische Konzeption im Dienste dominikanischer Studien-bedürfnisse* (Münster: Landschaftsverband Westfalen-Lippe, 1996).

134 On Henry's historiographic activity, see Rosemarie Schlemmer, 'Die Bedeutung Heinrichs von Herford für die Westfälische Geschichtsschreibung', *Jahresbericht des historischen Vereins für die Gradschaft Ravensberg 1962–1963*, 65 (1964), pp. 125–66.

135 Small sections of the *Catena aurea entium* have been published in critical edition to date: Enrico di Herford, *Catena aurea entium. Tabula quaestionum I–VII*, ed. by L. Sturlese (Pisa: Scuola Normale Superiore, 1987); Id., *Catena aurea entium. Tabula quaestionum VIII–X*, ed. by A. Palazzo (Pisa: Scuola Normale Superiore, 2004); Henricus de Hervordia, *Catena aurea entium. Liber VI (De mineralibus)*, ed. M. Loconsole (CPTMA, 7. 4) (Hamburg: Meiner, 2023); Id., *Catena aurea entium. Liber VII Ansae 1–2 (De plantis)*, ed. M. Panarelli (CPTMA, 7. 5) (Hamburg: Meiner, 2023).

136 Henricus, *Chronicon*, pp. 273–74: '[…] epydimia tam ingens, atrox et seva violenter incanduit […]'. The interpretation of the plague outburst as a deluge of fire is noteworthy: '[…] tam ingens, tam pestifer ignis epydimialis conflagravit' (p. 274). To depict the devastation produced by the plague, Henry evokes images that were widespread in historical and literary sources (e.g. in Boccaccio's *Decameron*): people were abandoned by their loved ones, towns and the countryside were left empty, and cemeteries were overflowed. On the relationship between the medical treatises (i.e., the *consilia* of Gentile da Foligno and Giovanni della Penna) and Boccaccio's depiction of plague-stricken Florence, see Shona Kelly Wray, 'Boccaccio and the doctors: medicine and compassion in the face of plague', *Journal of Medieval History*, 30 (2004), pp. 301–22 and the literature quoted therein; Marafioti suggests an influence of the *Decameron* on later plague treatises, see Martin Marafioti, 'Post-*Decameron* Plague Treatises and the Boccacian Innovation of Narrative Prophylaxis', *Annali d'Italianistica* 23 (2005), *Literature & Science*, pp. 69–87.

137 Henricus, *Chronicon*, p. 277, pp. 280–81.

138 Henricus, *Chronicon*, p. 285; Ovidius, *Metam.* VII. 523–613. Kay Peter Jankrift, 'The Language of Plague and its Regional Perspectives: The Case of Medieval Germany', in *Pestilential complexities: understanding medieval plague*, pp. 53–58, argues that the concept of universality applied to epidemics in medieval records never refers to the "whole world", but to a specific region: this would be clear from the re-use of previous sources' descriptions of past epidemics that were confined to limited areas. This very same mechanism is also at work with Henry of Herford: in this regard, Jankrift alludes to Henry's mention of famine and mortality 'throughout the world' in 1003: pp. 55–56.

apocalyptic images, and naturalistic explanations. Laura A. Smoller has claimed that 'perhaps nowhere [i.e., in the plague literature] is this overlap and ambiguity between the natural and the supernatural more apparent than in the chronicle of Heinrich of Herford'.[139] In this work, we find a catalogue of several "miraculous" and supernatural events, which we might read as the consequence of the distress tormenting a plague-stricken society: fire fallen down from the sky; a rain of owls and snakes lasting several days;[140] devils haunting and killing people;[141] a lamb with two heads being born;[142] monsters, portents, and ghosts seen across Germany;[143] terrible visions sparking fear.[144] Moreover, Henry regards the appearing of the flagellants as a prefiguration of the coming of the Antichrist.[145] He describes them as being 'without a head' (*sine capite*) because they were lacking a leader (*caput*) to unite and guide them.[146] In this way, Henry hints at the famous Cedar of Lebanon prophecy (*quasi prophetice*), which had been circulating since around 1240, but in the fourteenth century had been redated to 1347 and was widely interpreted as foreshadowing the disaster of the plague.[147] Furthermore, Henry informs us that a Dominican named friar Robert (of Uzès?) had prophesized the great pestilence as God's punishment for human sins in 1317, thirty-three years before the plague outburst.[148]

This supernatural interpretation of the events related to the plague pandemic makes Henry of Herford far removed from Albert's scientific study of the pestilences. Despite this general difference, Albert's presence in the *Chronicon* remains nonetheless strong in several ways.

In the wake of Albert, Henry has recourse to scientific theories predicated on astrology and natural philosophy. The two-headed lamb is a monstrous birth due to

139 Smoller, 'Of Earthquakes, Hail, Frogs, and Geography', p. 177 (p. 178: 'No longer are these portents seen through the lens of an either/or dichotomy, either as natural events or as supernatural apocalyptic signs'. She examines Henry's *Chronicon* at pages 168–71, 177–82.

140 Henricus, *Chronicon*, p. 269: '[...] ignis de celo cadens [...] pluit aliquot diebus bufones et serpentes'.

141 Henricus, *Chronicon*, pp. 269–70.

142 Henricus, *Chronicon*, p. 270: 'Item hoc anno [scil. 1346] in Sosato opido Westphalie natus est agnus cum duobus capitibus'.

143 Henricus, *Chronicon*, p. 277: 'Principium autem regni Karoli istius multum videtur memorabile propter monstra et portenta et singularia plurima, quae tunc apparuerunt [...] Et fantasmata per diversas Theutonie partes et portenta varia similiter apparebant'; see also p. 279.

144 Henricus, *Chronicon*, pp. 277–78.

145 Henricus, *Chronicon*, p. 277: 'Gens sine capite flagellariorum adventum Antichristi prenuntiavit'.

146 Henricus, *Chronicon*, p. 280: 'Ex eodem anno gens sine capite [...] exsurgunt, cruciferos se vel flagellarios appellantes. Dicebantur quasi prophetice sine capite, vel quia ad litteram caput non habebant, quo unirentur vel dirigerentur [...]'.

147 Robert E. Lerner, *The Powers of Prophecy. The Cedar of Lebanon Vision from the Mongol Onslaught to the Dawn of the Enlightment* (Berkeley-Los Angeles-London: University of California Press, 1983), pp. 114–22 (p. 110).

148 Henricus, *Chronicon*, p. 233: 'Item frater Robertus ordinis predicatorum domus Avinionensis, genere quidem nobilis, sed sanctitate et devotione nobilior, pestilentiam generalem predixit ad annos 30, priusquam fieret'.

astral influence causing the seed to produce a form different from its quality.[149] On this subject, Henry adduces the scientific explanations of monstrous and spontaneous generation found in Albert the Great's commentaries on the *Physica* and the *Met.*[150] Moreover, in line with Albert's emphasis on conjunctionist astrology, Henry quotes the passage from Gherard of Cosvelde's tractate stating that an astral configuration had foreshadowed the flagellant movement.[151]

It is also worth noting that Henry, like Albert, bases some of his accounts on first-person observations. For instance, Henry recounts an event occurred in the town of Hameln near Minden, which was similar to Albert's anecdote about the events in Padua. There are only a few differences: the well of Albert's anecdote becomes a pit in the *Chronicon*; a fourth man is added to the three referred to by Albert.[152] These changes suggest that Henry is describing an event that occurred in reality. In other words, Henry, like Conrad a few years earlier, adapts a real fact to the narrative frame of Albert's anecdote.

As regards the origin of the poisonous vapour, Henry relates two widespread opinions. According to some, a basilisk snake was living in a small cavity inside the pit, infecting through sight or with its breath whatever got close to it. It should be noticed that the ability of the basilisk to infect through sight, which is documented in Albert's works, was absent in Conrad. Others thought that the earth had become poisonous because long before the pit had been used as a latrine. Henry admits that nobody knew what the truth was ('Quid autem esset in veritate, penitus a nullo sciebatur').

149 For the interpretations of this anomalous generation given in the course of histoy, see Sergey Ivanov, 'It's Raining Calves: History and sources of a spurious citation from Avicenna in Albert the Great's *Meteorology*', *Mediterranean. International journal on the transfer of knowledge*, 5 (2020), pp. 1–49.

150 Henricus, *Chronicon*, 270. See Albertus Magnus, *Physica. Pars 1 Libri 1–4*, ed. by Paul Hossfeld (Alberti Magni Opera omnia, 4. 1) (Münster i.W.: Aschendorff, 1987), II. 3. 3, p. 138, 33–46; *Met.*, II. 1. 21. p. 58, 26–38; III. 3. 20. pp. 171, 80–172, 3. On Albert's abnormal births, see Luke Demaitre and Anthony A. Travill, 'Human Embriology and Development in the Works of Albertus Magnus', in *Albertus Magnus and the Sciences*, pp. 405–40 (pp. 432–39); Theodor Wolfram Köhler, Homo animal nobilissimum. *Konturen des spezifisch Menschlichen in der naturphilosophischen Aristoteleskommentierung des dreizehnten Jahrunderts* (Leiden-Boston: Brill, 2008), pp. 387–411; Gabriella Zuccolin, *I gemelli nel medioevo. Questioni filosofiche, mediche e teologiche* (Como-Pavia: Ibis, 2019), pp. 144–57; Irven M. Resnick, 'Albert the Great on Nature and the Production of Hermaphrodites: Theoretical and Practical Considerations', *Traditio*, 74 (2019), pp. 307–34.

151 Henricus, *Chronicon*, pp. 283–84.

152 Henricus, *Chronicon*, pp. 285–86: 'Quarto anno Karoli in opido Hamelen supra Mindam in metis Westphalie et Saxonie pestis quedam singularis oboritur. Siquidem fovea fodiebatur, purgabatur et eruderabatur in area civis cujusdam ibidem. Fossor existens in imo, subito, nescitur a quo tactus, corruit et exspiravit. Alius descendit ad extrahendum primum jam frigidum, et ipse quoque mox extinctus est. Fama per opidum et terram diffunditur. Omnes admiratione metuque percelluntur. Lues quidem videbatur, sed causa non apparuit. Tertius cautius agere volens, fune forti cingitur circa corpus, per quem de fovea, cum opus esset, extraheretur. Ad medium fovee descendens pervenit, totoque corpore stupidus esse cepit et rigere. Signum dat. Semivivus extrahitur, aliquamdiu sic permanens. Post reviviscens, tempore longo decubuit, et tandem sanatur. Quartus descendens in foveam similiter ut primi duo periclitatur. Quidam opinabantur, in aliqua cavernula fovee serpentem basiliscum habitare, qui visu et anhelitu suo, quidquid sibi propinquat, dicitur vitiare; aliis putantibus, terram in fovea qualitatem aliquam venenosam contraxisse, quia prius et tempore multo latrina fuerit in eodem loco. Quid autem esset in veritate, penitus a nullo sciebatur'. See also, Smoller, 'Of Earthquakes, Hail, Frogs, and Geography', pp. 181–82.

Henry's failure to find the cause of the *lues* in Hameln is the clearest sign of his distance from Albert's scientific discourse on pestilences.

Significantly, while Albert — and Conrad in his wake — saw a connection between the intoxication produced by a well and the processes leading to the earthquake, which causes a pestilence, Henry does not. This is even more more significant if one considers that Henry's *Chronicon* also describes the terrible consequences of the 1348 earthquake of Carinthia.[153] Yet Henry does not claim the existence of a natural cause-and-effect relationship between the earthquake, which he dates to 1345,[154] and the plague epidemic, considering the earthquake to be an extraordinary harbinger, but not a cause, of the epidemic to come.

Henry also deals with plague and epidemics in the *Catena aurea entium*. This work is a collection of extracts from different sources (Albert the Great, Thomas Aquinas, Peter of Auvergne, Aristotle, Avicenna, Latin poets, *Timaeus*, medical literature, etc.) adduced to answer thousands of questions. Albert's works are the key sources for all the issues of natural philosophy addressed by Henry; therefore, it is hardly surprising to find almost all Albert passages pertaining to pestilences being cited by Henry too. Besides Albert, Henry draws on several other sources on pestilential vapours, poisons, pestilences, and contagious diseases. For instance, he deals with the impact of seasonal changes on diseases several times, drawing upon Hippocras, Galen, Constantine the African, and Pseudo-Aristotle's *Problemata* (V. 1. 127; II. 5. 13; X. 4. 118bis). Moreover, the section devoted to fevers and contagious diseases (X. 4) is based on medical literature (Galenus, Rogerius Salernitanus, Isaac Israeli's *De febribus*, Iohannes de Sancto Paulo, etc.). It is noteworthy that plague does not feature among the topics discussed in this section, with the only exception of question 119bis, which is however a mere cross-reference to previous questions (V. 1. 136; V. 2. 7). By contrast, leprosy is given particular attention as the subject of six questions. The reliance on Albert's natural philosophy and the other medical sources gives the examination of pestilences in the *Catena autea entium* a scientific tone that distances it from the tendency to the supernatural typical of the *Chronicon*.

To properly assess Henry's dependence on Albert's theory of pestilences in the *Catena*, a careful analysis of all the questions where Albert's texts are quoted would be required. Here a few remarks will suffice. In the *Catena*, all of Albert's main views about epidemics re-emerge: the distinction between astrological and physical causes of miasmatic contamination (IV. 3. 43); the role played by poisonous vapours and their origin from marshes and stagnant waters (II. 4. 25; II. 4. 33); the notion that the tainted air is more harmful to the human body than food and drink. As far as Henry's style of quotation is concerned, he either transcribes literally or paraphrases passages from Albert's works (II. 4. 25; II. 4. 33). A comparison between the questions of the *Catena* and the original passages quoted reveals that sometimes Henry slightly, but

153 Henricus, *Chronicon*, pp. 268–69.

154 Henry's account of the earthquake comes from correspondence between the convent of Friesach in Carinthia and the prior of the Dominican province of Germany: Rohr, 'Man and Natural Disaster', p. 140, n. 26. The inaccuracy of the dating may be due to the use of second-hand sources.

significantly, modifies his source. For instance, question II. 4. 25 explains why places that are very humid and not very warm are poisonous and pestiferous by quoting a passage from Albert's *DNL* (1. 13).[155] In this case, however, Henry mentions two swampy regions, the March of Brandeburg and Frisia, confirming his tendency to accommodate his sources — especially Albert quotations — within the framework of his own experience (II. 4. 33; IV. 4. 91). Moreover, Henry's quotation omits the last part of Albert's passage, the one that explains the relationship between the pestilential vapours and their natural environment (humid areas) in terms of the connaturality of the *locatum* with its *locus* ('locus et locatum connaturalitatem multam habent').

5. Conclusion

Albert's analysis of pestilences was conditioned by ineliminable historical limitations. Having died in 1280, about 70 years before a devastating plague pandemic — the so-called Black Death broke out in Europe in 1347–48 — he did not have the chance to experience and study plague in reality. As a consequence, he did not use the words *pestis* o *pestilentia* to refer to plague in the proper sense, caused by the bacterium *Yersinia pestis*, but to unspecified epidemics and contagious diseases, leprosy, miasmatic contamination, or malaria-like illness. Moreover, Albert's pages on pestilences mainly had a bookish origin, rather than being grounded in personal experience and observation.

However, despite all these objective limitations, his analyses deserve careful attention from the historian of philosophy and of medicine. Albert based his investigation into the causes and, in a few cases, the clinical progress of the disease on a solid scientific basis, relying on the conceptual resources of Aristotelian natural philosophy, the Hippocratic-Galenic and Avicennian medical tradition, and world astrology (i.e., the theory of conjunctions). His study of pestilences was thus a part of an all-encompassing attempt to explain all natural phenomena in scientific terms, without the need of a fideistic recourse to God's will. This was not tantamount to denying God's causality or His miraculous interventions, but to expelling supernatural factors from the realm of philosophical and scientific enquiry.

Moreover, his rigorous scientific approach was one of the reasons why Albert's analyses were widely echoed in the fourteenth-century plague treatises. Confronted with the unprecedented nature of the devastating pandemic of plague of their time, the authors of these tractates could only devise prophylactic remedies and therapeutic

155 Henricus de, *Catena aurea entium*, II. 4. 25. Erfurt, Universitätsbibliothek, cod. Ampl. F 371, fol. 81rb: 'Cur loca multum humida et parum calida sunt venenosa et pestifera ut Marchia Brandeburgensis et Frisia et similiter loca paludosa. Responsio Alberti ibidem: Quia loca talia plus habent humidi, quam calor consumere possit, et ideo calor idem adhuc plus multiplicat ipsum et vapores multos elevans corrumpit et loca pestifera facit. Et iterum in locis illis fiunt tonitrua et coruscationes et corrumpunt et inficiunt multum, ita quod inducunt in homines et alia animalia gravem mortem. Quod est quia aer humidus fit et corruptus et venenosus et penetrat indigestus ad interiora vitalium et perimit subito. Et loca paludosa similiter talia sunt'.

measures with a limited effectiveness. When it came to understanding the origin and the process of the dissemination of plague, the etiological models established by Albert played a major role. His analyses were a constant reference point for the fourteenth-century *Pesttraktate*. Indeed, they were the basis for the late-medieval discourse on plague — a discourse destined to remain basically unchanged for several centuries, until Alexandre Yersin discovered the bacterium *Yersinia pestis* in 1894, thus making clear the chain of contagion and the actual mechanism of transmission of the disease. It is ironical that in the fourteenth century Albert's concepts, which had been set forth to account for various pestilences and infections, but not for plague, were massively used for the construction of the etiological and nosological identity of this 'new' destructive disease.

Bibliography

Ad preseruandum a pestilencia regimen bonum, ed. by Karl Sudhoff, *Archiv für Geschichte der Medizin*, 11, 1/2 (1918), no. 113, pp. 72–73.

Aethicus Ister, *Cosmographia*, ed. by Michael W. Herren (Publications of the Journal of Medieval Latin, 8) (Turnhout: Brepols, 2011).

Albert the Great, *On the Causes of the Properties of the Elements (Liber de causis proprietatum elementorum)*, trans. with introduction and notes by Irven M. Resnick (Milwaukee: Marquette University Press, 2010).

Albertus Magnus, *De vegetabilibus libri VII*, ed. by Ernst Heinrich Friedrich Meyer and Karl Friedrich Wilhelm Jessen (Berlin: Typis et impensis Georgii Reimeri, 1867).

———, *De mineralibus*, ed. by Auguste Borgnet (Alberti Magni Opera omnia, 5), (Paris: Vivès, 1890).

———, *Commentarii in IV Sententiarum (dist. I–XXII)*, ed. by Auguste Borgnet (Alberti Magni Opera omnia, 29) (Paris: Vivès, 1894).

———, *Commentarii in IV Sententiarum dist. XXIII–L*, ed. by Auguste Borgnet (Alberti Magni Opera omnia, 30) (Paris: Vivès, 1894).

———, *Enarrationes in primam partem Evangelii Lucae (I–IX)*, ed. by Auguste Borgnet (Alberti Magni Opera omnia, 22) (Paris: Vivès, 1894).

———, *Enarrationes in secundam partem Evangelii Lucae (X–XXIV)*, ed. Auguste Borgnet (Alberti Magni Opera omnia, 23) (Paris: Vivès, 1894).

———, *De animalibus libri XXVI nach der Cölner Urschrift*, ed. by Hermann Stadler, 2 vols (Münster i.W.: Aschendorff, 1916–1920).

———, *Quaestiones super De animalibus*, ed. by Ephrem Filthaut (Alberti Magni Opera omnia, 12) (Münster i.W.: Aschendorff, 1955).

———, *De anima*, ed. by Clemens Stroick (Alberti Magni Opera omnia, 7. 1) (Münster i.W.: Aschendorff, 1968).

———, *De fato*, ed. by Paul Simon (Alberti Magni Opera omnia, 17. 1) (Münster i.W.: Aschendorff, 1975).

———, *De natura loci*, ed. by Paul Hossfeld (Alberti Magni Opera omnia, 5. 2) (Münster i.W.: Aschendorff, 1980).

———, *De causis proprietatum elementorum*, ed. by Paul Hossfeld (Alberti Magni Opera omnia, 5. 2) (Münster i.W.: Aschendorff, 1980).

———, *Physica. Pars 1 Libri 1–4*, ed. by Paul Hossfeld (Alberti Magni Opera omnia, 4. 1) (Münster i.W.: Aschendorff, 1987).

———, *De causis et processu universitatis a prima causa*, ed. by Winfried Fauser (Alberti Magni Opera omnia, 17. 2) (Münster i.W.: Aschendorff, 1993).

———, *Meteora*, ed. by Paul Hossfeld (Alberti Magni Opera omnia, 6. 1) (Münster i.W.: Aschendorff, 2004).

Alphontius Cordubensis, *Epistola et regimen de pestilentia*, ed. by Karl Sudhoff, *Archiv für Geschichte der Medizin*, 3, 3 (1909), pp. 223–26.

ps.-Aristoteles, *De causis proprietatum elementorum*, ed. by. Paul Hossfeld, in Albertus Magnus, *De causis proprietatum elementorum*, ed. by Paul Hossfeld (Münster i.W.: Aschendorff, 1980) (Alberti Magni Opera omnia, 5.2).

Avicenna , *Liber canonis* (Venetiis: 1507; repr. Hildesheim: Georg Olms Verlag, 2003).

———, *Liber de anima seu Sextus de naturalibus IV–V*, ed. by Simone Van Riet (Louvain-Leiden: Éditions Orientalistes-Brill, 1968).

Biblia Sacra iuxta Vulgatam versionem, ed. Robert Weber and others, 2 vols (Stuttgart: Deutsche Bibelgesellschaf, 1969).

Blasius Brascinonensis, *Pestschrift*, ed. Karl Sudhoff, *Archiv für Geschichte der Medizin*, 17, 1/3 (1925), no. 273, pp. 103–118.

Boccaccio, Giovanni, *Decameron*, ed. Vittore Branca, vols 2 (Torino: Einaudi, 2014[4]).

Causa epidemiae et preservatio eiusdem, ed. by Karl Sudhoff, *Archiv für Geschichte der Medizin*, 5, 1/2 (1911), no. 23, pp. 42–46.

Compendium de epidimia per collegium Facultatis medicorum Parisius ordinatum, ed. by H. Émile Rébouis, in Rébouis, Hippolyte Émile, *Étude historique et critique sur la peste* (Paris: Alphonse Picard–Croville-Morant & Foucart, 1888), pp. 70–145.

Eckhart, *Expositio s. evangelii secundum Iohannem*, ed. by Karl Christ and others (*Die lateinischen Werke*, Bd. 3) (Stuttgart-Berlin-Köln: Kohlhammer, 1994).

Enrico di Herford, *Catena aurea entium. Tabula quaestionum I–VII*, ed. by Loris Sturlese (Pisa: Scuola Normale Superiore, 1987).

———, *Catena aurea entium. Tabula quaestionum VIII–X*, ed. by Alessandro Palazzo (Pisa: Scuola Normale Superiore, 2004).

Gabriel de Mussi, *Historia de morbo*, ed. by August Wilhelm Henschel, 'Document zur Geschichte des schwarzen Todes', *Archives für die gesammte Medicin*, 2 (1842), pp. 45–59.

Galenus, *Commentarii in Hippocratis Epidemiorum libros*, ed. Karl Gottlob Kühn, vol. 17.1 (Leipzig: 1828).

Henricus de Hervordia, *Liber de rebus memorabilioribus sive Chronicon*, ed. August Potthast (Gottingae: Sumptibus Dieterichianis, 1959).

———, *Catena aurea entium. Liber VI (De mineralibus)*, ed. Mario Loconsole (CPTMA, 7. 4) (Hamburg: Meiner, 2023).

———, *Catena aurea entium. Liber VII Ansae 1–2 (De plantis)*, ed. Marilena Panarelli (CPTMA, 7. 5) (Hamburg: Meiner, 2023).

Iohannes de Rupescissa, *De consideratione quintae essentiae* (Basel: 1561).

Isidorus Hispalensis, *Etymologiarum sive originum libri XX*, ed. Wallace Martin Lindsay, (Oxford: Clarendon, 1911).

Jacme d'Agramont, 'Regimen of Protection Against Epidemics or Pestilences and Mortality', trans. by María Luisa Duran-Reynals and Charles-Edward A. Winslow, *Bulletin of the History of Medicine*, 23 (1949), pp. 57–89.

———, *Regiment de preservació de pestilència* (Lleida, 1348), intr. by Jon Arrizabalaga, Luis García Ballester, and Joan Veny, ed. by Joan Veny (Barcelona: Enciclopèdia Catalana, 1998).

Konrad von Megenberg, *Tractatus de mortalitate in Alamannia (De epidimia magna)*, ed. by Sabine Krüger, in Krüger, Sabine, 'Krise der Zeit als Ursache der Pest? Der Traktat De mortalitate in Alamannia des Konrad von Megenberg', in *Festschrift für Hermann Heimpel zum 70. Geburtstag am 19. September 1971*, 2 Bd., ed. by Mitarbeitern des Max-Planck-Instituts für Geschichte (Göttingen: Vandenhoeck & Ruprecht, 1972), pp. 866–68.

———, *Werke. Ökonomik (Buch III)*, ed. by Sabine Krüger (Monumenta Germaniae Historica. Staatsschriften des späteren Mittelalters III, 5. 3) (Stuttgart: Anton Hiersemann, 1984).

Ovidius, *Metamorphoses*, ed. William S. Anderson (Leizpig: Teubner, ^{4}1988).

Paulus Diaconus, *Historia Langobardorum*, ed. Georg Waitz (Monumenta Germaniae Historica. Scriptores rerum Langobardicarum et Italicarum sec. VI–IX) (Hannover: Hahn, 1988; repr. of ed. Hannoverae, impensis bibliopolii Hahniani 1878).

Petrarca, Francesco, *Prose*, ed. Pier Giorgio Ricci, Enrico Carrara, and Enrico Bianchi (Milano-Napoli: Ricciardi, 1955).

Petrus Lombardus, *Sententiae in IV libris distinctae*. T. II, *Liber III et IV*, Editiones Collegii S. Bonaventurae Ad Claras Aquas (Grottaferrata: 1981).

Practicus de Montepessulano, Tractatus de epidemia, in *Documents inédits sur la grande peste de 1348*, in L.-A. Joseph Michon, *Documents inédits sur la grande peste de 1348 (Consultation de la Faculte de Paris, consultation d'un praticien de Montpellier, description de Guillaume de Machaut)* (Paris: J.-B. Baillière et fils, 1860), pp. 71–81.

Quaestiones, ed. Karl Sudhoff, *Archiv für Geschichte der Medizin*, 11, 1/2 (1918), no. 107, pp. 52–55.

Raimundus Chalmelli de Vivario, *De peste*, ed. by Robert Hoeniger, in Id., *Der schwarze Tod in Deutschland: ein Beitrag zur Geschichte des vierzehnten Jahrhunderts* (Berlin: Grosse, 1882), pp. 159–77.

Symon de Covino, *De judicio Solis in conviviis Saturni*, ed. by Emile Littré, 'Opuscule relatif à la peste de 1348, composé par un contemporain', *Bibliothèque de l'école des chartes*, 2 (1841), pp. 206–43.

Utrum mortalitas, que fuit hijs annis, fit ab ultione divina propter iniquitates hominum vel a cursu quodam naturali, ed. by Karl Sudhoff, «Pestschriften aus den ersten 150 Jahren nach der Epidemie des "schwarzen Todes" 1348. XI. Ausarbeitungen über die Pest vor der Mitte des 15. Jahrhunders entstanden im niederen Deutschland», *Archiv für Geschichte der Medizin*, 11, 1/2 (1918), no. 106, pp. 44–51.

Villani, Giovanni, *Nuova Cronaca*, ed. Giuseppe Porta (Milano-Parma: Fondazione Pietro Bembo-Ugo Guanda, 1991).

Villani, Matteo, *Cronica con la continuazione di Filippo Villani*, ed. Giuseppe Porta (Milano-Parma: Fondazione Pietro Bembo-Ugo Guanda, 1995).

***

Aberth, John, *From the Brink of the Apocalypse: Confronting Famine, War, Plague, and Death in the Later Middle Ages* (New York-London: Routledge, 2001).

———, *The Black Death. The Great Mortality of 1348–1350. A Brief History with Documents* (New York: Palgrave Macmillan, 2005).

———, *Doctoring the Black Death: Medieval Europe's Medical Response to Plague.* (Lanham–Boulder–New York–London: Roman and Littlefield, 2021).

Alexander, Robert McNeill, 'The Evolution of the Basilisk', *Greece and Rome,* 10 (1963), pp. 170–81.

Arrizabalaga, John, 'Facing the Black Death: perceptions and reactions of university medical practitioners', in *Practical Medicine from Salerno to the Black Death,* ed. by Luis García-Ballester and others (Cambridge: Cambridge Universtiy Press, 1994), pp. 237–88.

Barker, Hannah, 'Laying the Corpses to Rest: Grain, Embargoes, and *Yersinia pestis* in the Black Sea, 1346–48', *Speculum,* 91/1 (2021), pp. 97–126.

Bazin-Tacchella, Sylvie, and others (eds.), *Air, miasmes et contagion. Les épidémies dans l'Antiquité et au Moyen Âge* (Langres: Dominique Guéniot, 2001).

———, 'Rupture et continuité du discours médical à travers les écrits sur la peste de 1348: Le *Compendium de epidemia* (1348) et ses adaptations françaises. La relation de peste contenue dans la *Chirurgia Magna* de Guy de Chauliac (1363)', in Bazin-Tacchella, Sylvie, and others (eds.), *Air, miasmes et contagion. Les épidémies dans l'Antiquité et au Moyen Âge* (Langres: Dominique Guéniot, 2001), pp. 105–56.

Benedictow, Ole J., *The Black Death 1346–1353. The complete history* (Woodbridge: Boydell Press, 2004).

Bergdolt, Klaus, *Der Schwarze Tod in Europa. Die Große Peste und das Ende des Mittelalters* (München: Beck, 1994).

Berlioz, Jacques, *Catastrophes naturelles et calamités au Moyen Age* (Firenze: Sismel-Edizioni del Galluzzo, 1998).

Biraben, Jean-Noël, *Les hommes et la peste en France dans les pays européens et méditerranéens,* 2 vols (Paris-La Haye: Mouton, 1975–76).

Bjork, Robert E., *Catastrophes and the Apocalyptic in the Middle Ages and the Renaissance* (Turnhout: Brepols, 2019).

Bonini, Francesca, 'Forms of *Pronosticatio* in the Plague Tractate by Augustine of Trento', in *Prophecy and Prophets in the Middle Ages,* ed. by Alessandro Palazzo and Anna Rodolfi (Firenze: Sismel-Edizioni il Galluzzo, 2020), pp. 215–34.

———, 'The Plague Tractate by Augustine of Trento', *Studi Filosofici,* 43 (2020), pp. 53–74.

———, 'Plague and Astrology in the Fourteenth Century: The Plague Tractate by Augustine of Trento', *Bulletin de Philosophie Médiévale,* 63 (2022), pp. 383–472.

Borst, Arno, 'Das Erdbeben von 1348. Ein historischer Beitrag zur Katastrophenforschung', *Historische Zeitschrift,* 233 (1981), pp. 529–69.

Brody, Saul Nathaniel, *The Disease of the Soul. Leprosy in Medieval Literature* (Ithaca-London: Cornell University Press, 1974).

Buchillet, Dominique, 'Epidemic Diseases in the Past: History, Philosophy, and Religious Thought', in *Encyclopedia of Infectious Diseases: Modern Methodologies,* ed. by Michel Tibayrenc (Hoboken: John Wiley and Sons, 2007), pp. 517–24.

Byrne, Joseph P., *Encyclopedia of the Black Death* (Santa Barbara, California-Denver, Colorado-Oxford: ABC-CLIO, 2012).

Campbell, Anna Montgomery, *The Black Death and Men of Learning* (New York: Coloumbia University Press, 1931).

Carmichael, Ann G., 'Universal and Particular: The Language of Plague, 1348–1500', in *Pestilential complexities: understanding medieval plague, Medical History. Supplement*, 27 (London: Wellcome Trust Centre for the History of Medicine at UCL, 2008), pp. 17–52.

Cerrito, Amalia, *Albert the Great (c. 1193-1280) and the Configuration of the Embryo: Virtus Formativa* (London: Palgrave Macmillan, 2023).

Chandelier, Joël, 'Définition et terminologie des épidémies dans la médicine latine de la fin du Moyen Âge', in *Épidémies, épizooties. Des représentations anciennes aux approches nouvelles*, ed. by François Clément (Rennes: Presses universitaires de Rennes, 2017), pp. 29–42.

Chase, Melissa P., 'Fevers, Poisons and Apostemes: Authority and Experience in Montpellier Plague Treatises', *Annals of the New York Academy of Sciences*, 441 (1985), pp. 153–69.

Cipolla, Carlo Maria, *Miasmi e umori* (Bologna: Il Mulino, 1989).

———, *Il pestifero e contagioso morbo. Combattere la peste nell'Italia del Seicento* (Bologna: Il Mulino, 2012).

Cohn, Samuel K., Jr., 'The Black Death and the Burning of the Jews', *Past and Present*, 196 (2007), pp. 3–36.

Collard, Franck, *Les écrits sur les poisons* (Turnhout: Brepols, 2016).

Comba, Rinaldo, 'Il rilevamento demografico: prima e dopo la peste nera', in *La peste nera: dati di una realtà ed elementi di una interpretazione.* Atti del XXX Convegno storico internazionale, Todi, 10–13 ottobre 1993 (Spoleto: Centro italiano di studi sull'Alto Medioevo, 1994), pp. 155–73.

Conrad, Lawrence I., and Wujastyk , Dominik (eds.), *Contagion. Perspectives from Pre-Modern Societies* (London-New York: Routledge, 2000).

Coville, Alfred, 'Écrits contemporains sur la peste de 1348 à 1350', in *Histoire littéraire de la France*, t. 37 (Paris: Imprimerie Nationale, 1938), pp. 325–90.

Cremades Rodríguez, Francisco José, *Traducció al castellà del* Regiment de preservació a epidèmia o pestilència e mortaldats *de Jacme d'Agramont* (Tesi doctoral, Universitat d'Alacant, 2009).

———, ———, *El Regiment de preservació de pestilència (1348) de Jacme d'Agramont. Història del manuscrit guardat a Verdú, context i versió en català actual* (Tàrrega-Lleida: Museu Comarcal de l'Urgell-Tàrrega, 2016).

Crisciani, Chiara, and Pereira, Michela, 'Black Death and Golden Remedies. Some Remarks on Alchemy and the Plague', in Paravicini Bagliani, Agostino, and Santi, Francesco (eds.), *The Regulation of Evil. Social and Cultural Attitudes to Epidemics in the Late Middle Ages* (Firenze: Sismel-Edizioni del Galluzzo, 1998), pp. 7–39.

Cunningham, Andrew, 'Transforming Plague: The Laboratory and the Identity of Infectious Disease', in *The Laboratory Revolution in Medicine*, ed. by Andrew Cunningham and Perry Williams (Cambridge: Cambridge University Press, 1992), pp. 209–44.

Dameron, George, 'Identificazione di un killer. Recenti scoperte scientifiche e storiche sulla natura della peste nera', in *Boccaccio 1313–2013*, ed. by Francesco Ciabattoni, Elsa Filosa, and Kristina Marie Olson (Ravenna: Longo, 2015), pp. 57–70.

de Asúa, Miguel, 'War and Peace: Medicine and Natural Philosophy in Albert the Great', in *A Companion to Albert the Great. Theology, Philosophy, and the Sciences*, ed. by Irven M. Resnick (Leiden-Boston: Brill 2013), pp. 269–97.

Demaitre, Luke, and Travill, Anthony A., 'Human Embriology and Development in the Works of Albertus Magnus', in *Albertus Magnus and the Sciences. Commemorative Essays 1980*, ed. by James Weisheipl (Toronto: Pontifical Institute of Medieval Studies, 1980), pp. 405–40.

Demaitre, Luke, *Leprosy in Pre-Modern Societies. A Malady of the Whole Body* (Baltimore: Johns Hopkins University Press, 2007).

Derbes, Vincent J., 'De Mussis and the Great Plague of 1348. A Forgotten Episode of Bacteriological Warfare', *Journal of the American Medical Association*, 196. 1 (1996), pp. 59–62.

Draelants, Isabelle, 'Phénomènes célestes et tremblements de terre au Moyen Âge: enquête sur l'historiographie médiévale dans les limites de la Belgique actuelle (600–1200)', in *Les catastrophes naturelles dans l'Europe médiévale et moderne*, ed. by Bartolomé Bennassar (Toulouse: Presses universitaires du Midi, 1996), pp. 187–222.

Ducos, Joëlle, 'L'air corrompu dans les traités de peste', in Bazin-Tacchella, Sylvie, and others (eds.), *Air, miasmes et contagion. Les épidémies dans l'Antiquité et au Moyen Âge* (Langres: Dominique Guéniot, 2001), pp. 87–104.

Eisenberg, Merle, and Mordechai, Lee, 'The Justinianic Plague and Global Pandemics: The Making of the Plague Concept', *American Historical Review*, 125 (2020), pp. 1632–67.

Gibbs, Frederick W., *Poison, Medicine, and Disease in Late Medieval and Early Modern Europe* (London-New York: Routledge, 2019).

Gobbi, Domenico, *Agostino da Trento. Astrologia e medicina* (Trento: Civis, 2009).

Goldstein, Bernard R., and Pingree, David, 'Levi ben Gerson's Prognostication for the Conjunction of 1345', *Transactions of the American Philosophical Society*, 80. 6, (1990) pp. 1–60.

Gottfried, Robert S., *The Black Death. Natural and Human Disaster in Medieval Europe* (New York-London-Toronto-Sydney: The Free Press, 1983), pp. 92–111.

Gottschall, Dagmar, 'Scienza in volgare: Corrado di Megenberg e la peste del 1348', in *Filosofia in volgare nel medioevo*. Atti del convegno della Società italiana per lo studio del pensiero medievale (S.I.S.P.M.). Lecce, 27–29 settembre 2002, ed. by Nadia Bray and Loris Sturlese (Louvain-la-Neuve: FIDEM, 2003), pp. 107–31.

———, *Konrad von Megenbergs* Buch von den natürlichen Dingen*: ein Dokument deutschsprachiger Albertus Magnus-Rezeption im 14. Jahrhundert* (Leiden-Boston: Brill, 2004).

———, 'Conrad of Megenberg and the Causes of the Plague: a Latin Treatise on the Black Death Composed ca. 1350 for the Papal Court in Avignon', in *La vie culturelle, intellectuelle et scientifique à la cours des papes d'Avignon*, ed. by Jacqueline Hamesse (Turnhout: Brepols, 2006), pp. 319–32.

Graus, F., *Pest — Geissler — Judenmorde. Das 14. Jahrhundert als Krisenzeit* (Göttingen: Vandenhoeck & Ruprecht, 1987; 2. durchges. Aufl.).

Green, Monica H. (ed.), *Pandemic Disease in the Medieval World: Rethinking the Black Death* (Kalamazoo–Bradford: ARC Medieval Press, 2015).

———, 'The Four Black Deaths', *American Historical Review*, 125 (2020), pp. 1601–31.

Grmek, Mirko D., 'Le concept d'infection dans l'Antiquité et au Moyen Age, les anciennes mesures sociales contre les maladies contagieuses et la fondation de la première quarantaine à Dubrovnik (1377)', *Rad Jugoslavenske Akademije Znanosti i Umjetnosti*, 384 (1980), pp. 9–55.

Hammerl, Christa, *Das Erdbeben vom 25. Jänner 1348 — Rekonstruktion des Naturereignisses* (Phd diss.: University of Vienna, 1992).

Hecker, Justus Friedrich Karl, 'The Black Death in the fourteenth century', *Wissenschaftliche Annalen der gesammten Heilkunde*, 29 (1834), pp. 219–39.

Herlihy, David, *The Black Death and the Transformation of the West*, ed. and introd. by Samuel K. Cohn, Jr. (Cambridge, Mass.-London: Harvard University Press, 1997).

Hissette, Roland, '*Le Symbolum Parisinum*: approche de trois commentaires médiévaux et évocation de doctrines significatives d'Albert le Grand', in *Il commento filosofico nell'Occidente latino (secoli XIII–XV)*, ed. by Gianfranco Fioravanti and others (Turnhout: Brepols, 2002), pp. 469–98.

Horden, Peregrine, 'Disease, dragons and saints: the management of epidemics in the Dark Ages', in *Epidemic and ideas. Essays on the historical perception of pestilence*, ed. by Terence Ranger and Paul Slack (Cambridge: Cambridge University Press, 1992), pp. 45–76.

Horrox, Rosemary (trans. and ed. by), *The Black Death* (Manchester-New York: Manchester University Press, 1994).

Jacquart, Danielle, 'Theory, Everyday Practice and Three Fifteenth-Century Physicians', *Osiris*, 6 (1990), pp. 140–60.

———, 'La perception par les contemporains de la peste de 1348', in *L'homme face aux calamités naturelles dans l'Antiquité et au Moyen Âge.* Actes du 16ème colloque de la Villa Kérylos à Beaulieu-sur-Mer les 14 & 15 octobre 2005 (Paris: Académie des Inscriptions et Belles-Lettres, 2006), pp. 237–47.

———, 'Les multiples facettes des relations entre empoisonnement et peste dans les explications médicales de la fin du Moyen Âge', in *Poison. Knowledge, Uses, Practices*, ed. by Caterina Mordeglia and Agostino Paravicini Bagliani (Firenze: Sismel-Edizioni del Galluzzo, 2022), pp. 223–48.

Jankrift, Kay Peter, 'The Language of Plague and its Regional Perspectives: The Case of Medieval Germany', in *Pestilential complexities: understanding medieval plague, Medical History. Supplement*, 27 (London: Wellcome Trust Centre for the History of Medicine at UCL, 2008), pp. 53–58.

———, *Im Angesicht der 'Pestilenz'. Seuchen in westfälischen und rheinischen Städten (1349–1600)* (Stuttgart: Steiner Verlag, 2020).

Jarcho, Saul, *The Concept of Contagion in Medicine, Literature and Religion* (Malabar: Krieger Publishing Company, 2000).

Ivanov, Sergey, 'It's Raining Calves: History and sources of a spurious citation from Avicenna in Albert the Great's *Meteorology*', *Mediterranean. International journal on the transfer of knowledge*, 5 (2020), pp. 1–49.

Keil, Gundolf, 'Seuchenzüge des Mittelalters', in *Mensch und Umwelt im Mittelalter*, ed. by Bernd Herrmann (Stuttgart: Deutsche Verlags-Anstalt, 1986), pp. 109–28.

Köhler, Theodor Wolfram, Homo animal nobilissimum. *Konturen des spezifisch Menschlichen in der naturphilosophischen Aristoteleskommentierung des dreizehnten Jahrunderts* (Leiden-Boston: Brill, 2008).

Krause, Katja, 'Grenzen der Philosophie. Albert der Großen Kommentar zu De animalibus und die Medizin', *Documenti e Studi sulla Tradizione Filosofica Medievale*, 30 (2019), pp. 265–93.

Krüger, Sabine, 'Krise der Zeit als Ursache der Pest? Der Traktat De mortalitate in Alamannia des Konrad von Megenberg', in *Festschrift für Hermann Heimpel zum 70. Geburtstag am 19. September 1971*, 2 Bd., ed. by Mitarbeitern des Max-Planck-Instituts für Geschichte (Göttingen: Vandenhoeck & Ruprecht, 1972), pp. 839–83.

La peste nera: dati di una realtà ed elementi di una interpretazione. Atti del XXX Convegno storico internazionale, Todi, 10–13 ottobre 1993 (Spoleto: Centro italiano di studi sull'Alto Medioevo, 1994).

Lerner, Robert E., 'The Black Death and Western European Eschatological Mentalities', *The American Historical Review*, 86 (1981), pp. 533–52.

———, *The Powers of Prophecy. The Cedar of Lebanon Vision from the Mongol Onslaught to the Dawn of the Enlightment* (Berkeley-Los Angeles-London: University of California Press, 1983), pp. 114–22.

Little, Lester K. (ed.), *Plague and the End of Antiquity. The Pandemic of 541–750* (Cambridge: Cambridge University Press, 2007).

———, 'Plague Historians in Lab Coats', *Past and Present*, 213 (November 2011), pp. 267–90.

Luongo, Alberto, *La peste nera. Contagio, crisi e nuovi equilibri nell'Italia del Trecento* (Roma: Carocci, 2022).

Marafioti, Martin, 'Post-*Decameron* Plague Treatises and the Boccacian Innovation of Narrative Prophylaxis', *Annali d'Italianistica* 23 (2005), *Literature & Science*, pp. 69–87.

Matheus, Michael, 'L'uomo di fronte alle calamità ambientali', in *Le calamità ambientali nel Tardo Medioevo europeo: realtà, percezioni, reazioni*. Atti del XII convegno del Centro di Studi sulla civiltà del tardo Medioevo S. Miniato, 31 maggio — 2 giugno 2008, ed. by Michael Matheus and others (Firenze: Firenze University Press 2010), pp. 1–20.

McCormick, Michael, 'Gregory of Tours on Sixth-Century Plague and Other Epidemics', *Speculum*, 96/1 (2021), pp. 38–96.

Michon, L.-A. Joseph, *Documents inédits sur la grande peste de 1348 (Consultation de la Faculte de Paris, consultation d'un praticien de Montpellier, description de Guillaume de Machaut)* (Paris: J.-B. Baillière et fils, 1860).

Naphy, William, and Spicer, Andrew, *Plague. Black Death and Pestilence in Europe* (Stroud: Tempus Publishing Limited, 2004).

Naso, Irma, 'Individuazione diagnostica della "Peste nera". Cultura medica e aspetti clinici', in *La peste nera: dati di una realtà ed elementi di una interpretazione*. Atti del XXX Convegno storico internazionale, Todi, 10–13 ottobre 1993 (Spoleto: Centro italiano di studi sull'Alto Medioevo, 1994), pp. 351–81.

Nutton, Vivian, 'The Seeds of Disease: An Explanation of Contagion and Infection from the Greeks to the Renaissance', *Medical History*, 27 (1983), pp. 1–34.

——— (ed.), *Pestilential complexities: understanding medieval plague, Medical History. Supplement*, 27 (London: Wellcome Trust Centre for the History of Medicine at UCL, 2008).

Palazzo, Alessandro, 'Astrology and Politics: the Theory of Great Conjunctions in Albert the Great', in *Stars, Kingdoms, Beliefs, and Masses. Political Astrology in the Mediterrenean Area from the Middle Ages to the Renaissance*, ed. by Marienza Benedetto and others, *Quaestio*, 19 (2019), pp. 173–203.

———, 'Deluges, the Great Year, and Great Conjunctions in Albert the Great's Aristotelian Paraphrases', *Giornale critico della filosofia italiana*, s. VII, vol. XVII, a. C (CII), fasc. 3 (2021), pp. 495–520.

———, 'Forms and Models of Contagion According to Albert the Great. Pestilence, Leprosy, the Basilisk, the Menstruating Woman, and Fascination', *Quaestio*, 23 (2023), pp. 221–251.

Palazzotto, Dominick, *The Black Death and medicine: a report and analysis of the tractates written between 1348 and 1350* (PhD dissertation, University of Kansas, 1973).

Palmer, Richard, 'The Church, Leprosy and Plague in Medieval and Early Modern Europe', in *The Church and Healing*. Papers Read at the Twentieth Summer Meeting and the Twenty First Winter Meeting of the Ecclesiastical History Society, ed. William J. Sheils (Oxford: Basil Blackwell, 1982), pp. 79–99.

Paravicini Bagliani, Agostino, and Santi, Francesco, *The Regulation of Evil. Social and Cultural Attitudes to Epidemics in the Late Middle Ages* (Firenze: Sismel-Edizioni del Galluzzo, 1998).

Pfeiffer, Jens, 'Macht der Sterne oder Miasmen der Erde: Heinrich von Mügeln und Konrad von Megenberg über die Pest von 1348', in Artes *im Mittelalter*, ed. by Ursula Schaefer (Berlin: Akademie Verlag, 1999), pp. 110–23.

Piché, David, *La condamnation Parisienne* (Paris: Vrin, 1999).

Rébouis, Hippolyte Émile, *Étude historique et critique sur la peste* (Paris: Alphonse Picard–Croville-Morant & Foucart, 1888), pp. 34–46.

Resnick, Irven M., 'Albert the Great on Nature and the Production of Hermaphrodites: Theoretical and Practical Considerations', *Traditio*, 74 (2019), pp. 307–34.

Robert, Aurélien, 'Contagion morale et transmission des maladies: histoire d'un chiasme [XIIIe-XIXe siècle]', *Tracés. Revue de Sciences humaines*, 21 (*Contagions*) (2011), pp. 41–60.

Rohr, Christian, 'Man and Natural Disaster in the Late Middle Ages: The Earthquake in Carinthia and Northen Italy on 25 January 1348 and its Perception', *Environment and History*, 9 (2003), pp. 127–49.

Schlemmer, Rosemarie, 'Die Bedeutung Heinrichs von Herford für die Westfälische Geschichtsschreibung', *Jahresbericht des historischen Vereins für die Gradschaft Ravensberg 1962–1963*, 65 (1964), pp. 125–66.

Schumann, Klaus Peter, 'Wundergeschichten des Mindener Dominikaners Heinrich von Herford', *Mitteilungen des Mindener Geschichtsvereins*, 55 (1983), pp. 87–102.

———, *Heinrich von Herford. Enzyklopädische Gelehrsamkeit und universalhistorische Konzeption im Dienste dominikanischer Studien-bedürfnisse* (Münster: Landschaftsverband Westfalen-Lippe, 1996).

Scott, Susan, and Duncan, Christopher, *Biology of Plagues. Evidence from Historical Population* (Cambridge: Cambridge University Press, 2001).

———, and ———, *Return of the Black Death: the world's greatest serial killer* (Chichester: Wiley, 2004).

Shipperges, Heinrich, 'Das medizinische Denken bei Albertus Magnus', in *Albertus Magnus. Doctor Universalis 1280/*1980, ed. by Gerbert Meyer and Albert Zimmermann (Mainz: Matthias-Grünewald-Verlag, 1980), pp. 279–94.

Sies, Rudolf, *Das 'Pariser Pestgutachten' von 1348 in altfranzösischer Fassung* (Würzburger medizinhistorische Forschungen, 7) (Hannover: Pattensen, 1977).

Singer, Dorothea Waley, 'Some Plague Tractates (Fourtheenth and Fifteenth Centuries)', *Proceedings of the Royal Society of Medicine*. Section of the History of Medicine, 9 (1916), pp. 159–212.

Siraisi, Nancy, 'The Medical Learning of Albertus Magnus', in *Albertus Magnus and the Sciences. Commemorative Essays 1980*, ed. by James Weisheipl (Toronto: Pontifical Institute of Medieval Studies, 1980), pp. 379–404.

Slack, Paul, 'Responses to Plague in Early Modern Europe: The Implications of Public Health', *Social Research*, 55 (1988), pp. 433–53.

Smoller, Laura A., 'Of Earthquakes, Hail, Frogs, and Geography: Plague and the Investigation of the Apocalypse in the Later Middle Ages', in *Last Things. Death and the Apocalypse in the Middle Ages*, ed. by Caroline Walker Bynum and Paul Freedman (Philadelphia: University of Pennsylvania Press, 2000), pp. 156–87, pp. 316–37.

Snowden, Frank M., *Epidemics and Society: From the Black Death to the Present* (New Haven: Yale University Press, 2019).

Stearns, Justin K., *Infectious Ideas. Contagion in Premodern Islamic and Christian Thought in the Western Mediterranean* (Baltimore: The Johns Hopkins University, 2011), pp. 91–105.

Stok, Fabio, 'Il lessico del contagio', in *Atti del Seminario Internazionale di Studi 'Letteratura scientifica e tecnica greca e latina'* (Messina 29–31 ottobre 1997), ed. by Paola Radici Colace and Antonino Zumbo (Messina: Edizioni Dr Antonino Sfameni, 2000), pp. 55–89.

Sudhoff, Karl, 'Pestschriften aus den ersten 150 Jahren nach der Epidemie des "schwarzen Todes" 1348. III', *Archiv für Geschichte der Medizin*, 5 (1912), pp. 62–69.

———, 'Pestschriften aus den ersten 150 Jahren nach der Epidemie des "schwarzen Todes" 1348. XI Ausarbeitungen über die Pest vor der Mitte des 15. Jahrhunderts entstanden im niederen Deutschland', *Archiv für Geschichte der Medizin*, 11, 1/2 (1918), pp. 44–92.

———, 'Pestschriften aus den ersten 150 Jahren nach der Epidemie des "schwarzen Todes" 1348. XVIII. Pestschriften aus Frankreich, Spanien und England', *Archiv für Geschichte der Medizin*, 17, 1/3 (1925), pp. 12–139.

Thorndike, Lynn, 'A pest tractate before the black death', *Sudhoffs Archiv für Geschichte der Medizin*, 23 (1930), pp. 346–56 (repr. with additions as 'Augustine of Trent; a pest tractate before the black death', in Lynn Thorndike, *A History of Magic and Experimental Science*, vol. 3 [New York: Columbia University Press, 1934], pp. 224–32).

Touati, François-Olivier, 'Contagion and Leprosy: Myth, Ideas and Evolution in Medieval Minds and Societies', in *Contagion. Perspectives from Pre-Modern Societies*, pp. 179–201.

Toubert, Pierre, 'La Peste Noire (1348), entre histoire et biologie moléculaire', *Journal des Savants*, 1 (2016), pp. 17–31.

Twigg, Graham, *The Black Death: a biological reappraisal* (London: Batsford, 1984).

Varanini, Gian Maria, 'Presentazione', in *Le calamità ambientali nel Tardo Medioevo europeo: realtà, percezioni, reazioni*. Atti del XII convegno del Centro di Studi sulla civiltà del tardo Medioevo S. Miniato, 31 maggio — 2 giugno 2008, ed. by Michael Matheus and others (Firenze: Firenze University Press 2010), pp. VII–X.

Weber, Jan Philipp, *Die Jugendpogrome zur Zeit des Schwarzen Todes 1348–1350. Was waren die Ursachen?* (München: Grin Verlag, 2019).

Weill-Parot, Nicolas, 'La rationalité médicale à l'épreuve de la peste: médecine, astrologie et magie (1348–1500)', *Médiévales*, 46 printemps (2004), pp. 73–88, https://journals.openedition.org/medievales/884

Wheelis, Mark, 'Biological Warfare at the 1346 Siege of Caffa', *Emerging Infectious Diseases*, 8 (2002), pp. 971–75.

Winslow, Charles-Edward A., and Duran-Reynals, María Luisa, 'Jacme d'Agramont and the first of the plague tractates', *Bulletin of the History of Medicine*, 22 (1948), pp. 747–65.

Wray, Shona Kelly, 'Boccaccio and the doctors: medicine and compassion in the face of plague', *Journal of Medieval History*, 30 (2004), pp. 301–22.

Ziegler, Philip, *The Black Death* (London: Collins, 1969).

Zuccolin, Gabriella, *I gemelli nel medioevo. Questioni filosofiche, mediche e teologiche* (Como-Pavia: Ibis, 2019).

DIANA DI SEGNI

4. Latin-into-Hebrew Treatises on the Black Death*

▼ **ABSTRACT** When the first epidemics of the Black Death struck Europe, a specific genre of medical literature on the plague developed. Among the medical manuals circulating at the time, a certain number were also written in Hebrew. Some of them were original works composed by Jewish physicians; other texts were translations of Arabic and Latin works into Hebrew. The phenomenon of Latin-into-Hebrew translations has long been disregarded, as it was considered marginal compared to the Arabic-into-Hebrew movement; this paper sheds light on this lesser-known aspect of the intercultural exchanges involving Hebrew, by focusing on plague treatises. The corpus of medical literature on the plague that was translated from Latin into Hebrew includes works by Gentile da Foligno, Francesco Zanelli of Bologna, John of Burgundy, Petrus de Tossignano, Antonio Guaineri of Pavia, and Valescus de Taranta. The aim of the paper is to offer a general overview of these texts, as until now only incomplete or erroneous information is available.

1.

When the first epidemics of the Black Death struck Europe between 1348 and 1353, a specific genre of medical literature developed and became widely influential.[1]

* This research was funded by the Department of Philosophy "Piero Martinetti" of the University of Milan under the Project "Departments of Excellence 2018-2022" awarded by the Ministry of University and Research (MUR).

1 For a general overview on the Black Death, see Anna Montgomery Campbell, *The Black Death and Men of Learning* (New York: Columbia University Press, 1931); Philip Ziegler, *The Black Death* (London: Collins, 1969; repr. 1991); Jean-Nöel Biraben, *Les hommes et la peste en France et dans les pays européens et méditerranéens*, 2 vols (Paris-La Haye: Mouton, 1975–76); *The Black Death*, trans. and ed. by Rosemary Horrox (Manchester-New York: Manchester University Press, 1994); Jon Arrizabalaga, 'Facing the Black Death: Perceptions and reactions of university medical practitioners', in *Practical Medicine from Salerno to the Black Death*, ed. by Luis García-Ballester and others (Cambridge: Cambridge University Press, 1994), pp. 237–88. See also chapter 3 of this volume.

Epidemics and Pandemics, ed. by Michele Nicoletti and Alessandro Palazzo (Turnhout: Brepols, 2024), pp. 105–130
BREPOLS PUBLISHERS 10.1484/M.STPH-EB.5.136408

Treatises devoted to the plague gathered scientific explanations for the pestilence, practical advice to avoid an infection, and possible remedies to treat the disease.[2] Among the various medical manuals circulating at the time, a certain number of those dedicated to the causes, treatment, and prevention of the plague were also written in Hebrew.[3] Original works composed by Jewish physicians as well as translations of Arabic and Latin texts into Hebrew formed a corpus of handbooks focused on the cure of the pestilence. Among the treatises written directly in Hebrew, we find the *Tractatulus de pestilentia* by Abraham Ben Solomon Ḥen;[4] the *Ma'amar be-qaddaḥot divriyyot u-minei qaddaḥot* ('Treatise on pestilential fevers and other kinds of fevers') by Abraham Caslari;[5] the *Be'er la-Ḥay* ('Well of life') by Isaac Ben Todros;[6] and the anonymous *Ha-ma'amar be-qaddaḥot ha-dever* ('Treatise on pestilential fever').[7]

The fact that medical literature in Hebrew flourished was first and foremost a result of the influence of works written in foreign languages, so that translations played a fundamental role in shaping Jewish medical libraries.[8] If in general Arabic-into-Hebrew translations were more frequent, the field of medicine represents an exception: especially in the fourteenth century, the number of Latin-into-Hebrew translations of medical treatises increased considerably.[9] This tendency reflects the

---

2 For a brief presentation of the most famous treatises, see Dorothea Waley Singer, 'Some Plague Tractates (Fourteenth and Fifteenth Centuries)', *Proceedings of the Royal Society of Medicine*. Section of the History of Medicine, 9 (1916), pp. 159–212. For a more detailed analysis, see Karl Sudhoff, 'Pestschriften aus den ersten 150 Jahren nach der Epidemie des 'Schwarzen Todes' 1348', *Archiv für Geschichte der Medizin*, 4 (1910–11), pp. 191–222, pp. 389–424; 5 (1911–12), pp. 36–87, pp. 332–96; 6 (1912–13), pp. 313–79; 7 (1913–14), pp. 57–114; 8 (1914–15), pp. 175–214, pp. 236–86; 9 (1915–16), pp. 53–78; pp. 117–67; 11 (1918–19), pp. 44–92, pp. 121–76; 14 (1922–23), pp. 1–25, pp. 79–105, pp. 129–68; 16 (1924–25), pp. 1–76, pp. 77–188; 17 (1925), pp. 12–139, pp. 241–91.

3 For a survey of this literature, see Ron Barkai, 'Jewish Treatises on the Black Death (1350–1500): A Preliminary Study', in *Medicine from the Black Death to the French Disease*, ed. by Roger French and others (London: Routledge, 2020), pp. 6–25.

4 See Gerrit Bos and Guido Mensching, 'The Black Death in Hebrew Literature: Abraham Ben Solomon Ḥen's *Tractatulus de pestilentia*', *Jewish Studies Quarterly*, 18 (2011), pp. 32–63.

5 See Herman Pinkhof, *Abraham Kashlari over Pestachtige Koortsen.* Hebreeuwsch met Nederlandsche Vertaling. Naar het te Leiden voorhanden handschrift, benevens een bericht over vier andere 14e eeuwsche Hebreeuwsche handschriften, handelende over de pest (Amsterdam: 1891).

6 See David Ginzburg, 'Be'er la-Ḥay: The Plague Treatise of R. Isaac ben Todros' [Hebrew], in *Jubelschrift zum neunzigsten Geburtstag des Dr L. Zunz*, (Berlin: Gershel, 1884), pp. 91–126.

7 The text is transmitted in the following manuscripts: Berlin, Staatsbibliothek Preussischer Kulturbesitz, Or. Qu. 836, fols 123–129, see Moritz Steinschneider, *Die Handschriften-Verzeichnisse der Königlichen Bibliothek zu Berlin: Verzeichniss der hebräischen Handschriften*, 2 vols (Berlin: Buchdruckerei der Königl. Akademie der Wissenschaften, 1878–1897), vol. 2, no. 232, p. 84.

8 For a general overview, see Carmen Caballero-Navas, 'Medicine among Medieval Jews. The Science, the Art, and the Practice', in *Science in medieval Jewish cultures*, ed. by Gad Freudenthal (Cambridge: Cambridge University Press, 2011), pp. 320–42. On translations, see Luis García-Ballester and others, 'Jewish Appreciation of Fourteenth-Century Scholastic Medicine', *Osiris*, (2nd series), 6 (1990), pp. 85–117; Lola Ferre, 'Hebrew Translations from Medical Treatises of Montpellier', *Korot*, 13 (1998), pp. 21–36. On the use of Hebrew in medical writings, see Harry Friedenwald, 'The use of the Hebrew language in medical literature', *Bulletin of the Institute of the History of Medicine*, 2 (1934), pp. 77–111.

9 See Gad Freudenthal, 'Arabic and Latin Cultures as Resources for the Hebrew Translation Movement. Comparative Considerations, Both Quantitative and Qualitative', in *Science in medieval Jewish cultures*, pp. 73–105.

needs of Jewish physicians, who sought for the most advanced knowledge that was available at the time, but whose access to contemporary scientific developments was hampered due to their lack of familiarity with the Latin language and to the fact that they were excluded from universities. The phenomenon of Latin-into-Hebrew translations has long been disregarded, as it was considered marginal compared to the Arabic-into-Hebrew movement.[10] The present paper sheds light on this lesser-known aspect of the intercultural exchanges involving Hebrew, by focusing on a specific genre within medical literature, namely plague treatises. The number of texts devoted to the pestilence that has been translated from Latin in the fourteenth and fifteenth centuries is a clear indicator of the interest that Jewish physicians had in the information at disposal of their Christian colleagues as well as of the shift towards Latin sources rather than Arabic ones. Often, these translations feature a preface written by the translator, which is of fundamental importance in order to understand the motivations that led to such an endeavour.

The corpus of medical literature on the plague that was translated from Latin into Hebrew includes works by Gentile da Foligno, Francesco Zanelli of Bologna, John of Burgundy, Petrus de Tossignano, Antonio Guaineri of Pavia, and Valescus de Taranta.[11] The aim of the present paper is to offer a general overview of these texts, as until now only incomplete or erroneous information is available.[12] Most references to those writings are found in scholarship that dates back to the nineteenth century and needs to be updated. Thanks to various ongoing projects dedicated to the digitalization of manuscripts, documents were recently made accessible, which enabled the identification of previously unknown sources. This contribution thus presents newly discovered data and organizes research material in a coherent way, by relating different pieces of information that were hitherto spread in various sources.

10 See Alexander Fidora and others, 'Latin-into-Hebrew: Introducing a Neglected Chapter in European Cultural History', in *Latin-into-Hebrew: Texts and Studies*, vol. 1, ed. by Alexander Fidora and others (Leiden-Boston: Brill, 2013), pp. 1–10.

11 We also know of translations from Latin into Judeo-Spanish, such as the treatise *Preservatio contra pestilenciam*, written in 1370 by the physician Jean de Tournemire, see Barkai, 'Jewish Treatises on the Black Death', p. 7. Moreover, there are also translations from vernacular languages into Hebrew, such as the treatise *Hanhagat ha-dever* (*Regimen of the Plague*), based on Valescus de Taranta's work on the plague, see below, n. 82.

12 The groundbreaking work by Ron Barkai is fundamental in order to approach the topic of plague treatises in Hebrew; however, it contains some imprecisions: it, e.g., dates the *'Etzer elohi ma'mar be-'ipush ha-avir ve-ha-dever* to the year 1399 (see Barkai, 'Jewish Treatises on the Black Death', p. 7), while the manuscript Paris, Bibliothèque nationale de France, héb. 1191, fols 141r–145v mention the year 22 — for which it has been suggested to read 122, corresponding to the year 1362. Moreover, Barkai attributes the translation of Francesco Zanelli's work to Samuel ben Jacob (see Barkai, 'Jewish Treatises on the Black Death', p. 9), while in the manuscript Paris, Bibliothèque nationale de France, héb. 1124, fols 135r–139v the translation is attributed to Joshua of Bologna. Barkai also erroneously states that Antonio Guaineri's *Tractatus de peste* was not translated into Hebrew (see Barkai, 'Jewish Treatises on the Black Death', p. 8). Further, the list of translated treatises does not mention the anonymous Hebrew translation of Petrus de Tossignano's *Tractatus de peste*.

2.

In general, fourteenth and fifteenth-century plague treatises focus on three main aspects, namely on the causes of the epidemics, on the necessary measures to prevent contagion, and on the treatment of the disease itself. Understanding the causes of the pestilence was a crucial point often tackled by the authors. Two main causes were acknowledged: a metaphysical one — the divine will, which identifies God as the last cause — and a physical one.[13] Since remote physical causes are identified with the celestial spheres, numerous works feature an astrological *excursus*, in which the influence of the celestial bodies on the epidemics as well as on the cure is examined.[14] Following the theory of the great conjunctions, formulated in the nineteenth century by Albumasar, who considered the conjunction between the major planets (Saturn, Jupiter, and Mars) as the cause for political and natural calamities, the faculty of medicine in Paris adopted a similar explanation for the Black Death in 1348.[15] The conjunction of Saturn, Jupiter and Mars that was observable in 1345 was seen as the cause for the miasmas that corrupted the air and thus facilitated the spread of the malady.[16]

Since the corruption of the air was believed to be the result of excessive heat and humidity, the most commonly suggested remedies were fumigations and scents that were supposed to improve the quality of the air. According to traditional ancient medicine, opposites are cured with opposites, so that it was considered necessary to use cold and dry ingredients to balance heat and humidity. A detailed prophylactic regime to avoid illness, involving advice on diet and life habits, was often described. Finally, a number of compounds and their recipes are presented, such as ointments and lotions, which were prescribed in the case of an actual infection. Indeed, if corrupted air enters into the bodies through the pores, the blood becomes corrupted as well, acquiring the characteristics of the air, in this case heat and humidity.

One of the most ancient treatises, dating back to 1348, was composed by Gentile da Foligno, who eventually died of the plague in that same year.[17] Apart from the

---

13 See Campbell, *The Black Death*, p. 34 ff.; Arrizabalaga, 'Facing the Black Death', pp. 248–64.

14 See *The Black Death*, ed. by Horrox, p. 167.

15 On the theory of the great conjunctions, see Lynn Thorndike, *A History of Magic and Experimental Science*, vol. 1 (New York: Columbia University Press, 1923), pp. 648–51; Richard Lemay, *Abu Ma'shar and Latin Aristotelianism in the Twelfth century* (Beirut: American University of Beirut, 1962); Bernard R. Goldenstein, 'A Prognostication based on the Conjunction of Saturn and Jupiter in 1166 [561 AH]', in *Studies in the History of the Exact Sciences in Honour of David Pingree* (Leiden-Boston: Brill, 2004), pp. 735–57; Tullio Gregory, 'I cieli, il tempo, la storia', in Id., *Speculum naturale. Percorsi del pensiero medievale* (Roma: Storia e Letteratura, 2007), pp. 69–91; Graziella Federici Vescovini, *Le Moyen Âge magique. La magie entre religion et science aux* XIII*e et* XIV*e siècles* (Paris: Vrin, 2011), pp. 248–77; Alessandro Palazzo, 'Astrology and Politics: the Theory of Great Conjunctions in Albert the Great', in *Quaestio*, 19 (2019), *Stars, Kingdoms, Beliefs, and Masses. Political Astrology in the Mediterrenean Area from the Middle Ages to the Renaissance*, ed. by Marienza Benedetto and others, pp. 173–203.

16 See Arrizabalaga, 'Facing the Black Death', p. 253; *The Black Death*, ed. by Horrox, pp. 173–76. On conjunctions, see also section 3.3. of chapter 3 of this volume.

17 On Gentile da Foligno, see Lynn Thorndike, 'Gentile da Foligno and fourteenth-century medicine', in *History of magic and experimental science*, vol. 3 (New York: Columbia University Press, 1934), pp. 233–52;

most famous *Consilium contra pestilentiam*,[18] Gentile wrote various *Consilia* about the pestilence:[19] the *Consilium in epidemia magna dum accidit Perusii*,[20] the *Consilium in pestilentia que accidit Ianue*,[21] which is followed in the manuscripts and in the prints by a *Consilium aliud*, whose incipit reads: 'Manifestum videtur quod causa terribilis mortis'.[22] Moreover, the manuscript tradition also testifies to a short *Sumarium de peste*,[23] a *Consilium magistri Gentilis super pestilentiam*,[24] some *Considerationes aliorum medicorum circa easdem pestilencias*,[25] and a *Prognosticatio*.[26]

Id., '*Consilia* and more works in manuscript by Gentile da Foligno', *Medical History*, 3 (1959) pp. 8–19; Roger French, *Canonical Medicine. Gentile da Foligno and Scholasticims* (Leiden-Boston-Köln: Brill, 2001). On Gentile's treatises on the Black Death, see Sudhoff, 'Pestschriften', *Archiv für Geschichte der Medizin*, 5 (1911), pp. 332–40; Sudhoff raises doubts about the date of composition and suggests an earlier date (p. 336).

18 The incipit reads: 'Quoniam gloriosus et excelsus Deus de largitate sua'. The text is found in the manuscripts Città del Vaticano, Biblioteca Apostolica Vaticana, Pal. lat. 1147, fols 124r–136v; Firenze, Biblioteca Medicea Laurenziana, Plut. 90 sup. 90, fols 63r–94r. Moreover, it is printed in Gentilis de Fulgineo, *Consilium contra pestilentiam* (Pataviae: per Laurentium Canozium, *c.* 1472–75); Gentilis de Fulgineo, *Consilium contra pestilentiam* (Colle in Valle Elsae: per Bonuum Gallum, *c.* 1478–79); Gentilis de Fulgineo, *Consilium contra pestilentiam, Tractatus de resistentiis* (Venetiis?: *c.* 1500).

19 Thorndike raises the question whether these are different versions or extracts from one *consilium*, see Thorndike, 'Gentile da Foligno', p. 244.

20 The incipit reads: 'Nulla videtur precessisse temporibus memorabilibus'. The work is transmitted in the manuscripts Città del Vaticano, Biblioteca Apostolica Vaticana, Pal. lat. 1260, fols 97r-v; Città del Vaticano, Biblioteca Apostolica Vaticana, Pal. lat. 1264, fols 302r-v. The work is divided in two; on fol. 302v, the following incipit is found: 'Gentilis de Fulgineo cum venerabili collegio magistrorum in preservationem et defensionem a tanta pestilentia'. It is not clear whether the latter text is the second paragraph of the Perugian *Consilium* or an independent *Consilium*. The text is printed in Gentilis de Fulgineo, *Consilia* (Papiae: per Antonium Carcanum, *c.* 1486); *Consilia Cermisoni. Consilia Gentilis. Recepte Gentilis de febribus. Tractatulus de balneis Gentilis* (Venetiis, per O. Scottum, 1495).

21 The incipit reads: 'Illustrissimis amicis nostris de Ianua'. The *Consilium* is found in the manuscripts Città del Vaticano, Biblioteca Apostolica Vaticana, Pal. lat. 1260, fols 96v–97r; Città del Vaticano, Biblioteca Apostolica Vaticana, Pal. lat. 1264, fols 301r; München, Bayerische Staatsbibliothek, Clm 77, fols 117r–118r; Basel, Universitätsbibliothek, A.VI.6, fols 296v–298r; Leipzig, Universitätsbibliothek, ms. 1178, fols 53r–54r. It is printed in Gentilis de Fulgineo, *Consilia* (Papiae: per Antonium Carcanum, *c.* 1486); *Consilia Cermisoni. Consilia Gentilis. Recepte Gentilis de febribus. Tractatulus de balneis Gentilis* (Venetiis: per O. Scottum, 1495).

22 Thorndike, '*Consilia* and more works in manuscript', p. 14, suggests that this second *Consilium* should be considered the second paragraph of the Genoese *Consilium*. It is found in Città del Vaticano, Biblioteca Apostolica Vaticana, Pal. lat. 1264, fols 301v–302r; Città del Vaticano, Biblioteca Apostolica Vaticana, Vat. lat. 1043, fols 374r-v; Leipzig, Universitätsbibliothek, ms. 1178, fol. 54r. This *Consilium* is also present in the already mentioned printed editions.

23 Città del Vaticano, Biblioteca Apostolica Vaticana, Vat. lat. 8690, fol. 152.

24 The incipit reads: 'Emergentis et inexcogitati considerantes eventus periculum et fragilitatis previsionis humane oportet'. It is transmitted in Wien, Österreichische Nationalbibliothek, ms. 2317, fols 34v–35r.

25 The incipit reads: 'Circa causam huius pestilencie variatur consideracio magistrorum'. The work is not explicitly ascribed to Gentile, but Sudhoff noted numerous similarities with the other *Consilia* (cf. Sudhoff, 'Pestschriften', *Archiv für Geschichte der Medizin*, 5 (1911), pp. 36–87 (pp. 83–87). The text is found in the manuscript Würzburg, Universitätsbibliothek, M.p.misc.f. 6, fols 63r–64r.

26 The title is *Prognosticatio magistri Gentilis in quadam pestilentia scilicet tempore magne mortalitatis*. The incipit reads: 'Egritudines erunt febres continue'. The text is found in the manuscript Città del Vaticano, Biblioteca Apostolica Vaticana, Pal. lat. 1264, fol. 303r.

An anonymous Hebrew translation bears the title *'Etzah 'al ha-dever* ('Advice on the Plague'), and the authorship of the text is ascribed to Gentile da Foligno.[27] The work is transmitted in the manuscript Wien, Österreichische Nationalbibliothek, Cod. hebr. 59, fols 224v–225v.[28] Both Steinschneider and the Vienna catalogue hypothesize that the author of the translation might have been Joshua the Physician from Bologna, since in the same Vienna manuscript two other *Advices* on the plague translated from Latin are included, and Joshua from Bologna is identified as the translator in the latter. The title in the manuscript is somehow puzzling because it mentions that the *Advice* had been sent to Pisa — so that it coincides neither with the Genoese nor with the Perugian *Advice*.[29] However, it seems that the text kept in the Vienna manuscript is the translation of that *Consilium aliud*, which followed the Genua *Consilium* in the manuscripts and in the prints. Indeed, in the incipit, the city of Pisa is mentioned, together with Genua and Naples, which are also referred to in the Hebrew text: 'Manifestum videtur quod causa terribilis mortis, que manifesta fuit prius apud Januam, deinde venit Pisas et Plumbinum et Massam et que est nunc Neapolim, sit venenosa putredo circa partes cordis et pulmonis'.[30] The Hebrew text states the same, but it replaces the cities of Piombino and Massa with Catalonia.[31]

The text is quite short and deals mostly with health regimen. After a brief introduction, mentioning the causes, the author describes the disease as being an affection of the heart and the lungs. The main remedy involves the purification of the air with scented herbs and the use of vinegar. Dietary advice for healthy people to prevent the infection is given and recipes to treat it are mentioned. In case one has contracted the malady, bloodletting is prescribed. Regarding the recommendations for ill patients, Gentile suggests to separate them from the healthy ones and to place them in a higher location than the others. Moreover, the importance of washing hands numerous times is stressed. The work ends with a series of recipes.

A pupil of Gentile da Foligno, the physician Francesco Zanelli (also known as Giannelli) of Bologna,[32] who taught at the University of Perugia from 1351, composed a *Consilium* on the plague himself and commented on a *Consilium ad evitandum pestilencie periculum* by the Neapolitan physician Giovanni della Penna.[33] Both texts refer to topics treated by Gentile. Indeed, Giovanni della Penna also wrote another *Consilium*, specifically with the aim of rejecting Gentile's opinions: 'Consilium magistri Johannis

---

27 See Moritz Steinschneider, *Die hebräischen Übersetzungen des Mittelalters und die Juden als Dolmetscher* (Berlin: Kommissionsverlag des Bibliographischen Bureaus, 1893), p. 791.

28 See Arthur Zacharias Schwarz, *Die hebräischen Handschriften der Nationalbibliothek in Wien* (Wien-Prag-Leipzig: Strache, 1925), no. 175, pp. 193–94.

29 Probably for this reason, Steinschneider considered the possibility of reading Perugia instead of Pisa: see Steinschneider, *Die hebräischen Übersetzungen*, p. 791.

30 Città del Vaticano, Biblioteca Apostolica Vaticana, Pal. lat. 1264, fol. 301v.

31 Wien, Österreichische Nationalbibliothek, Cod. hebr. 59, fol. 224v:
דבר ברור הוא ונראה המיתה האכזרית אשר נולדה בתחלה בגינואה, ובקטלונייא ואחר זה בפישה ועתה היא בנפולי הוא עפוש ארסיי בסביבות הלב והריאה.

32 On Franciscus de Zanellis, see Giuseppe Ermini, *Storia dell'Università di Perugia*, 2 vols (Firenze: Leo S. Olschki, 1971), vol. 1, p. 176, pp. 178–80.

33 See Sudhoff, 'Pestschriften', *Archiv für Geschichte der Medizin*, 16 (1925), pp. 162–67.

dela Penna in magna pestilentia post magnam promulgationem dictorum consiliorum et specialiter in mente dicti magistri Gentilis'.[34]

In the manuscript Breslau, Universitätsbibliothek, Cod. III F 6, fols 191v–195, both *Consilia* by Giovanni della Penna and Francesco Zanelli are found, with the information that the text was presented by Francesco to the University of Perugia: 'Consilium magistri Francisci de Bononia super eadem peste, cuius oppositum suprascriptum consilium et illud reprobans, quod consilium fuit publicatum per eundem reverendum magistrum Franciscum coram universitate Perusiensis studi sub anno Domini 1364 tempore Urbani pape V'.[35] The text is preceded by Giovanni della Penna's *Consilium ad evitandum pestilencie periculum*, against which Zanelli argues.[36]

The *'Etzah 'al ha-dever* ('Advice on the plague') transmitted in the manuscripts Paris, Bibliothèque nationale de France, héb. 1124, fols 135r–139v and Wien, Österreichische Nationalbibliothek, Cod. hebr. 59, fols 227v–232v is attributed to Francesco Zanelli of Bologna.[37] In the third part, the refutation of the *Advice* by Giovanni della Penna is found.[38] As stated in the colophon, the *'Etzah 'al ha-dever* has been translated by Joshua the physician of Bologna.[39] It thus seems that this *Advice* is the translation of the Latin text, as it is found in the Breslau manuscript, in which the two *Consilia*, that of Francesco Zanelli and that of Giovanni della Penna, are transmitted together, with a reference to the refutation of the latter by the former. Indeed, the incipit of the Hebrew text reads:
כאשר השגנו מדברי גאלינו

34 The work is found in the manuscript Leipzig, Universitätsbibliothek, ms. 1178, fols 54r–57r. See Sudhoff, 'Pestschriften', *Archiv für Geschichte der Medizin*, 5 (1911), pp. 341–48. The incipit is: 'Licet presentis pestilentie pravitas'.

35 See fol. 192r. See Breslau, Universitätsbibliothek, *Katalog rękopisów dawnej Biblioteki Uniwersyteckiej we Wrocławiu*, t. 7 (III F 1–30) p. 8, available at https://www.bibliotekacyfrowa.pl/dlibra/publication/10035?tab=1&language=en#description (last accessed 14/02/2022); see Sudhoff, 'Pestschriften', *Archiv für Geschichte der Medizin*, 16 (1922–23), p. 162. I suggest the reading 'Perusiensis' instead of 'Parysiensis'. The incipit of the text reads: 'Sicut colligitur ex dictis gloriosissimi Galieni'.

36 The incipit reads: 'Prima et communis regula est non sinere approximare homines venientes a regionibus'. The same text is transmitted also in the manuscript Wiesbaden, Nassauische Landesbibliothek, cod. 61, fols 51r–52r: see Sudhoff, 'Pestschriften', *Archiv für Geschichte der Medizin*, 16 (1925), pp. 162–67. Francesco Zanelli and Giovanni della Penna had another controversy on the *animatio seminis*: see *Documenti per la storia dell'Università di Perugia*, ed. by Adamo Rossi, *Giornale di erudizione artistica*, 5 (1876), p. 313; Francesco Puccinotti, *Storia della medicina*, 3 vols (Livorno: Wagner, 1850), vol. 2, p. 2, pp. 348–51.

37 The name is transcribed according to its variant 'de Giannelli': די גאנילי (the Parisian catalogue suggests to read it as Ganili or Gagnali; the Vienna catalogue retains the name in Hebrew). See *Catalogue des manuscrits hébreux et samaritains de la Bibliothèque imperiale* (Paris: Imprimerie Impériale, 1866) p. 208; Schwarz, *Die hebräischen Handschriften*, pp. 193–94. See Steinschneider, *Die hebräischen Übersetzungen*, p. 790.

38 The name is therefore neither to be read as Gioan Delfina, as suggested by Steinschneider (*Die hebräischen Übersetzungen*, p. 790), nor is the author to be identified with Joannes Platearius, as suggested by the catalogue of the *National Library of Israel*, available at https://web.nli.org.il/sites/NLIS/en/ManuScript/Pages/Item.aspx?ItemID = PNX_MANUSCRIPTS990001315510205171 (last accessed 19/01/2022).

39 See Stefano Arieti, 'Medici ebrei a Bologna tra XV e XVI secolo', in *Verso l'epilogo di una convivenza: gli ebrei a Bologna nel XVI secolo*, ed. by Maria Giuseppina Muzzarelli (Firenze: Giuntina, 1996), pp. 235–43, (p. 238); Mauro Perani, 'La cultura ebraica a Bologna nella testimonianza dei manoscritti' in *La cultura ebraica a Bologna tra Medioevo e Rinascimento* (Firenze: Giuntina, 2002), pp. 29–70 (p. 63).

One of the most widespread and popular treatises devoted to the Black Death was the *De epidemia*, or *De pestilentia*, probably written in 1365 by John of Burgundy.[40] The author, also known as John à la Barbe, was a professor of medicine between 1330 and 1370 in Liège. In his *De epidemia*, John declares that he wrote two other works on the plague, the *De causis et natura corrupti aeris* and the *De distinctione morborum epydimialium ab aliis morbis*, mentioning their respective incipits. However, only the third treatise is preserved, while the former two have not been found until now.

The popularity of the work is testified by its manuscript dissemination, which counts more than a hundred copies, as well as by its translations into numerous languages, including English, French, Dutch, and Hebrew.[41] As it was often the case with widespread manuals, the text underwent a series of modifications, abbreviations, and interpolations during its transmission, and it was, at some point, even attributed to the faculty of medicine of Bologna. The work is known in at least two main versions, a long and a short one; in the latter, the astrological introduction is absent.[42] As stated by its author, the aim of the writing is to help simple people take care of themselves in difficult times.

Various parts of the short version of John of Burgundy's *De epidemia* were translated into Hebrew, forming two different manuals with a slightly different content: the *'Etzer elohi ma'mar be-'ipush ha-avir ve-ha-dever* ('Divine help: A treatise on the corruption of the air and the plague') and the *'Etzah 'al ha-dever* ('Advice on the plague').[43] Both translations are partial and extract only few passages from the original text; in particular, the *Divine help* focuses on prophylaxis, while the *Advice on the plague* also gives instructions for treatment.

The *'Etzer elohi* is transmitted in two manuscripts: Paris, Bibliothèque nationale de France, héb. 1191, fols 141r–143r, and Moscow, Russian State Library, Günzburg 1481, fols 19–20r.[44] The title is probably a reference to the incipit of the text: 'Ego Johannes de Burgundia divino auxilio invocato preservationem et curam epidemie enucleare intendo'.[45] As it is stated in the colophon, the *Divine Help* was translated by Benjamin of Carcassonne — known only for this translation —, who explains his

---

40 See Sudhoff, 'Pestschriften', *Archiv für Geschichte der Medizin*, 5 (1911), pp. 58–69; *The Black Death*, ed. by Horrox, pp. 184–93; Lister M. Matheson, 'John of Burgundy: Treatises on Plague', in *Sex, Aging, and Death in a Medieval Medical Compendium. Trinity College Cambridge MS R.14.52, Its Texts, Language, and Scribe*, ed. by M. Teresa Tavormina, (Tempe: Arizona Center for Medieval and Renaissance Studies, 2006), pp. 569–606; Kari Anne Rand, 'A Previously Unnoticed Fragment of John of Burgundy's Plague Tract and Some Connected Pest Regimens', *Notes and Queries*, 53 (2006), pp. 295–97.

41 See Lister M. Matheson, '*Médecins sans Frontières?*: The European Dissemination of John of Burgundy's Plague Treatise', *A Quarterly Journal of Short Articles, Notes and Reviews*, 18 (2005), pp. 19–30.

42 See Matheson, '*Médecins sans Frontières?*', p. 19.

43 See Steinschneider, *Die hebräischen Übersetzungen*, pp. 803–04. Moreover, see Dorothea Waley Singer and Reuben Levy, 'Plague Tractates', *Annals of Medical History*, 4 (1917), pp. 394–411.

44 For the description of the Parisian manuscript, see https://archivesetmanuscrits.bnf.fr/ark:/12148/cc8073s (last accessed 24/01/2022). For the Günzburg manuscript, see Moritz Steinschneider, 'Eine medizinische hebräische Handschrift', *Magazin für die Wissenschaften des Judenthums*, 12 (1885), pp. 182–214. The Günzburg manuscript corresponds to the Parisian copy, but it mentions the city of Montpellier instead of Liège.

45 See Sudhoff, 'Pestschriften', *Archiv für Geschichte der Medizin*, 5 (1911), p. 62.

motivations to make the text accessible to a Jewish audience. According to him, the treatise was extensively used by Christian physicians, but it was kept hidden; he then acquired a copy to translate it into Hebrew, so that Jewish physicians would profit from a manual that was widespread among their colleagues. It is reported that the work had been composed in the year 22; scholars suggested to read it as 122, which would correspond to the year 1362 (even though the work is supposed to have been written in 1365).[46] Moreover, a previous work is mentioned, whose incipit might correspond to the *De causis et natura corrupti aeris,* also cited in the Latin version of the treatise.[47]

The *Divine help* translates only part of John of Burgundy's short version of *De epidemia,* and it focuses on the corruption of the air as the cause for the pandemics, as well as on practical remedies to prevent and treat the disease. Indeed, it was assumed that the reason for the spreading of the plague into numerous countries was the air that had been corrupted by the miasmas. However, the pestilence was also considered to be the result of the concomitance of bad bodily humors. Depending on the variety of humors, corrupted air generates different illnesses, which are not lethal for every human being. The explanation for the high mortality is the mixture of bad humors with which human bodies were filled before contracting the malady. Making reference to Galen, John of Burgundy maintains that the disease strikes only those bodies that are susceptible to corruption, which is why a series of precautions is necessary to keep the bodies clean and purged. However, this does not apply to bodies whose *complexio* is opposite to that of corrupted air, because they are considered to be able to remain healthy anyway.

Even though in the short version of the *De epidemia* the astrological *excursus* at the beginning is absent, a section on astrology is introduced before the discussion of the remedies. When administering a treatment, the physician must be aware of the astrological conditions, since a medicine taken in the wrong moment will not achieve the expected, and sometimes even the opposite, result. This section refers to Hippocrates regarding the central role played by astrology within the field of medicine, and to Avicenna and Averroes about the importance of knowing the proximate and remote causes, with celestial bodies being the primary causes of things.

In the last part, a list of recommendations is provided, for instance, containing the suggestions to abstain from excessive eating and intercourse. Moreover, it is advised to avoid bathing, as it opens the pores through which the corrupted air may enter the body. The *Divine help* continues with a series of dietary instructions, listing food that should be avoided — such as fruits and honey — and food that is allowed — such as vinegar and light food. Finally, suggestions concerning the climate are provided: if the weather is humid and rainy, a fire should be lit in the room. The text then abruptly stops (the Parisian manuscript presents a *lacuna*) and four recipes follow.

---

46 See Steinschneider, *Die hebräischen Übersetzungen*, p. 804. For the discussion of this point, see *infra*, n. 53.

47 According to the Latin version, the incipit of this lost work reads: 'Deus Deorum dicens'; in Hebrew: אלי אלי.

The *'Etzah 'al ha-dever* has a similar content, yet it slightly diverges from the previous treatise, as it translates other fragments of John of Burgundy's *De epidemia*. The text is transmitted in the manuscripts Paris, Bibliothèque nationale de France, héb. 1124, fols 133v–135r;[48] and Wien, Österreichische Nationalbibliothek, hebr. 59, fols 225v–227v.[49] The name of the translator is unknown; since the same two manuscripts transmit Francesco Zanelli's *Advice on the plague*, which was translated by Joshua of Bologna, it has been proposed that the author of the translation could be the same.[50] From a linguistic point of view, the numerous vernacular terms used by the translator seem to support the thesis that its origin is Italian. The physician who wrote the original version is called Gioan de Cenobarba, and in the colophon the date 1399 is found.[51]

In the *Advice on the plague*, the focus lies more on curing the disease rather than on its prevention. Therefore, the description of how the illness spreads in the body is more detailed with regard to the different organs involved; moreover, instructions for bloodletting are provided. When the corrupted air enters the body, the main organs — the heart, the brain, and the liver — try to depurate themselves from the poisonous miasmas, which cause different symptoms according to the organ that is involved the most. Consequently, bloodletting has to be performed choosing the vein according to the location of the symptoms.

As for the prophylactic treatment, dietary instructions for infirm people are described: patients must avoid excessive eating and should drink infusions, in particular water with vinegar. Recipes for unguents are provided, specifically for a powder called *Zinwar*, which is said to have been used by Arab emperors.[52]

The treatise includes a short astrological epilogue, in which the cause for the pestilence is considered to be the conjunction that occurred 22 years before, whose consequences were still noticeable.[53]

At this point, the *'Etzah 'al ha-dever* deals with the topic of prophylaxis, and thus rejoins the previous treatise, repeating the same preventive measures already featured

48 See *Catalogue des manuscrits hebreux et samaritains de la Bibliothèque imperiale*, p. 208.

49 See Schwarz, *Die hebräischen Handschriften*, pp. 193–94.

50 See Steinscheinder, *Die hebräischen Übersetzungen*, p. 804; Schwarz, *Die hebräischen Handschriften*, p. 193.

51 Steinscheinder, *Die hebräischen Übersetzungen*, p. 804, suggests that the word דצינו should be considered a translation of 'dictus', so that the name would be 'Gioan called Barba'.

52 The Hebrew זינואר translates the Latin 'bethazaer': 'dicitur pulvis imperialis, quia imperatores gentilium eo utebantur [...] et dicitur in lingua Arabiae Bethzaer, id est a morte liberans'. In Petrus de Tussignano's *Tractatus de peste*, the same remedy is called Bezaar and the etymology is linked to the Hebrew language: 'Et dicitur lingua hebrayca Bezaar quod interpretatur a morte liberans': see Petrus de Tussignano, *Tractatus de peste* (Venetiis: *c.* 1472).

53 The astrological epilogue is not present in the Latin text published by Sudhoff, but one might compare the indication given in the French version of the *De epidemia*: 'Item ne croie nulz que ceste pestilence soit pour la raison de Saturne & de iupiter pour la coniunccion qui se fist deulz & dautres lan passe cest assauoir en lan LXV. aincois dient des reliques de lautre coniunccion autresfoiz faite de lan XLV dont les traces apperent encore en effect': see Singer, 'Some plague tractates', p. 209. Given the correspondence with the French version, it seems more appropriate to read the indication as 22 years ago, rather than in the year 22, which — following the conjecture made by Steinschneider regarding the date of the composition of the *Divine help* — would be the year 1362.

in the *Divine Help*. However, it also adds certain recommendations that were absent in the former work, such as the use of a sponge soaked in vinegar or sprinkling the house with water, vinegar, and rose water. The book ends with the recipe for the pill of Rhazes.

The translation method adopted for the *Advice on the plague* is different from that of the *Divine Help*, as vernacular terms transcribed in Hebrew characters appear often. Vernacular words are frequently used for herbal terminology, such as סנבוקו (*sanbuco*), קמומילא (*camomilla*), גינסיאנה (*gensiana*), אוזילא קרודא (*osella cruda*), as well as for medical vocabulary, such as בשליקא and צפילקא (*basilica* and *cefalica*, referring to the veins), גלנדולי (*glandule*), שפינא (*safena*). However, also generic terms not pertaining to a technical terminology appear, such as קומוני (*comune*), טישאנה (*tisana*), אינפידילי (*infedeli*), גראטיקולא (*graticola*), קונדיטי (*conditi*).[54]

The master Petrus de Tossignano, who taught medicine in Bologna and Padua, composed a widely spread work titled *Tractatus de peste* in 1398. Numerous manuscripts as well as a fifteenth-century print of this treatise have survived.[55] A reworked version of the text was published in 1491 in Venice, under the title *Consilium pro peste evitanda*, with a dedication to Gian Galeazzo Visconti.[56] In secondary literature, the text transmitted by the manuscript tradition has been considered the same as that printed in the 1491 edition.[57] However, numerous differences can be noticed between the manuscript version — which corresponds mostly to the *c.* 1472 print — and the 1491 print.[58] This suggested the assumption that Petrus wrote two different works. Both these suppositions — namely that the 1491 print and the manuscripts correspond and that the author wrote two different works — seem to be incorrect. A comparison between the two versions indeed reveals a close proximity, but also noticeable differences, which can only be explained through a reworked

54 See the notes in Singer, 'Plague Tractates', pp. 402–05.

55 I have been able to identify the following manuscripts transmitting the *Tractatus de peste*: Città del Vaticano, Biblioteca Apostolica Vaticana, Pal. lat. 1260, fols 99va-104vb; Città del Vaticano, Biblioteca Apostolica Vaticana, Pal. lat. 1144, fols 228r–239v; Città del Vaticano Biblioteca Apostolica Vaticana, Vat. lat. 2482, fols 97r–106v; Città del Vaticano, Biblioteca Apostolica Vaticana, Vat. lat. 5373, fols 25r–36r; Berlin, Staatsbibliothek zu Berlin – Preußischer Kulturbesitz, Ms. lat. qu. 371, fols 273r–286v; Kraków, Biblioteka Jagiellonska, ms. 782, fols 273r–278v; Leipzig, Universitätsbibliothek, ms. 1175, fols 109r–119r; Leipzig, Universitätsbibliothek, ms. 1198, fols 207–215; Venezia, Biblioteca Marciana, lat. XIV 289 [4615], fols 30r–43r; Roma, Biblioteca Vallicelliana, ms. F 93, fols 145r–150r; Roma, Biblioteca Angelica, ms. 1283, fols 33r–53v; Roma, Biblioteca Angelica, ms. 1377, fols 51v–73v; Firenze, Biblioteca Riccardiana, ms. 1177, fols 183–190. The work has been printed in Venice around 1472. On Petrus de Tussignano, see Sudhoff, 'Pestschriften', *Archiv für Geschichte der Medizin*, 5 (1911), pp. 390–95; Giuseppe Mazzini, *Vita e opera di maestro Pietro da Tossignano* (Roma: Leonardo da Vinci, 1926); Singer, 'Some plague tractates', pp. 187–89; Augusto De Ferrari, 'Curialti, Pietro', in *Dizionario biografico degli Italiani*, 31 (Roma: Istituto della Enciclopedia Italiana, 1985), pp. 432–34.

56 The treatise was printed in 1491 in Venice with the *Fasciculus medicinae* by Iohannes de Ketham: *Fasciculus medicinae, auctore Johanne de Ketham* (Venetiis: per J. et G. de Gregoriia, 1491; 1495; 1500; 1513).

57 See Mazzini, *Vita e opera di maestro Pietro da Tossignano*, p. 84. However, Mazzini mentions some major differences between the two versions (see p. 90).

58 Sudhoff speaks of "recht erheblichen Abweichungen der beiden Drucke untereinander und der Handschriften von den Drucken": see Sudhoff, 'Pestschriften', *Archiv für Geschichte der Medizin*, 5 (1911), p. 392.

version made either by its author or by the editor. Moreover, in the manuscript tradition, the writing is transmitted with different titles, which has led to some confusion over the number of handbooks that Petrus devoted to the pestilence.[59] It is still not clear whether de Tossignano wrote two further treatises on the plague, namely the *De remediis ac pestilentie curatione* and the *Tractatus de pestilentia*, or whether it is the same work with different titles.[60]

Probably in the fifteenth century, an anonymous author translated the *Tractatus de peste* into Hebrew.[61] The work is transmitted in the manuscript Paris, Bibliothèque nationale de France, hébr. 1195, fols 98r–113r.[62] With regard to the abovementioned ambiguity with the *Consilium pro peste evitanda*, Steinschneider has noted a difference between the Latin and Hebrew incipit;[63] however, the incipit of the Hebrew translation coincides with that of the *Tractatus de peste*, which reads: 'Dixit Galienus primo de ingenio circa finem. Decet nos nil negligentie habere in ostendendo sanitatis ingenio […]'. The translation copied in the Parisian manuscript starts with the following words: אמר גלינוס בראשון מתחבולת הרפואה בדרך למור שלא נתרשל בשום.

The treatise is divided into four chapters: the first chapter deals with the investigation of the causes of the plague; the second describes a prophylactic regimen; in the third chapter, eleven common doubts concerning the pestilence are explained and answered; finally, therapeutic measures are discussed.

It is noteworthy that, in considering the causes, Petrus de Tussignano mentions contact and warns not to touch objects that have been touched by a sick person; moreover, he stresses the importance of moving away from places where the pandemic has spread and of not letting anyone enter the city who comes from an infected area. Since transmission happens more often within social gatherings, the author recommends to isolate patients and to prohibit public meetings. The explanation of the causes appears to be similar to that given by John of Burgundy, but Petrus is more focused on the notion of contagion. Apart from contact, the author mentions multiple other factors concurring in the transmission, one of the most relevant causes being the patient's predisposition. Referring to Aristotle and Avicenna concerning this point, he states that it is necessary to keep the body dry in order to avoid the infection. Celestial causes also play a fundamental role, since they are responsible for the corruption of the air, while the proximate cause is the mixture of miasmas with

---

59 See for instance the database *Mirabile* http://www.mirabileweb.it/author/petrus-de-tussignano-m-8-4-1407-author/23161 (last accessed 24/01/2022) which lists the *Consilium pro peste vitanda*, the *De peste*, and the *Tractatus de pestilentia*. However, the manuscripts listed under the title *Consilium pro peste vitanda* and *Tractatus de pestilentia* actually transmit the *Tractatus de peste*.

60 According to secondary literature, the *De remediis ac pestilentie curatione* is found in the ms. Città del Vaticano, Biblioteca Apostolica Vaticana, Vat. lat. 1180, while the *Tractatus de pestilentia* is transmitted in the mss. Napoli, Biblioteca nazionale "Vittorio Emanuele III", VII D 35, fols 75–81 and Firenze, Biblioteca nazionale centrale, Magl. XV.185, fols 149r–168r: see *I manoscritti datati della Biblioteca nazionale centrale di Firenze*, vols 4, ed. by Michelangiola Marchiaro and Stefano Zamponi, vol. 4 (Firenze: Sismel – Edizioni del Galluzzo, 2018), p. 69. It was impossible for me to personally check this information.

61 See Steinschneider, *Die hebräischen Übersetzungen*, p. 818.

62 See *Catalogue des manuscrits hébreux et samaritains de la Bibliothèque impériale*, p. 220.

63 Steinschneider, *Die hebräischen Übersetzungen*, p. 818.

venomous air — such as that originating from corpses. Finally, Petrus distinguishes between particular and common pestilential disease; the particular disease infects singular individuals and is not caused by corrupted air, while the illness is defined as common if it occurs in a specific area, according to the climatic conditions of the place, and is then called endemic.

In the second chapter, the regimen is treated, and special attention is devoted to the three organs that, if infected, cause the death of the body, namely the heart, the brain, and the liver. A series of hygienic remedies, such as adopting a suitable diet, are prescribed in order to keep the body dry and purged. Regarding life habits, it is advised not to sleep during the day nor after meals, and even the best sleeping position is indicated. Excessive physical exercise is to be avoided, as well as coitus and baths. De Tussignano suggests to listen to nice stories in order to cheer oneself up and prevent sadness — especially political conversations, on the other hand, are to be avoided. Finally, the *rectificatio* of the air through herbal fumigations is considered to be of great help.

The next chapter is devoted to eleven doubts. In particular, certain questions seem to be of particular interest, such as why pandemics occur mostly in autumn, although the air is not as humid as in summer, or why birds, which usually fly in the higher sky, fly closer to the earth during epidemics and vice versa. Moreover, the varying virulence with which the disease attacks different bodies is the main topic of the next doubts concerning differences in mortality. Even if the cause for the plague is universal, it has been observed that, within the same family, one person dies and the rest survives, or that a strong young man dies and an old woman survives.

Finally, therapeutic measures against the malady are prescribed, focusing especially on symptoms like fever, dysentery, and the swelling of glands. Bloodletting is treated at length, and different kind of boils are described. Since they contain a contagious poison, it is recommended to the surgeon who treats them to use vinegar. Further, advice concerning the purification of the air in the room of the patient as well as a list of recipes are presented.

Antonio Guaineri of Pavia, born at the end of the fourteenth century, studied medicine in Padua and Pavia — where he was also active as a lecturer — and was then hired as a physician at the Savoy court in Piedmont.[64] According to his own statements, Guaineri experienced two epidemics during his life, in 1402 and in 1416.[65] Mostly working in the field of *medicina pratica*, he devoted two of his writings to the pestilence, namely the *Tractatus de peste* and the *Liber de febribus*, even though the latter does not specifically focus only on the plague. The *Tractatus de peste* addresses the matter in its entirety: from causes to treatment, it deals with signs and medicines,

---

64 On Antonio Guaineri, see Daniela Mugnai Carrara, 'Guaineri, Antonio', in *Dizionario Biografico degli Italiani*, vol. 60 (Roma: Istituto della Enciclopedia Italiana, 2003), https://www.treccani.it/enciclopedia/antonio-guaineri_(Dizionario-Biografico)/ (last accessed: 27.06.2022). Danielle Jacquart, 'Theory, Everyday Practice, and Three Fifteenth-Century Physicians', *Osiris* 6 (1990), pp. 140–60; Ead., 'De la science à la magie: le cas d'A. Guainerio, médecin italien du XVe siècle', *Littérature, médecine et société*, 9 (1988), pp. 137–56.

65 See Jacquart, 'Theory, Everyday Practice', p. 142.

with the purification of the air, dietary instructions and advice on sleep, with exercise and sexual intercourse. The second treatise focuses more on curing the disease, giving instructions for bloodletting, sharing recipes for pills and bezoars as well as for remedies against fever and boils. The *Tractatus* also includes a section on poisons, which is sometimes transmitted separately as an independent work.[66] The writing is dedicated to Filippo Maria Visconti, duke of Milan.

The violence of the pestilence and the exceptional nature of this disease compared to other illnesses is accurately described in the prologue to the work:

> Persepe animadvertens hoc mortale hominum genus innumeris casibus additum [*coni.* subiectum] et infinita mortis varietate facile corrumpi, nullamque ex omnibus moriendi causis acerbiorem fieri atque acutiorem hac ipsa amarissima et prope modum crudelissima peste que tanto impetu tantaque latenti voracitate in nostra viscera descendit [...][67] (Very often observing that the mortal mankind is subject to innumerable circumstances and easily corrupted by an infinite variety of deaths, and that none of all these causes of death is more unpleasant and more severe than this very bitter and extremely cruel plague that, with such strong force and such latent insatiability, descends in our bowels [...]).

Following the tradition of etymologies, the treatise starts with an exposition of the terminological distinctions between different words used, such as *pestis, pestilentia, febris pestilentialis, lues, contagium, epidemia, mortalitas*. In general, Antonio Guaineri mostly avoids astrological explanations, even though divine causes are acknowledged as the primary causes for the epidemics. To demonstrate the divine origin of the plague, Guaineri reminds of the numerous apparitions of the Virgin and of the saints that foretold the pandemics; for this reason, the author suggests to pray, especially to the saints. Concerning the different treatment options, special attention is devoted to the bezoars. As opposed to Petrus de Tussignano, Guaineri does not investigate the notion of contagion in such great detail; indeed, it is advised not to talk to a person that comes from an infected area, but it is also recommended to move sick patients elsewhere, to let them breathe uncorrupted air. The idea of contagion through

---

66 See Sudhoff, 'Pestschriften', *Archiv für Geschichte der Medizin*, 16 (1925), pp. 77–188 (pp. 117–118). The text is transmitted in the following manuscripts: Città del Vaticano, Biblioteca Apostolica Vaticana, Pal. lat. 1098, fols 289v–368r; Città del Vaticano, Biblioteca Apostolica Vaticana, Pal. lat. 1214, fols 5r–70r; Città del Vaticano, Biblioteca Apostolica Vaticana, Pal. lat. 1195, fols 194v–216r; Wien, Schottenkloster, cod. 268, fols 93r–172r; Leipzig, Universitätsbibliothek, ms. 1167, fols 1r–55r; München, Bayerische Staatsbibliothek, Clm. 184, fols 162–207; Neustift, Augustiner-Chorherrenstift, cod. 748, fols 90v–137v; Breslau, Universitätsbibliothek, cod. III T 11; Oxford, Bodleian Library, Canon. Misc. 451, fols 127r–159; Vendôme, Bibliothèque municipale, ms. 107, fols 53r–152v; Bonn, Universitäts- und Landesbibliothek, S 480, fols 78r–121v; Paris, Bibliothèque nationale de France, lat. 6981, fols 129v–198v; Firenze, Biblioteca Riccardiana 878, fols 103r–119v; Venezia, Biblioteca Nazionale Marciana, lat. VII. 47 (3380). The work has been printed separately (Venetiis: Rainald von Nimwegen, *c.* 1486–87) and together with other works in 1481 and 1488 (Papiae: Antonius Carcanus), in 1497 (Venetiis: Octavianus Scotus), in 1500 (Venetiis: Johann Hamann), in 1508 (Venetiis: Iacobus Pentius), in 1517 (Venetiis: Luccantonius de Giunta), in 1518 (Papiae: Bernardinus de Garaldo) and in 1525 (Lugduni: Jacob Myt).

67 Antonius Guainerius, *Tractatus de peste* (Venetiis: Rainald von Nimwegen, *c.* 1486–87), fol. 1.

contact only plays a minor role when compared to the notion of the corruption of the air as the cause for the malady.

A short part of the *Tractatus de peste* was translated into Hebrew by an anonymous writer, with the title *Ma'amar be-dever* ('Treatise on the plague'). Today, this translation is transmitted in the manuscript Moscow, Russian State Library, Günzburg 1122, fols 35r–37r.[68] The codex contains a fragment of a larger text, whose structure, however, does not seem to correspond to that of the *Tractatus de peste*, even though the work is explicitly attributed to Antonio Guaineri. In the introduction to the Hebrew translation, two parts are mentioned: the first one deals with the pestilence and the second with poisons — exactly as in the Latin version. Nonetheless, the division of the chapters does not seem to correspond to the original. In the Hebrew version, the first part is divided into four chapters, dealing with the use of laxatives to protect against the disease, some kinds of bezoar, external means — such as stones — and the treatment of boils. In the Günzburg manuscript, the text is interrupted in the middle of the second chapter. The interest of the translator clearly seems to be on the practical side, as the selection of chapters to be translated shows. The first part of the original version, which deals with the causes and precautions, is missing, to the benefit of the exposition about healing methods, mentioned in the second treatise of the Latin text.

After the *Tractatus de peste*, in 1434, Antonio Guaineri composed the already mentioned *Liber de febribus*, which was dedicated to Antonio Magliano, one of his former teachers at the University of Pavia.[69] Even though it did not specifically focus on the plague, a chapter of the second treatise is devoted to the regimen in times of pestilence.

The *Liber de febribus* was translated under the title *Ha-klal me-ha-qaddaḥot* ('The whole knowledge on fevers') by Solomon ben Moses Shalom 'Sephardi', who seems

68 See Steinschneider, *Die hebräischen Übersetzungen*, p. 800.

69 On the *De febribus*, see Sudhoff, 'Pestschriften', *Archiv für Geschichte der Medizin*, 16 (1925), pp. 77–188 (pp. 117–118); Lynn Thorndike, *A History of Magic and Experimental Science*, vol. 4 (New York: Columbia University Press, 1953), pp. 670–77. The work is transmitted in the following manuscripts: Città del Vaticano, Biblioteca Apostolica Vaticana, Pal. lat. 1194, fols 75r–107r; Città del Vaticano, Biblioteca Apostolica Vaticana, Pal. lat. 1195, fols 1r–47v; Città del Vaticano, Biblioteca Apostolica Vaticana, Pal. lat. 1221, fols 51r–86r; Città del Vaticano, Biblioteca Apostolica Vaticana, Vat. lat. 2482, fols 168r–216r; Oxford, Bodleian Library, Canon. Misc. 426, fols 187r–228; Vendôme, Bibliothèque municipale, ms. 107, fols 1r–52v; Wien, Schottenkloster, cod. 268, fols 31r–91r; Firenze, Biblioteca Riccardiana, ms. 1177, fols 212v–241v; Firenze, Biblioteca Riccardiana, ms. 2153, fols 105r–135v; Leipzig, Universitätsbibliothek, ms. 1167, fols 128–163; Bonn, Universitäts- und Landesbibliothek, S 480, ff. 21r–76v; Bruxelles, KBR, ms. 3204–18; Hildesheim, Stadtarchiv, Best. 52 Nr. 344, fols 122r–165r; Kraków, Biblioteka Jagiellonska, ms. 810, fols 203r–249v; Neustift, Augustiner-Chorherrenstift, cod. 748, fols 1v–40v; Venezia, Biblioteca Nazionale Marciana, lat. VII 47 [3380]; Wolfenbüttel, Herzog August Bibliothek, Extrav. 112.1, fols 8r–40r; Paris, Bibliothèque nationale de France, lat. 6981, fols 1r–51v; Paris, Bibliothèque nationale de France, NAL 1253, fols 1r–77v; München, Bayerische Staatsbibliothek, Clm. 205, fols 11r–59r. The work has been printed several times: separately in 1474 (Neapoli: Bertholdus Rihing; Pataviae or Venetiis: Conradus de Padeborn); together with other treatises in the editions already mentioned, see above, n. 66.

to have been active as a translator between 1473 and 1486.[70] The text is transmitted in the following manuscripts: Parma, Biblioteca Palatina, Ms. Parm. 2263, fols 19r–101r;[71] Berlin, Staatsbibliothek, Or. Qu. 511, fols 89r–157r — which is a direct copy of the Parma manuscript;[72] Paris, Bibliothèque nationale de France, hébr. 1131, fols 161r–217r;[73] Paris, Bibliothèque nationale de France, hébr. 1134, fols 73r–119r.[74]

The work is preceded by the translator's prologue, in which the author is identified as Antonio of Pavia. Moreover, Solomon ben Moses Shalom apologizes for the use of vernacular terms, explaining that the equivalent Hebrew terms were obsolete; only readers with a profound knowledge of the ancient language would be able to understand these, which is why he adopted the vernacular language.[75] Because of these difficulties, he asks the reader not to correct his work, as it was often the case. Finally, he mentions the translation of a work titled *Pandetti* and of the *Consilia medica* by Bartolomeo Montagnana.

Another anonymous translation of the same text was completed in 1483, by the son or at the request of a certain Gedalia. The work is found in the manuscript Leiden, University Library, Or. 4778, fols 23v–78r.[76] The name of the author is absent in the incipit, but the content of the three parts seem to correspond to Guaineri's *De febribus*. Contrary to the previous translation, some words, which were translated in the former version, are given in the original language, such as שינוקא אינפלאטיווא (*synocha inflativa*) or פוטרידא (*putrida*).

The writing is divided into three parts. The first part has only one chapter, which is devoted to ephemeral fever; the second part discusses the humors and is divided into five treatises, the last of which deals with pestilential fevers. More specifically, the sixth chapter of the fifth treatise discusses the signs and treatments of the plague. Finally, the third part examines fever of the limbs and is divided into three chapters.

70 See Steinschneider, *Die hebräischen Übersetzungen*, p. 799. Solomon ben Moses Shalom also translated the *Medical advice* by Bartolomeo Montagnana. Moreover, he was the copyist of a manuscript for David Kalonymos in 1473.

71 See Giuliano Tamani, 'Inventario dei manoscritti ebraici di argomento medico della biblioteca Palatina di Parma', *La Bibliofilia*, 69 (1967), pp. 245–76 (pp. 254–255, no. 9); *Hebrew manuscripts in the Biblioteca Palatina in Parma: catalogue*, ed. by Benjamin Richler, Malachi Beit-Arié (Jerusalem: Hebrew University of Jerusalem-Jewish National and University Library, 2001), p. 450. The manuscript was copied in 1486 by Raphael ben Ephraim da Modena.

72 See Steinschneider, *Die Handschriften-Verzeichnisse der Königlichen Bibliothek zu Berlin*, vol. 1, no. 62, pp. 39–42. The copyist was Samuel ben Menachem from Soliano (?); in 1585, the manuscript was in Spezzano.

73 See *Catalogue des manuscrits hébreux et samaritains de la Bibliothèque impériale*, p. 210.

74 See *Catalogue des manuscrits hébreux et samaritains de la Bibliothèque impériale*, p. 211. At the end of the work, a list of questions and answers on fever as well as fragments taken from different medical writings are added.

75 See Jean-Pierre Rothschild, 'Motivations et méthodes des traductions en hébreu du milieu du XIIe à la fin du XVe siècle', in *Traduction et traducteurs au Moyen Âge. Actes du colloque international du CNRS organisé à Paris*, ed. by Geneviève Contamine (Paris: Éditions du CNRS, 1989), pp. 279–302 (p. 290).

76 See Moritz Steinschneider, *Catalogus Codicum Hebraeorum Bibliothecae Academiae Lugduno-Batavae* (Leiden: Brill, 1858), p. 156; Albert van der Heide, *Hebrew Manuscripts of Leiden University Library* (Leiden: Bibliotheca Universitatis Leidensis, 1977), p. 34.

In general, the text extensively refers to Avicenna; moreover, it reveals an interest in magic, even with a certain criticism towards popular beliefs: in a passage mentioning a recipe to restore youth, taken from Ovid's *Metamorphoses*, the author strongly criticizes superstitious beliefs and especially the legend of the android fabricated by Albert the Great.[77]

The chapter on pestilential fever starts with a reference to Antonio Guaineri's previous treatise, the *Tractatus de peste*. The author states that this chapter is a brief summary of the *Tractatus de peste*, which he advises to consult for more information. As in the longer version, the chapter mostly deals with the cause of the pestilence, which is identified with the corruption of the air generated not only by celestial influence, but also by corpses or infected water. Moreover, in reference to Avicenna, the author maintains that putrid air is found also in the depth of the earth and that, consequently, the vegetation that grows on the corrupted spot is infected as well. When human beings eat animals fed on this vegetation, they are also corrupted. After the section on the causes, Guaineri devotes numerous paragraphs to the signs of fever according to the different kinds of pestilential fevers, quoting Gentile da Foligno as an authority on the topic. Numerous recommendations are prescribed: in order to purify and reduce humidity, it is suggested to use willow leaves and vinegar. Advice on diet, bloodletting and recipes for medicines and remedies are given. Finally, the author suggests listening to pleasant melodies or songs.

The physician Valescus de Taranta (Vasco de Taranta), born in Portugal, was active in the medical school in Montpellier and was the first physician of Charles VI of France.[78] In 1418, he composed the work *Practica*, which is also known under the title *Philonium*.[79] The writing is divided into seven books and treats different medical subjects, not only being a compilation of ancient sources, but also a documentation based on personal experience as a physician. Moreover, he also wrote the short

77 See *Liber de febribus*, III, 3 (Pataviae or Venetiis: Conradus de Padeborn, 1474), fol. 48v: 'Et si in hoc experiri volueris, Ovidium lege similiter et receptam, quam tu invenies in VII Methamorphoseos circa principium, illam partem memorie mandes, tamen hoc non plus repugnat quam Albertus Magnus fecerat caput ex succis herbarum ex tali constellatione, quod velut homo loquebatur, ut isti fratres predicatorum asserunt, sed quantum ad hoc naturaliter sit possibile, considera. Sed, o bone Deus, quamdiu poteris istos ribaldos fratres infatuire. Sed obmissis istis fratribus garulantibus ad curam est de cetero transeundum, in qua proposui satis breviter et succincte pertransire'. On this legend by Albert the Great, see Alessandro Palazzo, 'Le apparizioni angeliche e demoniache secondo Alberto il Grande e Ulrico di Strasburgo', *Giornale critico della filosofia italiana*, 85 (2006), pp. 237–253 (p. 251).

78 See *Dictionnaire historique de la médecine ancienne et moderne*, vol. 1 (Paris: Imprimerie de Trouvé et Compagnie, 1828), pp. 259–60.

79 *Practica Valesci de Tharanta que alias Philonium dicitur* (Lugduni: Yohann Trechsel, 1490); it was printed again: in Lugduni: Nicolas Wolff, 1500; Lugduni, 1401 (i.e. 1501); Venetiis, 1502; Lugduni, 1516. It was later printed under the title *Philonium pharmaceuticum et chirurgicum de medendis omnibus* (Francofurti: Nikolaus Basse, 1599; Francofurti-Lipsiae: J. A. Kästneri, 1680).

treatise *De epidemia et peste,*[80] which was soon translated into Catalan by Joan Villa, and the Castilian version was published in 1494.[81]

The vernacular version of the work was translated into Hebrew, bearing the title *Hanhagat ha-dever* ('Regimen of the Plague').[82] In the colophon, the translator explains his motivation for choosing this writing, stating that it was considered to be the best manual on the topic among Christians. A different version of Valescus' work is transmitted in another translation, known under the title *Ma'amar be-qaddaḥot* ('Treatise on fevers'); according to the colophon, in this case, the text was rendered from Latin into Hebrew. The treatise is found in the manuscript New York, Jewish Theological Seminary of America, Ms. 2661, fols 206r–215v, which was copied in Saragossa in 1488 by the copyist David Ha-Cohen. The *Ma'amar be-qaddaḥot* contains some excerpts from the *Philonium*, whose seventh book focuses on fevers. Indeed, the Hebrew text starts with an exposition on sweat, a topic that is treated in the sixteenth chapter of the seventh book of the *Philonium*. Further, the work features some extracts on epidemics.

The succinct treatise *De epidemia et peste* deals with the traditional topics of plague literature. Quoting Avicenna, it explains the astrological causes of epidemics and the time when they occur — mostly summer and autumn. Among the signs that predict the outbreak of the disease, there are comets, falling stars, and meteorological conditions. The author agrees with the traditional literature, blaming the corruption of the air, which might also be caused by stagnant and putrid water as well as by unburied corpses. Surprisingly, the mortality in places where the air is generally less good — such as prisons — is lower than in areas that are usually considered healthier. The most important prophylactic measures include the purification of the air in the house; it is recommended to keep stale water and latrines away from the dwelling and to close the windows as often as possible. Vinegar, rose water, and fumigations of aromatic herbs help purify the air in the house. To prevent infection, it is helpful to remove bad humors from the body, through purgation and bloodletting. It is not advised to perform hard physical exercise, as the acceleration of the breath facilitates the inhalation of corrupted air. Diet and sleep must also be regulated. Concerning the accidents of the soul, one must reach an equilibrium by avoiding extremes, such as rage, which provokes heat in the hearth, but also extreme happiness; a temperate feeling of joy should be encouraged. After having treated the prophylactic regimen, the author deals with remedies against the disease. He provides a series of recipes for

80 *Tractatus de epidimia et peste domini Valasti de Taranta* (*c.* 1474); later, it was published together with the works of Petrus de Abano and Arnaldus de Villanova: Mantuae: Johann Wurster, 1473; Mediolani: Christoph Valdarfer, 1475; Romae: Bartholomaeus Guldinbeck de Wila, 1475; Pataviae: Leonhard Achates, 1473; Pataviae, 1487. It is also included in the *Philonium*, under the title 'Capitula de epidimia'.

81 See Carlos Alvar, *Traducciones y traductores*, Materiales para una historia de la traducción en Castilla durante la Edad Media (Madrid: Centro de Estudios Cervantinos, 2010), p. 150.

82 See Steinschneider, *Die hebräischen Übersetzungen*, pp. 818–20. The work is found in the manuscripts New York, Jewish Theological Seminary of America, Ms. 2669, fols 1r–17v, and St Petersburg, The National Library of Russia, Ms. EVR I 336. In the colophon, it is stated that the translation has been made from the לשון לעז, which seems to indicate that the model was the vernacular version.

pills, instructions on how to treat fever and recommends ointments against boils. It is noteworthy that, on many occasions, Valescus refers not only to traditional medical literature, but also to his own knowledge, giving advice on the basis of his practical experience with the patients. The author, for instance, indicates which of the different traditional remedies were most useful according to his judgement.

Finally, a manuscript kept in Leeuwarden, Tresoar Friesland Historical and Literary Centre, Ms. PB 19, fols 194–196 transmits an anonymous translation titled *Hanagah divrit* [*sic*], a *Regimen sanitatis* in times of pestilence.[83] The Hebrew translator attributes it to an otherwise unknown Maestro Pablo, and the name is followed by the toponym שיפייא, whose identification however is problematic: possibly Sipaya, Sophia or Shpia. The original Latin text is not available and there is no information on it. The origin is certainly Spanish, since most medical terms are Spanish, transcribed with Hebrew letters; moreover, the author states that he lives in the city of Jaca and that the work is intended for the well-being of his town. The text is divided into three parts and transmits mostly recipes, featuring a few quotations from Arnaldus de Villa Nova.

3.

In conclusion, this overview allows for some interesting assumptions concerning medical literature in Hebrew. They outline the frame for the development of scientific learning in Hebrew, on the one hand, and of intercultural exchanges among scholars and physicians in Christian Europe, on the other. Attention has already been drawn to the fundamental historical testimonies that the prologues to the translations represent, which could be classified as an independent literary genre.[84] The methods of and motivations for the translation are often addressed in these prefaces, frequently accompanied by rhetorical apologies concerning the difficulty of the endeavor, which was due to the struggle of finding original texts as well as to terminological gaps in the Hebrew language. The use of the vernacular language transliterated in Hebrew characters stands out as a peculiar feature of this specific subgroup of medical literature.[85] These documents testify to the slow shift of the role of Romance languages from being a mediation instrument for oral exchanges in intercultural interactions to their development as independent languages with scientific authority. In their methodological considerations declared in the prologues, Jewish translators seem to be well aware of the differences between the Latin language of the

83 See Steinschneider, *Die hebräischen Übersetzungen*, p. 816; see also Adolf Neubauer, 'Handschriften in kleineren Bibliotheken', *Israelitische Letterbode*, 2 (1876–77), pp. 83–94 (p. 84).

84 See Rothschild, 'Motivations et méthodes des traductions en hébreu', p. 280.

85 For the use of vernacular language in Latin-into-Hebrew translations, see Cyril Aslanov, 'From Latin into Hebrew through the Romance Vernaculars: The Creation of an Interlanguage Written in Hebrew Characters', in *Latin-into-Hebrew*, vol. 1, pp. 69–84; Gerrit Bos and Guido Mensching, 'The Literature of Hebrew Medical Synonyms: Romance and Latin Terms and Their Identification', *Aleph*, 5 (2005), pp. 169–211.

original and the vernacular language that they often used to substitute the Hebrew.[86] This practice certainly responds to the concrete need to translate the names of the ingredients for medical preparations in an unequivocally understandable way as well as to communicate efficiently with non-Jewish patients. Moreover, it testifies to the widespread use of vernacular languages within Jewish communities, not only as a means to communicate with the outside world, but also as a scholarly instrument. These considerations are especially true for Italy, since a great number of the texts mentioned in the present paper were composed or translated there.[87] The significance of Italian centres of learning for medicine during the Middle Ages is reflected in the production of medical literature devoted to the Black Death — even if the epidemics equally struck other regions of the continent as well.

Besides the dynamics and interactions between Latin and vernacular languages, these treatises also testify to the shift from a context in which the main interest lay on scientific literature produced in Arabic to a setting in which scholarly reference texts were those written in Latin. If in the twelfth and thirteenth centuries Jewish translators were the vehicles for transmitting scientific and philosophical knowledge from Arabic into Latin — through the mediation of Hebrew and Romance languages — the direction changed towards Latin being the source language from the fourteenth century on. This transition went hand in hand with the decline of fluency in Arabic among Jews.[88] Of course, Latin plague treatises, as well as medical literature in general, relied on a *corpus* of translations from Arabic, hence counting it among the different intellectual languages at stake.

The motivations mentioned by the translators in their prologues resonate with a widespread *topos* of the translation genre: their endeavor was justified by the troubles that Jewish scholars faced when trying to gain access to a kind of knowledge that was not available to them.[89] While their Latin-speaking colleagues not only had the most up-to-date information, but also the most traditional and thus authoritative works at their disposal, Jewish physicians complained about the lack of first-hand sources. In the prologue of his work, the translator of Antonio Guaineri's *Liber de febribus*, Solomon ben Moses Shalom, refers to the contempt with which Christian scholars treated their Jewish colleagues, considering them unable to gain complete knowledge of fevers, which had to be based on ancient authorities, such as Galen and Hippocrates.[90] To avoid accusations of ignorance and to provide Jewish physicians with indispensable instruments to face the epidemics, translators undertook the effort

86 This was not always the case; often, Romance languages and Latin were not distinguished: cf. Aslanov, 'From Latin into Hebrew through the Romance Vernaculars'.

87 For an overview of the different places of translations, see Mauro Zonta, 'Medieval Hebrew Translations of Philosophical and Scientific texts. A chronological table', in *Science in medieval Jewish cultures*, pp. 17–73.

88 See Mauro Zonta, 'The Jewish Mediation in the Transmission of Arabo-Islamic Science and Philosophy to the Latin Middle Ages. Historical Overview and Perspective of Research', in *Wissen über Grenzen: Arabisches Wissen und Lateinisches Mittelalter*, ed. by Andreas Speer and Lydia Wegener (Miscellanea Mediaevalia, 33) (Berlin-New York: de Gruyter, 2006), pp. 89–105 (p. 105).

89 See Rothschild, 'Motivations et méthodes des traductions en hébreu', pp. 290–91.

90 See Parma, Biblioteca Palatina, Ms. Parm. 2263, fol. 19.

of obtaining a copy of the respective texts. Benjamin of Carcassonne, for instance, complains that John of Burgundy's work had been kept from the Jews by their Christian colleagues.[91] Further, the translators exposed themselves to criticism due to their terminological choices, as stated by Solomon ben Moses Shalom.

The interest in plague literature among Jewish physicians is also testified by a common phenomenon of translation movements, namely the re-translation of a text, as the case of Antonio Guaineri's *Liber de febribus* shows.[92] Furthermore, partial translations of John of Burgundy's *De epidemia* intersect, so that two Hebrew versions of some parts of the text exist. It is often not clear to what extent the translators were aware of the existence of another version of the same text. Besides the custom of 'double translations', original texts also exhibit a sort of duplication, due to the practice adopted by physicians who used to write and re-write their *consilia* more than once.[93] Gentile da Foligno composed numerous *consilia* on the plague, whose content overlaps and which address different recipients. Similarly, Petrus de Tossignano's *Consilium pro peste evitanda* seems to be a reworked version of his *Tractatus de peste*.

This overview can be seen as the starting point for more in-depth investigations of this topic, which might, first of all, explore the question of the sources. These would need to be examined in the framework of medical manuals, which often rely on each other, and in the context of medical schools. The reception of the Avicennian *Canon* has certainly played a major role in shaping these texts. However, the personal experience of the physicians is often not considered inferior with respect to the authorities, since they were aware of the fact that some of the ancient authors never experienced the pandemics. Secondly, each of the mentioned texts should be thoroughly analysed from a lexical perspective in order to better define the development of medical terminology in Hebrew — or in the vernacular used by Jewish physicians. The intersection of Latin and Hebrew not only shapes the language but also the profile of Jewish scholars living in medieval Europe, as the increasingly widespread use of the vernacular in medical contexts contributes to its development as a modern scientific language.

91 See Paris, Bibliothèque nationale de France, héb. 1191, fol. 142.

92 On this practice, see Jean-Pierre Rothschild, 'Traductions refaites et traductions révisées', in *Latin-into-Hebrew*, vol. 1, pp. 391–420.

93 On the *consilia* literature, see Jole Agrimi, Chiara Crisciani, *Les consilia médicaux* (Turnhout: Brepols, 1994).

Bibliography

Antonius Guainerius, *Tractatus de peste* (Venetiis: Rainald von Nimwegen, *c.* 1486–87).

Fasciculus medicinae, auctore Johanne de Ketham (Venetiis: per J. et G. de Gregoriia, 1491).

Gentilis de Fulgineo, *Consilium contra pestilentiam* (Pataviae: per Laurentium Canozium, *c.* 1472–75).

———, *Consilia* (Papiae: per Antonium Carcanum, *c.* 1486).

Practica Valesci de Tharanta que alias Philonium dicitur (Lugduni: Yohann Trechsel, 1490).

Tractatus de epidimia et peste domini Valasti de Taranta (*c.* 1474).

***

Agrimi, Jole, and Crisciani, Chiara, *Les consilia médicaux* (Turnhout: Brepols, 1994).

Alvar, Carlos, *Traducciones y traductores*, Materiales para una historia de la traducción en Castilla durante la Edad Media (Madrid: Centro de Estudios Cervantinos, 2010).

Arieti, Stefano, 'Medici ebrei a Bologna tra XV e XVI secolo', in *Verso l'epilogo di una convivenza: gli ebrei a Bologna nel XVI secolo*, ed. by Maria Giuseppina Muzzarelli (Firenze: Giuntina, 1996), pp. 235–43.

Arrizabalaga, Jon, 'Facing the Black Death: Perceptions and reactions of university medical practitioners', in *Practical Medicine from Salerno to the Black Death*, ed. by Luis García-Ballester and others (Cambridge: Cambridge University Press, 1994), pp. 237–88.

Aslanov, Cyril, 'From Latin into Hebrew through the Romance Vernaculars: The Creation of an Interlanguage Written in Hebrew Characters', in *Latin-into-Hebrew: Texts and Studies*, vol. 1, ed. by Alexander Fidora and others (Leiden-Boston: Brill, 2013), pp. 69–84.

Barkai, Ron, 'Jewish Treatises on the Black Death (1350–1500): A Preliminary Study', in *Medicine from the Black Death to the French Disease*, ed. by Roger French and others (London: Routledge, 2020), pp. 6–25.

Biraben, Jean-Nöel, *Les hommes et la peste en France et dans les pays européens et méditerranéens*, 2 vols (Paris-La Haye: Mouton, 1975–76).

Bos, Gerrit, and Mensching, Guido, 'The Literature of Hebrew Medical Synonyms: Romance and Latin Terms and Their Identification', *Aleph*, 5 (2005), pp. 169–211.

———, and ———, 'The Black Death in Hebrew Literature: Abraham Ben Solomon Ḥen's *Tractatulus de pestilentia*', *Jewish Studies Quarterly*, 18 (2011), pp. 32–63.

Caballero-Navas, Carmen, 'Medicine among Medieval Jews. The Science, the Art, and the Practice', in *Science in medieval Jewish cultures*, ed. by Gad Freudenthal (Cambridge: Cambridge University Press, 2011), pp. 320–42.

Campbell, Anna Montgomery, *The Black Death and Men of Learning* (New York: Columbia University Press, 1931).

Catalogue des manuscrits hébreux et samaritains de la Bibliothèque imperiale (Paris: Imprimerie Impériale, 1866).

De Ferrari, Augusto, 'Curialti, Pietro', in *Dizionario biografico degli Italiani*, 31 (Roma: Istituto della Enciclopedia Italiana, 1985), pp. 432–34.

Dictionnaire historique de la médecine ancienne et moderne, vol. 1 (Paris: Imprimerie de Trouvé et Compagnie, 1828).

Documenti per la storia dell'Università di Perugia, ed. by Adamo Rossi, *Giornale di erudizione artistica*, 5 (1876), p. 313.

Ermini, Giuseppe, *Storia dell'Università di Perugia*, 2 vols (Firenze: Leo S. Olschki, 1971).

Federici Vescovini, Graziella, *Le Moyen Âge magique. La magie entre religion et science aux XIII*[e] *et XIV*[e] *siècles* (Paris: Vrin, 2011).

Ferre, Lola, 'Hebrew Translations from Medical Treatises of Montpellier', *Korot*, 13 (1998), pp. 21–36.

Fidora, Alexander, and others, 'Latin-into-Hebrew: Introducing a Neglected Chapter in European Cultural History', in *Latin-into-Hebrew: Texts and Studies*, vol. 1, ed. by Alexander Fidora and others (Leiden-Boston: Brill, 2013), pp. 1–10.

French, Roger, *Canonical Medicine. Gentile da Foligno and Scholasticism* (Leiden-Boston-Köln: Brill, 2001).

Freudenthal, Gad, 'Arabic and Latin Cultures as Resources for the Hebrew Translation Movement. Comparative Considerations, Both Quantitative and Qualitative', in *Science in medieval Jewish cultures*, pp. 73–105.

Friedenwald, Harry, 'The use of the Hebrew language in medical literature', *Bulletin of the Institute of the History of Medicine*, 2 (1934), pp. 77–111.

García-Ballester, Luis, and others, 'Jewish Appreciation of Fourteenth-Century Scholastic Medicine', *Osiris*, (2nd series), 6 (1990), pp. 85–117.

Ginzburg, David, 'Be'er la-Ḥay: The Plague Treatise of R. Isaac ben Todros' [Hebrew], in *Jubelschrift zum neunzigsten Geburtstag des Dr L. Zunz*, (Berlin: Gershel, 1884), pp. 91–126.

Goldenstein, Bernard R., 'A Prognostication based on the Conjunction of Saturn and Jupiter in 1166 [561 AH]', in *Studies in the History of the Exact Sciences in Honour of David Pingree* (Leiden-Boston: Brill, 2004), pp. 735–57.

Gregory, Tullio, 'I cieli, il tempo, la storia', in Id., *Speculum naturale. Percorsi del pensiero medievale* (Roma: Storia e Letteratura, 2007), pp. 69–91.

Horrox, Rosemary (trans. and ed. by), *The Black Death* (Manchester-New York: Manchester University Press, 1994).

Jacquart, Danielle, 'De la science à la magie: le cas d'A. Guainerio, médecin italien du XVe siècle', *Littérature, médecine et société*, 9 (1988), pp. 137–56.

———, 'Theory, Everyday Practice, and Three Fifteenth-Century Physicians', *Osiris* 6 (1990), pp. 140–60.

Lemay, Richard, *Abu Ma'shar and Latin Aristotelianism in the Twelfth century* (Beirut: American University of Beirut, 1962).

Marchiaro, Michelangiola, and Zamponi, Stefano (eds.), *I manoscritti datati della Biblioteca nazionale centrale di Firenze*, vols 4, vol. 4 (Firenze: Sismel – Edizioni del Galluzzo, 2018).

Matheson, Lister M., '*Médecins sans Frontières?*: The European Dissemination of John of Burgundy's Plague Treatise', *A Quarterly Journal of Short Articles, Notes and Reviews*, 18 (2005), pp. 19–30.

———, 'John of Burgundy: Treatises on Plague', in *Sex, Aging, and Death in a Medieval Medical Compendium. Trinity College Cambridge MS R.14.52, Its Texts, Language, and Scribe*, ed. by M. Teresa Tavormina, (Tempe: Arizona Center for Medieval and Renaissance Studies, 2006), pp. 569–606.

Mazzini, Giuseppe, *Vita e opera di maestro Pietro da Tossignano* (Roma: Leonardo da Vinci, 1926).

Mugnai Carrara, Daniela, 'Guaineri, Antonio', in *Dizionario Biografico degli Italiani*, 60 (Roma: Istituto della Enciclopedia Italiana, 2003), https://www.treccani.it/enciclopedia/antonio-guaineri_(Dizionario-Biografico)/

Neubauer, Adolf, 'Handschriften in kleineren Bibliotheken', *Israelitische Letterbode*, 2 (1876–77), pp. 83–94.

Palazzo, Alessandro, 'Le apparizioni angeliche e demoniache secondo Alberto il Grande e Ulrico di Strasburgo', *Giornale critico della filosofia italiana*, 85 (2006), pp. 237–253.

———, 'Astrology and Politics: the Theory of Great Conjunctions in Albert the Great', in *Quaestio*, 19 (2019), *Stars, Kingdoms, Beliefs, and Masses. Political Astrology in the Mediterrenean Area from the Middle Ages to the Renaissance*, ed. by Marienza Benedetto and others, pp. 173–203.

Perani, Mauro, 'La cultura ebraica a Bologna nella testimonianza dei manoscritti' in *La cultura ebraica a Bologna tra Medioevo e Rinascimento* (Firenze: Giuntina, 2002), pp. 29–70.

Pinkhof, Herman, *Abraham Kashlari over Pestachtige Koortsen.* Hebreeuwsch met Nederlandsche Vertaling. Naar het te Leiden voorhanden handschrift, benevens een bericht over vier andere 14e eeuwsche Hebreeuwsche handschriften, handelende over de pest (Amsterdam: 1891).

Puccinotti, Francesco, *Storia della medicina*, 3 vols (Livorno: Wagner, 1850).

Rand, Kari Anne, 'A Previously Unnoticed Fragment of John of Burgundy's Plague Tract and Some Connected Pest Regimens', *Notes and Queries*, 53 (2006), pp. 295–97.

Richler, Benjamin, and Beit-Arié, Malachi (eds.), *Hebrew manuscripts in the Biblioteca Palatina in Parma: catalogue* (Jerusalem: Hebrew University of Jerusalem-Jewish National and University Library, 2001).

Rothschild, Jean-Pierre, 'Motivations et méthodes des traductions en hébreu du milieu du XIIe à la fin du XVe siècle', in *Traduction et traducteurs au Moyen Âge. Actes du colloque international du CNRS organisé à Paris*, ed. by Geneviève Contamine (Paris: Éditions du CNRS, 1989), pp. 279–302.

———, 'Traductions refaites et traductions révisées', in *Latin-into-Hebrew: Texts and Studies*, vol. 1, ed. by Alexander Fidora and others (Leiden-Boston: Brill, 2013), pp. 391–420.

Schwarz, Arthur Zacharias, *Die hebräischen Handschriften der Nationalbibliothek in Wien* (Wien-Prag-Leipzig: Strache, 1925).

Singer, Dorothea Waley, 'Some Plague Tractates (Fourteenth and Fifteenth Centuries)', *Proceedings of the Royal Society of Medicine*. Section of the History of Medicine, 9 (1916), pp. 159–212.

———, and Levy, Reuben, 'Plague Tractates', *Annals of Medical History*, 4 (1917), pp. 394–411.

Steinschneider, Moritz, *Catalogus Codicum Hebraeorum Bibliothecae Academiae Lugduno-Batavae* (Leiden: Brill, 1858).

———, *Die Handschriften-Verzeichnisse der Königlichen Bibliothek zu Berlin: Verzeichniss der hebräischen Handschriften*, 2 vols (Berlin: Buchdruckerei der Königl. Akademie der Wissenschaften, 1878–1897).

———, 'Eine medizinische hebräische Handschrift', *Magazin für die Wissenschaften des Judenthums*, 12 (1885), pp. 182–214.

———, *Die hebräischen Übersetzungen des Mittelalters und die Juden als Dolmetscher* (Berlin: Kommissionsverlag des Bibliographischen Bureaus, 1893).

Sudhoff, Karl, 'Pestschriften aus den ersten 150 Jahren nach der Epidemie des 'Schwarzen Todes' 1348', *Archiv für Geschichte der Medizin*, 4 (1910–11), pp. 191–222, pp. 389–424.

———, 'Pestschriften aus den ersten 150 Jahren nach der Epidemie des 'Schwarzen Todes' 1348', *Archiv für Geschichte der Medizin*, 5 (1911–12), pp. 36–87, pp. 332–96.

———, 'Pestschriften aus den ersten 150 Jahren nach der Epidemie des 'Schwarzen Todes' 1348', *Archiv für Geschichte der Medizin*, 6 (1912–13), pp. 313–79.

———, 'Pestschriften aus den ersten 150 Jahren nach der Epidemie des 'Schwarzen Todes' 1348', *Archiv für Geschichte der Medizin*, 7 (1913–14), pp. 57–114.

———, 'Pestschriften aus den ersten 150 Jahren nach der Epidemie des 'Schwarzen Todes' 1348', *Archiv für Geschichte der Medizin*, 8 (1914–15), pp. 175–214, pp. 236–86.

———, 'Pestschriften aus den ersten 150 Jahren nach der Epidemie des 'Schwarzen Todes' 1348', *Archiv für Geschichte der Medizin*, 9 (1915–16), pp. 53–78; pp. 117–67.

———, 'Pestschriften aus den ersten 150 Jahren nach der Epidemie des 'Schwarzen Todes' 1348', *Archiv für Geschichte der Medizin*, 11 (1918–19), pp. 44–92, pp. 121–76.

———, 'Pestschriften aus den ersten 150 Jahren nach der Epidemie des 'Schwarzen Todes' 1348', *Archiv für Geschichte der Medizin*, 14 (1922–23), pp. 1–25, pp. 79–105, pp. 129–68.

———, 'Pestschriften aus den ersten 150 Jahren nach der Epidemie des 'Schwarzen Todes' 1348', *Archiv für Geschichte der Medizin*, 16 (1924–25), pp. 1–76, pp. 77–188.

———, 'Pestschriften aus den ersten 150 Jahren nach der Epidemie des 'Schwarzen Todes' 1348', *Archiv für Geschichte der Medizin*, 17 (1925), pp. 12–139, pp. 241–91.

Tamani, Giuliano, 'Inventario dei manoscritti ebraici di argomento medico della biblioteca Palatina di Parma', *La Bibliofilia*, 69 (1967), pp. 245–76.

Thorndike, Lynn, *A History of Magic and Experimental Science*, vol. 1 (New York: Columbia University Press, 1923).

———, *History of magic and experimental science*, vol. 3 (New York: Columbia University Press, 1934).

———, *A History of Magic and Experimental Science*, vol. 4 (New York: Columbia University Press, 1953).

———, '*Consilia* and more works in manuscript by Gentile da Foligno', *Medical History*, 3 (1959).

van der Heide, Albert, *Hebrew Manuscripts of Leiden University Library* (Leiden: Bibliotheca Universitatis Leidensis, 1977).

Ziegler, Philip, *The Black Death* (London: Collins, 1969; repr. 1991).

Zonta, Mauro, 'The Jewish Mediation in the Transmission of Arabo-Islamic Science and Philosophy to the Latin Middle Ages. Historical Overview and Perspective of Research', in *Wissen über Grenzen: Arabisches Wissen und Lateinisches Mittelalter*, ed. by Andreas Speer and Lydia Wegener (Miscellanea Mediaevalia, 33) (Berlin-New York: de Gruyter, 2006), pp. 89–105.

———, 'Medieval Hebrew Translations of Philosophical and Scientific texts. A chronological table', in *Science in medieval Jewish cultures*, ed. by Gad Freudenthal (Cambridge: Cambridge University Press, 2011), pp. 17–73.

CONCETTA PENNUTO

5. Contagion and Pandemics

Plague in Early Modern Medical Thought

▼ **ABSTRACT** Beginning in the mid-fourteenth century, the second pandemic of plague afflicted Europe with regular outbreaks until the eighteenth century. Populations learned to live side-by-side with the disease, whereas physicians and public officials tried to understand the nature and behaviour of the plague in order to save lives and guarantee health. The notion of contagion, which was already developed in ancient sources and whose fields of application are not limited to medicine, was tested in everyday experience. The extreme danger associated with a disease like plague impelled practitioners to create means to protect themselves, but this was also a stimulus for them to meditate on their relation with patients and on their own responsibilities. Following a short historical introduction, I propose to analyse the notion of contagion on the basis of ancient and early modern sources, in order to underline the interaction between medical theory and practice. The social and ethical engagement of the practitioners is visible not only in the public health measures implemented, but also in the evolution of mentalities at the bedsides of plague-afflicted patients.

Since Antiquity, physicians have been confronted with outbreaks of contagious diseases, which compelled them to elaborate medical knowledge permitting them to understand the causes and behaviour of these transmissible afflictions. The word 'plague' (*pestis, loimos*) referred to maladies spread in the air by miasmas, as Hippocrates explained, and striking patients who did not adopt a healthy life-style, according to Galen. During the Renaissance, ancient theories of contagion were rethought and adapted in the light of everyday experience, for, from the fourteenth century, Europe was ravaged by the Black Death, that is, *Yersinia pestis*, which can take the forms of bubonic, pneumonic, and septicemic plague.[1] When contagion affects

1 On the different forms of *Yersinia pestis*, see Christian E. Demeure and others, '*Yersinia pestis* and the plague: an updated view on evolution, virulence determinants, immune subversion, vaccination, and diagnostics', *Genes & Immunity*, 20 (2019), pp. 357–70; Kathryn A. Glatter and Paul Finkelman, 'History of

Epidemics and Pandemics, ed. by Michele Nicoletti and Alessandro Palazzo (Turnhout: Brepols, 2024), pp. 131–166
BREPOLS PUBLISHERS 10.1484/M.STPH-EB.5.136409

a society, as Andrew T. Price-Smith has pointed out, many domains are impacted, including economics, politics, demography, productivity, fertility, and migrations, because of the direct or indirect threat to the interests of states and populations.[2] In fact, ever since the first epidemics of plague, physicians and public officials have conferred and worked together in the interest of public health to ensure the security of populations and prevent mortality, as is illustrated by the works of Carlo Cipolla on the fight against an invisible and deadly enemy.[3] Such collaboration proved potentially beneficial for the governance of society. Thus, many of the measures adopted during an outbreak of plague were maintained when the outbreak ceased. As the example of London shows, according to the study of Harold J. Cook, this could become a model for governments in introducing medical directives and schemes to preserve health and guarantee order.[4]

The social and political impact is not the only aspect of contagion that merits analysis. Obviously, contagion also affects medical knowledge, namely the search for the causes of transmissible diseases, their way of acting, and the therapies for them. In this context, the medical application of the word 'contagion', whose etymology implies the act of touching, is implicated in a cross-cultural melting pot of legal, philosophical-moral, religious, literary, and pathological references, as is illustrated by Vivian Nutton.[5] The public health and medical aspects of contagion thus give rise to a third level of thought in the context of transmissible disease. From an epistemological point of view, the scientific and cultural effects of the notion of contagion in medicine also have clinical repercussions, since the outbreak of a contagious disease transforms the manner of taking care of patients. This is not a simple technical point, which can be explained with reference to public health. It is an ethical and deontological subject, which particularly affected practitioners, as one can comprehend from reading Renaissance sources. Physicians and other practitioners, such as surgeons, became responsible for treating sick persons independently of their life-style, moral behaviour, and social status.

In approaching this set of problems, this article focuses on early modern medical thought during the outbreaks of the second pandemic of plague (fourteenth to eighteenth centuries), in four sections. After a brief introduction on the subject of pandemics, and plague in particular, the notion of contagion is analysed through a reflection on the evolution of medical thought at the intersection of different cultures and practices. Then, a short view of how physicians faced an outbreak of plague

---

the Plague: An Ancient Pandemic for the Age of Covid-19', *The American Journal of Medicine*, 134 (2021), pp. 176–81. See also chapter 3 of this volume.

2 Andrew T. Price-Smith, *Contagion and Chaos. Disease, Ecology, and National Security in the Era of Globalization* (Cambridge, Mass.–London, England: The MIT Press, 2009), pp. 16–18.

3 Carlo M. Cipolla, *Contro un nemico invisibile. Epidemie e strutture sanitarie nell'Italia del Rinascimento* (Bologna: Il Mulino, 1985).

4 Harold J. Cook, 'Policing the Health of London: the College of Physicians and the Early Stuart Monarchy', *The Society for the Social History of Medicine*, 2 (1989), pp. 1–33.

5 Vivian Nutton, 'Did the Greeks Have a Word for It? Contagion and Contagion Theory in Classical Antiquity', in *Contagion. Perspectives from Pre-Modern Societies*, ed. by Lawrence I. Conrad and Dominik Wujastyk (Aldeshot: Ashgate, 2000), pp. 137–62.

leads into the last section on the practitioner at the bedside of the patient. From my point of view, the study of the relationship between the practitioner and the patient still needs further investigation with respect to early modern medicine. This is perhaps one of the most durable contributions of the medical thought of such famous physicians and surgeons as Girolamo Fracastoro and Ambroise Paré, or of lesser known doctors, like Nicolas de Nancel, as one can appreciate when confronted with current pandemics.

1. The Plague and the Plagues: Histories of a Disease

In 2011, an article by Kirsten Bos and colleagues announced that it was now possible to obtain a draft genome of the infectious agent of the Black Death (1347–1351), that is, the pandemic of plague which struck Europe in the mid-fourteenth century and is now known by the name of bubonic plague, from its major sign: the bubo. By a genomic investigation conducted on 46 teeth and 53 bones of Black Death victims from the East Smithfield burial ground (London: 1348–49), the authors of this article were able to show not only that the bacterium *Yersinia pestis*, a recent evolution of the bacillus *Yersinia pseudotuberculosis*, was responsible for the pandemic of plague,[6] but also that this medieval plague 'was the main historical event that introduced human populations to the ancestor of all known pathogenic strains of *Y. pestis*', which originated in Asia.[7] Before and after the pandemic of the fourteenth century, other waves of pestilence are known, which may be related to *Y. pestis*. In fact, 18 *Y. pestis* isolates have been identified as belonging to the genomic area of plague.[8]

When studying contagion, pandemics, and epidemics, historians, philosophers, as well as biologists, are confronted with recurrent reports of plague, from Antiquity to the present day. Beginning in Antiquity, the world plague (*pestis*) became the name attributed to such epidemic scourges, which caused great mortality because of their speed of action and propagation, and their persistence in time and space. Plague thus became the most frightening disease to face for physicians, public officials, and patients. During Antiquity, many plagues are reported in literary, historical, religious, and medical sources, the most famous of which are 'the plague of Athens' (fourth Century BC) and 'the Antonine plague' (2nd Century AC).[9] Even if these plagues are

6 Kirsten I. Bos and others, 'A draft genome of *Yersinia pestis* from victims of the Black Death', *Nature*, 478 (2011), pp. 506–10. See also the results of the analysis of 100 skeletal remains in Verena J. Schuenemann and others, 'Targeted enrichment of ancient pathogens yielding the pPCP1 plasmid of *Yersinia pestis* from victims of the Black Death', *Proceedings of the National Academy of Sciences of the United States*, 108 (2011), pp. 746–52.

7 Bos and others, 'A draft genome', p. 508.

8 Michel Drancourt, 'Plague in the genomic area', *Clinical Microbiology and Infection*, 18 (2012), pp. 224–30.

9 On ancient plagues, see, for instance, Jean-Noël Biraben, *Les hommes et la peste en France et dans les pays européens et méditerranéens*, 2 vols (Paris-La Haye: Mouton, 1975–76), I, pp. 22–25; A. J. Holladay and J. C. Poole, 'Thucydides and the Plague of Athens', *The Classical Quarterly*, 29 (1979), pp. 282–300; James Longrigg, 'Epidemic, ideas and classical Athenian society', in *Epidemics and ideas. Essays on the historical perception of pestilence*, ed. by Terence Ranger and Paul Slack (Cambridge: Cambridge University Press,

not yet confirmed as epidemics of *Yersinia pestis*, the written production concerning them is still very important for understanding medical thinking and the notion of contagion, as we will see in the second section of this article. Moreover, during Antiquity other contagious diseases were known and considered particularly cruel, such as leprosy, a disease which ravaged Europe during the Middle Ages.[10]

It is at the end of the Antiquity that one finds evidence of the first great pandemic of the plague nowadays attributed to *Y. pestis*: the Justinian plague (541–750). Not only do the sources describe the symptoms and signs of bubonic plague, but biologists have been able to identify the infectious agent.[11] After this first pandemic of plague, two other pandemics are currently known: the one renowned as the Black Death, which started in the mid of the fourteenth century (1347–1351), as we have said, and persisted until the 1720s, when the last outbreak was named The Great Plague of Marseille (1720–1722); and the so-called 'third pandemic', which started in the nineteenth century and still persists at present.[12] The pandemic beginning with the Black Death and lasting 400 years, that is, the second pandemic, is the one which led physicians to elaborate complex theories on contagion and during which they also collaborated with officials to create effective means of combatting the mortality and the pathology, as well as of preventing the spread of the scourge. The second pandemic was not an endemic disease; rather, it came from Asia, as historians and biologists have demonstrated. Signaled in Armenia as coming from China or Africa, the plague travelled along the commercial routes, such as the silk road.[13] It entered Europe through Samarkand, where two great paths allowed travel to the West, via the Caspian Sea and Crimea. Along the route were Genoese merchants, who frequented towns for trading purposes, so the plague travelled to Constantinople, and, from there, to Sicily, Marseille, and all of Europe. At the start of the year 1348,

---

1992), pp. 21–44; Lisa Kallet, 'Thucydides, Apollo, the Plague, and the War', *The American Journal of Philology*, 134 (2013), pp. 355–82; R. P. Duncan-Jones, 'The Antonine Plague Revisited', *Arctos*, 52 (2018), pp. 41–72. See also chapter 1 of this volume on the Athenian plague.

10 Elinor Lieber, 'Old Testament "Leprosy", Contagion and Sin', in *Contagion. Perspectives from Pre-Modern Societies*, pp. 97–136; Françoise Bériac, 'A propos de la fin de la lèpre: XIIIe-XVe siècles', in *The Regulation of Evil. Social and Cultural Attitudes to Epidemics in the Late Middle Ages*, ed. by Agostino Paravicini Bagliani and Francesco Santi (Firenze: Sismel-Edizioni del Galluzzo, 1998), pp. 159–73; François-Olivier Touati, 'Contagion and Leprosy: Myth, Ideas and Evolution in Medieval Minds and Societies', in *Contagion. Perspectives from Pre-Modern Societies*, pp. 179–201; Luke Demaitre, *Leprosy in Premodern Medicine. A Malady of the Whole Body* (Baltimore: The Johns Hopkins University Press, 2007).

11 Lester K. Little, 'Life and Afterlife of the First Plague Pandemic', in *Plague and the End of Antiquity. The Pandemic of 541–750*, ed. by Lester K. Little (Cambridge: Cambridge University Press, 2007), pp. 3–32; Biraben, *Les hommes et la peste*, I, pp. 25–48.

12 Kirsten I. Bos and others, 'Eighteenth century *Yersinia pestis* genomes reveal the long-term persistence of an historical plague focus', *eLife* (2016), available at https://elifesciences.org/articles/12994#content (last accessed 26.9.2021). On the persistence of plague in Western Europe, see Ann G. Carmichael, 'Plague Persistence in Western Europe: A Hypothesis', in *Pandemic Disease in The Medieval World. Rethinking The Black Death*, ed. by Monica H. Green (Kalamazoo-Bradford: ArC Medieval Press, 2015), pp. 157–91; Meriam Guellil and others, 'A genomic and historical synthesis of plague in eighteenth century Eurasia', *Proceedings of the National Academy of Sciences of the United States of America*, 117 (2020), pp. 28328–35.

13 Biraben, *Les hommes et la peste*, I, pp. 49–52.

Western Europe was contaminated by the plague.[14] Once established in Europe, the plague continued to spread, causing recurrent outbreaks and evolution of the original infectious agent.[15] Outbreaks were linked to many sociological factors, such as journeys, trading, exchanges between maritime regions, wars, pilgrimages, and so on. Between the mid-sixteenth and the mid-seventeenth centuries, one can count a plague-wave about every ten years, with the persistence of the disease in many areas of Europe.[16]

From the first outbreak, physicians were confronted with a quite unknown disease, which killed thousands, even millions, of people in a very short time. As far as we know, the plague devastated China beginning in 1331 and killed millions of people; in Europe, historians highlight the demographic shock caused by the Black Death: in many regions, 50% to 70% of the population died of the plague.[17] Western physicians had no memory of the first pandemic (sixth–eighth centuries)[18] and had to search for both the causes and the treatments in contemporary and ancient medicine. One of the first medical reactions to the spread of the disease is the study made by the professors of medicine of the Sorbonne University in Paris in 1348. King Philippe de Valois (Philippe VI: 1328–50) asked the physicians of the faculty of medicine to study the scourge in order to find the appropriate means to fight against it.[19] The first words of the study underline the astonishment of the physicians, who had to look for the causes of this deadly disease.[20] According to medieval medical thought, the primal cause was found to lie in celestial constellations, especially in the 1345 conjunction of the three superior planets (Jupiter, Saturn, and Mars) in the zodiac sign of Aquarius.[21] This distant cause was echoed by a series of proximal causes linked to the influences of the stars, such as the corruption of the air, water, and food.[22]

14 Biraben, *Les hommes et la peste*, I, pp. 52–55.

15 Kirsten I. Bos and others, 'Eighteenth century *Yersinia pestis* genomes', pp. 5–7.

16 Edward A. Eckert, *The Structure of Plagues and Pestilences in Early Modern Europe. Central Europe, 1560–1640* (Basel: Karger, 1996).

17 Rinaldo Comba, 'Il rilevamento demografico : prima e dopo la peste nera', in *La peste nera: dati di una realtà ed elementi di una interpretazione* (Spoleto: Centro Italiano di Studi sull'Alto Medioevo, 1994), pp. 155–73; William Naphy and Andrew Spicer, *Plague. Black Death and Pestilence in Europe* (Wiltshire: Tempus, 2004), pp. 30–34; Stéphane Barry and Nobert Gualde, 'La Peste noire dans l'Occident chrétien et musulman 1346/1347–1352/1353', in *Epidémies et crises de mortalité du passé*, ed. by Dominique Castex and Isabelle Cartron (Pessac: Ausonius, 2007) pp. 201, 210–13.

18 A major problem was the language, since one of the most important sources for this pandemic was written in Greek: Procopius of Cesarea (Bella Persica, II, 22–23). See Evelyne Samama, 'Thucydide et Procope: Le regard des historiens sur les épidémies', in *Air, miasmes et contagion. Les épidémies dans l'Antiquité et au Moyen Age, ed. by Sylvie Bazin-Tacchella and others* (Langres: Dominique Guéniot, 2001), pp. 55–74.

19 H. Emile Rébouis, *Étude historique et critique sur la peste* (Paris: Alphone Picard–Croville-Morant et Foucart, 1888), p. 34.

20 *Compendium de epidimia per Collegium Facultatis medicorum Parisius ordinatum*, ed. by H. Emile Rébouis, in Id., *Étude historique et critique sur la peste*, p. 70.

21 *Compendium de epidimia*, pp. 76–80. On the astrological causes in French medical literature, see Joël Coste, *Représentations et comportements en temps d'épidémie dans la literature imprimée de peste (1490–1725). Contribution à l'histoire Culturelle de la peste en France à l'époque moderne.* Préface du professeur Yves-Marie Bercé (Paris: Honoré Champion Editeur, 2007), pp. 309–20.

22 *Compendium de epidimia*, pp. 80–84.

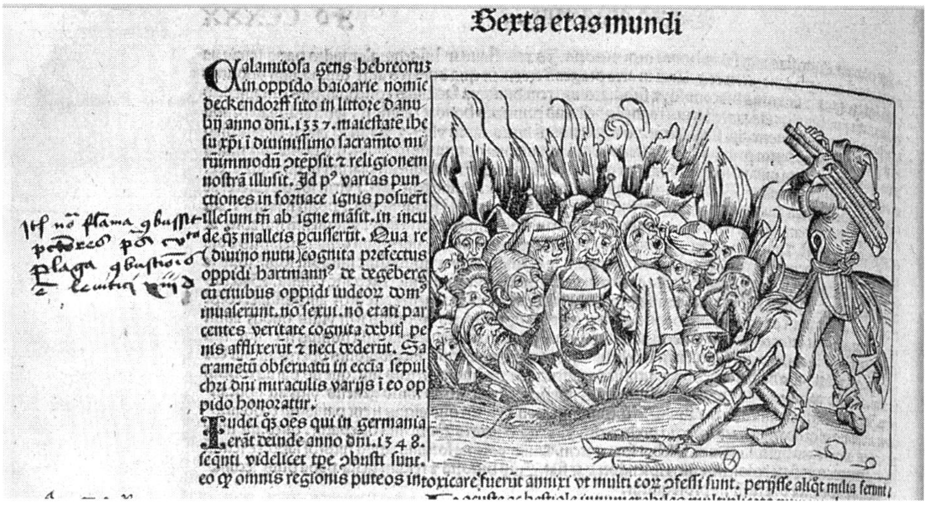

Figure 1. Hartmann Schedel, *Liber chronicarum* (Nuremberg: Anton Koberger, 1493), fol. 230v. © Wellcome collection

In the medical literature produced during the spread of the first outbreak and the following epidemic waves, these causes were discussed and the discussions enriched by reflections on eclipses, comets, terrestrial and meteorological cataclysms, like earthquakes and storms, as well as by considerations of wars and famine. Moreover, these secondary causes were frequently interpreted as a consequence of God's wrath, because of men's sins, religious heresies, the cohabitation with non-Christian people (Muslims and Jews) and persons already sick, such as lepers.[23] Jews were particularly targeted by the accusation of being responsible for the spread of the plague. They were suspected of working with lepers, Muslims, and the devil in order to poison wells, thus spreading the plague. Historians have recorded many massacres of Jewish people during outbreaks of pestilential diseases in Europe, in continuity with preceding persecutions:[24]

Historians underline similar reactions when syphilis started to spread in Europe, at the end of the fifteenth century. It was a new and unknown disease, which, moreover, affected the genitals. Thus, another target could be aimed at, namely prostitutes, and especially foreign prostitutes, who were considered 'to bring a variety of diseases, including plague', as Laura J. McGough has underlined.[25] During the sixteenth century in Venice, these 'loose women' had to be segregated from 'respectable women' and

23 See Biraben, *Les hommes et la peste*, II, pp. 7–17.

24 See Biraben, *Les hommes et la peste*, I, pp. 57–65; Naphy and Spicer, *Plague*, pp. 59–63; Anna Colet and others, 'The Black Death and Its Consequences for the Jewish Community in Tàrrega: Lessons from History and Archeology', in *Pandemic Disease in The Medieval World. Rethinking The Black Death*, pp. 63–96.

25 Laura J. McGough, 'Quarantining Beauty: The French Disease in Early Modern Venice', in *Sins of the Flesh. Responding to Sexual Disease in Early Modern Europe*, ed. by Kevin Siena (Toronto: Centre for Reformation and Renaissance Studies, 2005), p. 232.

placed in permanent quarantine: the island of Giudecca was chosen, where Jews already lived segregated in order to placate the wrath of God.[26]

2. Plague Contagion and Medical Theories

Ever since Antiquity, 'contagion', in medicine, has signified the transmission of a disease by both direct and indirect contact between one body and another.[27] In ancient Latin, *contagio* and *contagium* were formed from the association of *cum* (with) and *tangere* (to touch), thus indicating the contact, the relation, between two entities, the influence and communication of matter, especially corrupted and polluted matter. Ancient philosophers widened the semantic application of the word 'contagion': as Mirko D. Grmek has pointed out, in Cicero, *contagio* can refer to the relations between natural phenomena, thus translating the Greek word συμπάθεια.[28] As heirs to the ancient knowledge, Renaissance philosophers, physicians, and humanists underlined the semantic application of the word 'contagion' to the communication between entities. For instance, quoting ancient literary sources such as Virgil, Juvenal, Pollux, and Lucretius, the Latin dictionary of Ambrogio Calepino (1435–1510 *c.*), first published in 1502, finds the origin of the synonymous words 'contagium', 'contagio', and 'contages' in the association of 'con' and 'tago', from 'tango'. A contagion refers to a disease contracted by contact: 'morbus qui ex contactu contrahitur'.[29] This dictionary continued to be enriched and printed in the following decades by other humanists. In a late edition of the eighteenth century, the three words 'contages', 'contagio', and 'contagium' became three distinct entries. 'Contages' is described as synonymous with 'contagium', and both words indicate an infirmity transmitted by contact: 'male attaccaticcio [...] morbus, qui ex contactu contrahitur, a contingo'; the word 'contagio' is the one which could be translated, in Italian, by 'contagio, infezione' (contagion, infection).[30] The image of contact is distinctly expressed in the Latin dictionary of Robert Estienne (1503?-1559). At the entry 'Contactus, Contagium', one reads: 'Vide Contingo' (See 'to touch', 'to affect').[31] So, under the entry 'contingo', one can find 'contactus', 'contagium', 'contagio', and 'contages', with

26 McGough, 'Quarantining Beauty', pp. 211–37.

27 Danielle Gourevitch, 'Peut-on employer le mot d'*Infection* dans les traductions françaises de textes latin?', in *Mémoires V, Textes Médicaux Latins Antiques*, ed. by Guy Sabbah (Saint-Etienne: Publications de l'Université de Saint-Etienne, 1984), p. 49.

28 Mirko D. Grmek, 'Les vicissitudes des notions d'infection, de contagion et de germe dans la médecine antique', in *Mémoires V, Textes Médicaux Latins Antiques*, ed. by Guy Sabbah (Saint-Etienne: Publications de l'Université de Saint-Etienne, 1984), p. 54.

29 Calepinus (Impressum Rhegii Lingobardiae industria presbyteri Dionysii Berthochi impressoris, 1502), fol. m7v. On Ambrogio Calepino, see Thomas B. Deutscher, 'Ambrogio Calepino', in *Contemporaries of Erasmus*, vol. 1, ed. by Peter G. Bietenholz and Thomas B. Deutscher (Toronto-Buffalo-London: University of Toronto Press, 1985) p. 244.

30 Calepinus *hoc est Lexicon Latinum* (Patavii: Typis seminarii, 1741), p. 212.

31 *Dictionarium Latinogallicum* (Lutetiae: apud Iacobum Dupuys, excudebat Franciscus Stephanus, 1570), p. 311. On Robert Estienne, see Elizabeth Armstrong, *Robert Estienne, royal printer* (Cambridge: Cambridge University Press, 1954).

examples of contagion between bodies ('contagio cum corporibus'), gazes ('contagio aspectus'), minds ('contagio conscientiae'), crimes and evil ('malorum contagiones', 'sceleris contagio', 'turpitudinis contagio'), nature and terrain ('naturae contagio', 'terrena contagio'), and war ('contagio belli').[32]

In fact, the word 'contagion' covered quite large cultural fields, since the transmission of a disease was only one of the areas of its application. Religions, too, were concerned with contagion, namely with the contamination of a religion by another religious faith. In his study of contagion, Saul Jarcho shows how different religions were considered as infectious, with serious consequences for populations. For instance, in Antiquity, Jews could be expelled because they were accused of infecting Roman customs, just as Christians were considered to be superstitious. Fathers of the church, including Tertullian, established an analogy between fevers and heresies, implying the communicability of noxious physical and cultural conditions. The image of contagion in religious thought was also employed, however, to represent communication between God and humankind by the touch (*tactus*), as *The Creation of Man* by Michelangelo (1475–1564) illustrates.[33] The corruption of religion by 'false religion' and idolatry became a theme discussed by many philosophers into modern times,[34] as did the theme of superstition, which Paul-Henri Thiry d'Holbach (1723–89) considered a form of unholy contagion allied to tyranny and moral corruption.[35]

Yet religion and politics are not the only cultural and social fields in which the notion of contagion can be used to explain the dissemination of an idea and a condition. The quarantine of prostitutes and 'loose women' was presented not only as a sanitary decision, but also as a moral one, isolation being a means of social control, as also in the case of the confinement of Jews in ghettos.[36] In the same manner, the notion of the transmission of love, which figured in both ancient philosophy and medicine, was frequently cited as an example of the communication of a physical, moral, and psychological condition between two persons. Love can be contagious because the rays emitted by the beauty of the beloved person or object penetrate through the eyes and affect the imagination, as was theorized by Marsilio Ficino (1433–99) and other writers in early modern philosophical, medical, and literary thought. Moreover, if ocular contagion transmits love, it can also transmit affliction, through the evil eye.[37] Similarly, the contagion of love can become a pathological condition, namely

32 *Dictionarium Latinogallicum*, p. 316.

33 Saul Jarcho, *The Concept of Contagion in Medicine, Literature, and Religion* (Malabar: Krieger Publishing Company, 2000), pp. 27–41.

34 See, for instance, Matthew Day, 'The Sacred Contagion: John Trenchard, Natural History, and the Effluvial Politics of Religion', *History of Religions*, 50 (2010), pp. 144–161.

35 Paul-Henri Thiry d'Holbach, *La contagion sacrée ou Histoire naturelle de la superstition*, ed. by Jean Pierre Jackson (Paris: Coda, 2006).

36 Laura J. Mc Gough, *Gender, Sexuality, and Syphilis in Early Modern Venice* (New York: Palgrave Macmillan, 2011), pp. 112–15.

37 Donald Beecher, 'Windows on Contagion', in *Imagining Contagion in Early Modern Europe*, ed. by Claire L. Carlin (Houndmills: Palgrave, 2005), pp. 32–46.

lovesickness, acknowledged in medical treatises of the Renaissance as the result of a humoral and emotional mutation in the body of the beloved person.[38]

In general, emotions and physical conditions can be communicated by vapours or *species* exhaling from bodies, as early modern physicians stated. This is the case with laughter, which can become pathological.[39] Indeed, the notion and the term of contagion can be applied in many fields, more than this short survey offers, since political, cultural, philosophical, medical, and literary questions involve a metaphorical lexicon which illustrates an idea and a way of operating.[40] This way of operating can be transmitted by different means: sight and touch in the case of love, not only for the beloved but also for the lover;[41] touch and exhalations in the air, in the case of a transmissible disease.

Pollution of the air has been at the core of the notion of contagion since Antiquity. As Jacques Jouanna explains, in Hippocratic medicine one can find the word *miasma* — a word whose origin is not medical, since it indicated the action of staining. It was used to describe the spots of blood left after a crime or the impurity of a disease, as in the case of epilepsy.[42] In this sense, miasma is quite close to *infectio*, a word also coming from the lexicon of dyers (*infectores*), who transmitted colours to woven materials.[43] The notion of infusion in the act of colouring or staining allowed the link with medicine and health, because of the image of spot and dirtiness a *miasma* and an *infectio* can evoke. Thus, the notion of miasma could especially serve to identify the causal agent of a disease. In the case of a widespread disease, like a pestilent fever, the physician could make use of the image of miasma in the air to explain the pollution which infused the disease in many people at the same time and in different places. This situation was a quite difficult epistemological one for the physicians, who had to distinguish between the individual and the general disease. The latter could be explained by an external cause, like the polluted air; the former by an internal cause.[44] Accordingly, one can read in *Nature of man*:

38 Dominique Brancher, 'Du poème à la chair: La contagion érotique des traités médicaux (XVIe–XVIIe siècles), in *La contagion. Enjeux croisés des discours médicaux et littéraires (XVIe–XIXe siècle)*, ed. by Ariane Bayle (Dijon: Editions Universitaires de Dijon, 2013), pp. 25–40.

39 Dominique Bertrand, 'Contagious Laughter and the Burlesque: From the Literal to the Metaphorical', in *Imagining Contagion in Early Modern Europe*, ed. by Claire L. Carlin (Houndmills: Palgrave, 2005), pp. 177–194.

40 See Philippe Monneret, 'Epilogue linguistique. La contagion comme métaphore', in *La contagion. Enjeux croisés des discours médicaux et littéraires*, pp. 161–75.

41 Lise Wajeman, 'La contagion pétrifiante ou des dangers de l'agalmatophilie', in *La contagion. Enjeux croisés des discours médicaux et littéraires*, pp. 41–55.

42 Jacques Jouanna, 'Air, miasme et contagion à l'époque d'Hippocrate et survivance des miasmes dans la médecine posthippocratique', in *Air, miasmes et contagion*, pp. 9–11.

43 Gourevitch, 'Peut-on employer', p. 50.

44 Paul Demont, 'Notes sur le récit de la pestilence athénienne chez Thucydide et sur ses rapports avec la médecine grecque de l'époque classique', in *Formes de pensée dans la Collection hippocratique*. Actes du IV Colloque International Hippocratique, Lausanne 21–26 septembre 1981, ed. by François Lasserre and Philippe Mudry (Genève: Librairie Droz, 1983), p. 345.

> Diseases arise, in some cases from regimen, in other cases from the air by inspiration of which we live. The distinction between the two should be made in the following way. Whenever many men are attacked by one disease at the same time, the cause should be assigned to that which is most common, and which we all use most. This it is which we breathe in. For it is clear that the regimen of each of us is not the cause, since the disease attacks all in turn.[45]

Thus, in order to explain a widespread fever, namely a *loimos* (plague), like the Plague of Athens or the Antonine Plague, Hippocratic and Galenic physicians make use of the notion of miasma. A miasma could be an emanation from the stars to the earth, transmitted meteorologically, as well as one coming up from the earth, for instance after an earthquake, from swamps, or from decomposed corpses, as in the aftermath of wars.[46] In his work on the difference of fevers (*De differentiis febrium*), Galen (second century) utilized these arguments in characterizing the miasma as pollution by seeds of disease (λοιμοῦ σπέρματα).[47]

These physical phenomena could explain the origin of the infection of the air from a *miasma* or many *miasmata*, but the physician must also understand how they work. In the Hippocratic treatise *Breaths*, on can find the description of the particular way of acting of a pestilential fever, which is a common fever caused by the air: 'epidemic fever has this characteristic because all men inhale the same wind; when a similar wind has mingled with all bodies in a similar way, the fevers too prove similar'.[48] But this was too simple a theory, which could not explain why, in the case of a common disease like a widespread pestilential fever, someone survives or is not attacked by the disease, even if he or she breathes the same air. This question is a major one, which early modern physicians also tried to answer, and on which they elaborated theories of contagion based on their own experience.

In fact, the first physicians confronted with the plague, and early modern physicians generally, were imbued with ideas derived from Hippocratic and Galenic treatises. To answer this very important question, which could permit physicians to understand how really to save patients, they could read in Hippocrates that the reason why a common disease could strike one species of living beings but not all was that 'one body differs from another, one air from another, one nature from another and one nutriment from another'.[49] Galen went further in his treatise on the difference

---

45 Hippocrates, *Nature of man*, in Hippocrates, English trans. by William Henry Samuel Jones, vol. 4, The Loeb Classical Library, (Cambridge, Mass.-London: Harvard University Press-William Heinemann, 1959), Chap. 9, p. 25.

46 Jouanna, 'Air, miasme et contagion', p. 14.

47 Galen, *De differentiis febrium*, in Galenus, *Opera omnia*, ed. by D. Carolus Gottlob Kühn, vol. 7 (Lipsiae: Prostat in officina libraria Car. Cnoblochii, 1824), I. 6, p. 291. See Vivian Nutton, 'The Seeds of Disease: An Explanation of Contagion and Infection from the Greeks to the Renaissance', *Medical History*, 27 (1983), pp. 1–34.

48 Hippocrates, *Breaths*, in Hippocrates with an English trans. by William Henry Samuel Jones, vol. 2, The Loeb Classical Library, (Cambridge, Mass.-London: Harvard University Press-William Heinemann, 1959), Chap. 6, pp. 233–235.

49 Hippocrates, *Breaths*, p. 235.

of fevers, establishing a connection between the seeds of the pestilential disease and the suitableness and state of preparation of the body (τοῦ πάσχοντος ἐπιτηδειότης) to be struck. This preparation is to be found in men and women whose bodies are in an appropriate condition to receive those seeds and putrefy, because they are full of excrement, they live idly by participating in feasts and getting drunk, they suffer from plethora, they abuse their sexuality, and so on.[50] Galen offered to succeeding physicians a medical theory which could be supported by the laws of hygiene and the prevention of diseases. This theory was also a philosophical one, since it was based on the interaction between the agent (the seed) and the patient (the body) during their contact. It was an Aristotelian principle[51] which led Galen to explain the interaction between the agent and the patient as the result of a correspondence produced by the life-style of the sick person.

Medieval and early modern physicians appropriated this concept when they found themselves confronted with a common fever, even before the spread of the plague. In the *Conciliator*, Pietro d'Abano (1250–1316) was able to benefit from the Galenic theory of fevers transmitted to him by the *Canon* of Avicenna (970–1037) in elucidating the action of the pestilential fever (*febris pestilentialis*) as the action of an agent on a patient because of contact between the two.[52] Moreover, Galen's *De differentiis febrium* was known during the Middle Ages, thanks to the twelfth-century translation by Burgundio da Pisa (1110 *c.*-93).[53] Pietro quotes Galen's treatise on the difference of fevers when he comes to expound the functioning of putrid fever, and he introduces the notion of seed (*semen*) as the cause of the pollution of the air.[54] In continuity with this epistemological exposition of the way pollution spreads the disease, the physician Pietro da Tossignano (Pietro Curialti, second half the fourteenth century-1407), professor of medicine in the universities of Padova, Bologna, and Pavia,[55] describes plague as the putrefaction of the air because of noxious miasmas. His *Consilium pro peste evitanda* (1398) was edited and translated during the Renaissance within the *Fasciculus medicinae* of Johannes de Ketham (1415?-1470?), beginning with its first printed edition of 1491. In this Latin version, the corruption of the air is caused 'ex pulvere istorum vaporum malorum' (by the dust of these

50 Galen, *De differentiis febrium*, p. 291.

51 Aristotle, *On the Soul*, in Aristotle, *On the Soul, Parva naturalia, On Breath* with an English trans. by Walter Stanley Hett (Cambridge, Mass.-London: Harvard University Press-William Heinemann, 1935), II. 2, 414a11–12, p. 78 (Translation, p. 79: 'For it is upon that which is affected and in a given condition that the activity of what is producing an effect seems to operate').

52 Petrus Aponensis, *Conciliator controversiarum, quae inter philosophos et medicos versantur* (Venetiis: apud Iuntas, 1565), Diff. XCIIII, fol. 142r.

53 See Stefania Fortuna, De differentiis febrium *tradotto da Burgundio da Pisa*, in 'Galeno Latino. Catalogo della tradizione latina di Galeno: manoscritti ed edizioni', available at https://www.galenolatino.com/traduzioni.php?id = 1 (last accessed 26.9.2021).

54 Pietro d'Abano, Conciliator controversiarum, f. 143r.

55 See Augusto De Ferrari, 'Curialti, Pietro', in *Dizionario Biografico degli Italiani*, 31 (Roma: Istituto della Enciclopedia italiana, 1985), https://www.treccani.it/enciclopedia/pietro-curialti_(Dizionario-Biografico)/ (last accessed 26.11.2021).

noxious exhalations).[56] These noxious exhalations are at the origin of many common pestilential diseases. Among these, the epidemic disease ('infirmitas epidimialis') is the one which appears suddenly and strikes communities of people at the same time with many kinds of illness, such as anthrax accompanied by fevers, dysentery, bubonic plague, smallpox, and measles.[57] At the end of the fifteenth century, in his *Consilio contro la pestilenza* (1480), Marsilio Ficino comes back to the idea of noxious vapours as the vehicle of transmission of the plague, joining in a single image the poisonous exhalation ('vapore velenoso') of the air and its action by contact ('si appicca', it sticks).[58] Ficino explains that this poisonous exhalation can act on the bodies it touches only if these are suitable ('disposti') to receive it. Quoting Galen and Avicenna, he says that a body is suitable for the action of the plague if it is full of filth ('imbratti'), stinking humours, putrefying nourishment, warm and humid matter, unclean, with the heart weakened by intercourse and passions, and the pores of the flesh either too open or too closed.[59] The responsibility of the patient is represented in an image found in the *Vanquete de nobles cavalleros* by the physician Luis Lobera de Avila (1480–1560).[60] This work has chapters on the foods which can be dangerous during a pestilence, such as fruits. Especially interesting is the representation of a physician who abandons a patient and his entourage because the patient has not followed his advice not to eat fruit. The physician turns his back on the patient and he will not return, since the patient is responsible for his disease.[61]

Not all physicians agreed in attributing responsibility to the patient, especially in the case of a pestilential contagion. In his treatise on contagion, the physician Girolamo Fracastoro (1478–1553) develops a theory of the communication of the disease based on the action of analogy and sympathy among bodies. One should not forget that his *De contagione, contagiosis morbis et curatione* (1546) was published in the same volume as his treatise on sympathy and antipathy, *De sympathia et antipathia rerum*,

56 Pietro da Tossignano, '*Consilium pro peste evitanda*', in Johannes de Ketham, *Fasciculus medicine revisus per Georgium de Monteferrato* (Venetiis: per Joannem et Gregorium fratres de Forlivio, 1491), Chap. 1 'Diffinitio proprie pestilentie', fol. b6r. On the history of this book, see Tiziana Pesenti, *Il* Fasciculus medicinae, *ovvero le metamorfosi del libro umanistico* (Treviso: Antilia, 2001).

57 Pietro da Tossignano, '*Consilium pro peste evitanda*' (1491), Chap. 1 'Que sint infirmitates pestilentiales', fol. b6r: 'Infirmitas epidimialis est facta subito et in uno momento temporis, communis multitudine hominum, quia in tali epidimia egritudines apparent diverse. Nam aliquibus insunt carbunculi cum febre, aliquibus disinterie, aliquibus glandule vel apostemata, aliquando variole, aliquando morbili'.

58 Marsilio Ficino, *Consilio contro la pestilenza*, ed. Enrico Musacchio et con un saggio introduttivo di Giampaolo Moraglia (Bologna: Cappelli editore, 1983), Chap. 1 'Che cosa è pestilenza', pp. 55–56. On this treatise, see Teodoro Katinis, 'A Humanist Confronts the Plague: Ficino's *Consilio contro la Pestilentia*', *Modern Language Notes*, 125 (2010), pp. 72–83; Teodoro Katinis, 'Per la fortuna di Ficino nel Cinquecento: il caso dei *Dialoghi sopra le cause della peste universale* di Alessandro Puccinelli', *Bruniana et Campanelliana*, 26 (2020), pp. 453–66.

59 Ficino, *Consilio*, Chap. 3 'Come si distende la peste et in quali persone', pp. 58–59.

60 See Carlos José Hernando Sánchez, 'El banquete de damas y caballeros, la corte galante de Carlos V en Nápoles', *Bulletin hispanique*, 119 (2017), p. 444.

61 Luis Lobera de Avila, *Vanquete de nobles cavalleros e modo de bivir … et trata del regimiento curativo e preservativo de las fiebres Pestilenciales et de la Pestilencia* (Lutetiae Parisiorum: Georgii Iosse, S. D. [Augsburg: H. Steiner, 1530]), fols I4v-K1r.

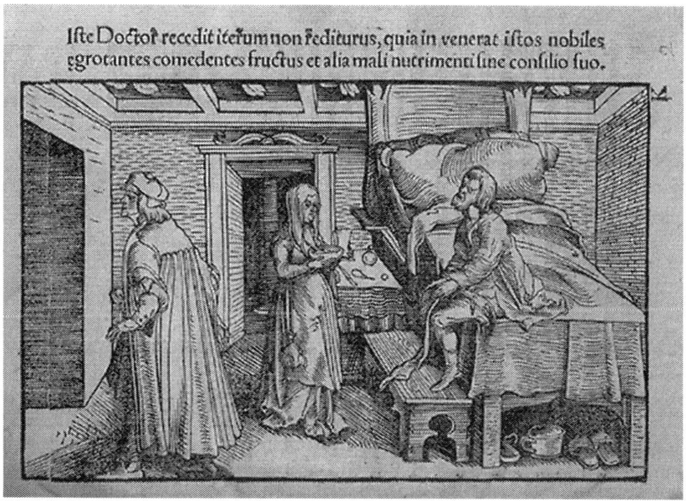
Iste Doctor recedit iterum non rediturus, quia in venerat istos nobiles
egrotantes comedentes fructus et alia mali nutrimenti sine consilio suo.

Figure 2. Luis Lobera de Avila, *Vanquete de nobles cavalleros e modo de bivir … et trata del regimiento curativo e preservativo de las fiebres Pestilenciales et de la Pestilencia* (Lutetiae Parisiorum: Georgii Iosse, S. D. [Augsburg : H. Steiner, 1530]), fol. K1r. © Wellcome Collection.

and that there are links between the two texts.[62] In fact, in his treatise on sympathy, Fracastoro establishes his medical theory on a philosophical basis by exploring similar natural phenomena (both physical and psychological), which function by natural inclination, *sympathia*, or natural repulsion, *antipathia*, like the attraction between the iron and the magnet, the repulsion between water and oil, the lion and the cock, cabbage and rue, as well as the communication of the yawn and the functioning of the emotions.[63] Contagion is merely one of these natural phenomena: 'inter quae et contagionum natura est'.[64] The notion of attraction and repulsion, sympathy and antipathy, is the basis of the theory of Fracastoro, who elucidates the harmony ('consensus')

62 Girolamo Fracastoro, *De sympathia et antipathia rerum liber unus. De contagione, contagiosis morbis et curatione libri tres* (Venetiis: apud heredes Lucaeantonii Iuntae Florentini, 1546). The bibliography on Fracastoro is very copious. See, for instance, Charles and Dorothea Singer, 'The Scientific Position of Girolamo Fracastoro (1478?-1553) with Especial Reference to the Source, Character and Influence of his Theory of Infection', *Annals of Medical History*, I (1917), pp. 1–34; Enrico Peruzzi, 'Antioccultismo e filosofia naturale nel *De sympathia et antipathia rerum* di Gerolamo Fracastoro', *Atti e memorie dell'Accademia Toscana di Scienze e Lettere* La colombaria, 45 (1980), pp. 41–131; Vivian Nutton, 'The Reception of Fracastoro's Theory of Contagion: The Seed That Fell among Thorns?', *Osiris*, 6 (1990), pp. 196–234; Amalia Perfetti, 'La *Syphilis sive de morbo gallico* de Jérôme Fracastor: exemple de la diffusion de Lucrèce en Italie dans la première moitié du XVIe siècle', *Revue d'histoire des sciences*, 55 (2002), pp. 263–72; *Girolamo Fracastoro fra medicina, filosofia e scienze della natura*, ed. by Alessandro Pastore and Enrico Peruzzi (Firenze: Leo S. Olschki, 2006); and, with a broader approach, Roger Teyssou, *La thérapeutique de Fracastor. Lexique des médicaments* (Paris: L'Harmattan, 2017).

63 For a catalogue of these natural phenomena, see Girolamo Fracastoro, *De sympathia et antipathia rerum Liber I*, Edizione critica, traduzione e commento a cura di Concetta Pennuto (Roma: Edizioni di Storia e Letteratura, 2008), Chap. 1, pp. 12–14.

64 Fracastoro, *De sympathia* (2008), p. 14.

and the discord ('dissensus') between bodies by citing the Aristotelian principle of the interaction of the agent and the patient that we have already found in Galen: 'Est praeterea rerum consensus et dissensus alius in agendo [...] Neque enim omnia in omnia agunt, sed certa solum in certa'.[65] This action is based on the conjunction of the agent and the patient because of the 'materiae aptitudo': 'Ergo in omni actione tria praecipue requiruntur [...]: Sunt autem facultas agentis, aptitudo materiae et applicatio conveniens'.[66]

Fracastoro defines contagion as 'an infection that passes from one thing to another' ('contagio sit quaedam ab uno in aliud transiens infectio').[67] Three kinds of contagion are possible: by direct contact, by a fomes, and at a distance.[68] In all of these cases, the vehicle of contagion are the seeds ('seminaria') emanating from the infected body to the second body, then from the second to the third, and so on. Fracastoro is quite close to the Galenic theory of contagion, since he makes use of a corpuscular theory of miasma. Moreover, the seeds cannot act and multiply if they do not find a suitable recipient body, namely a body with which they have harmony ('sympathia', 'consensus', 'analogia').[69] Nevertheless, according to Fracastoro, the suitability of the recipient body is not due to the life-style of the patient. He does not agree with Galen and his successors on this point. The 'analogia' among the bodies is a natural one: it is not based on the Galenic predisposition of the patient ('patientis aptitudo', τοῦ πάσχοντος ἐπιτηδειότης), but on the predisposition of the matter ('materiae aptitudo'), as he explains in the treatise on sympathy. In his theory of contagion, the shift from the patient to the matter allows Fracastoro to discharge the patient from responsibility for his contamination and that of others, since experience demonstrates that healthy people, even men and women who have a good (hygienic) style-life, also get sick of the plague. Fracastoro makes use of a paradoxical argumentation about the unsound predisposition of the patient: 'nam primo mirum videtur in decem millibus hominum, qui in pestilentia pereunt, eam esse praeparationem in omnibus, praesertim quod videmus innumeros exactissime sanos existentes, et nullo vitio humorum depravatos, concipere tamen contagionem illam ex sola conversatione cum pestilentia affecto, aut ex illius vestibus'.[70]

---

65 Fracastoro, *De sympathia* (2008), Chap. 11 'De analogia rerum in agendo', p. 74 ('In action, there is also another harmony and discord among things [...] In fact, all things do not act on all things, but only certain things on certain things').

66 Fracastoro, *De sympathia* (2008), p. 74 ('In every action, three main factors are necessary [...]: the capacity of the agent, the suitability of the matter, the right application').

67 Girolamo Fracastoro, *De contagione et contagiosis morbis et eorum curatione*, Translation and notes by Wilmer Cave Wright (New York–London: G. P. Putnam's Sons, 1930), I. 1 'Quid sit contagio?', pp. 2–3.

68 Fracastoro, *De contagione (1930)*, I. 2 'De prima contagionum differentia', p. 6.

69 Fracastoro, *De contagione (1930)*, I. 3–5, pp. 8–20; I. 8 'De analogia contagionum', p. 38.

70 Fracastoro, *De contagione (1930)*, II. 3 'De pestilentibus febribus', p. 80 (p. 81: 'for in the first place, it seems remarkable that this predisposition should exist in every one of ten thousand persons who die when there is a plague; especially when we see that countless persons who are perfectly healty and whose humors have suffered no depravity, nevertheless catch that contagion from merely associating with the plague-stricken, or from his clothes').

3. The Physician at Stake, the Officials in Action

Girolamo Fracastoro was an experienced physician, who specialized in contagious disease.[71] He reasoned on the basis, not of a theoretical paradigm, but of a realistic assessment and observation of natural phenomena. The contagion of a pestilent fever is independent of the state of a patient's body: a patient can have good or poor health before being struck by the plague:

> possunt enim esse in aliquo mensurate humores, potest abesse omnis obstructio, omnis plenitudo, pestilentia tamen ab alio concipi [...] quinimo illud fieri potest, ut in aliquo praeparatum sit aut phlegma aut cholera, ut putrescant ex praedictis principiis, minus tamen corripiantur a contagione, quam humor alius, quod analogia non sit ad illos.[72]

Fracastoro adopts a deontological approach, which might disturb the traditional Galenic physician, able to transfer to the patient responsibility for the failure of medicine. The Fracastorian physician remains with the patient, and tries to adapt therapies to the different conditions of the ill body. He must inquire into its previous state. Moreover, the physician has to fight against the disease, since its mortality depends also on its degree of aggressivity. As one reads in the third book of *De contagione*, the physician distinguishes between the 'truly pestilent' fevers, which are mostly fatal, and the 'malignant' fevers, which are often fatal. The therapy is determined by the interaction between the dangerousness of the disease and the condition of the matter of the patient's body, especially the degree of corruption of this matter.[73] Fracastoro furnishes arguments for the physicians who want to be at the bedside of patients and collaborate with the political authorities in order to eliminate the disease. As a matter of fact, in everyday life, there were physicians and surgeons committed to fighting the plague. As one may gather from Joël Coste's study of the French situation, the fight against the plague was conducted on four levels: medical practice, public administration, the community, and individuals.[74]

Physicians and surgeons practising during the many outbreaks of plague of the second pandemic left treatises in order to shed light on the disease and its treatment, as well as the ways of preventing contamination and death.[75] The experience of the plague was related in clinical observations, which describe the signs and the symptoms of the disease. According to the surgeon Ambroise Paré (1509?-90), a

---

71 See also chapter 6 of this volume on Fracastoro.

72 Fracastoro, *De contagione (1930)*, II. 3, pp. 82–84 (pp. 83–85: 'The humors in some individual may be in a normal condition, obstruction and plethora may be entirely lacking, and yet the plague may be contracted from another person. [...] In fact it may happen that, in an individual, either the phlegm or the bile is predisposed to putrefy [...], but that they nevertheless are not infected by the contagion so much as some other humor is infected, because the analogy with them is lacking').

73 Fracastoro, *De contagione (1930)*, III. 5 'De cura febrium pestilentum communi', p. 211.

74 Coste, *Représentations et comportements*, esp. Chapters 4–10.

75 Ann G. Carmichael, 'Universal and Particular: The Langage of Plague, 1348–1500', in *Pestilential Complexities: Understanding Medieval Plague*, ed. by Vivian Nutton (London: The Wellcome Trust Centre for the History of Medicine, 2008), pp. 17–52.

physician does not need much time to recognize that a person is sick: the pain and the 'tumour' in the armpit or the groin, together with the spots on the body, are the signs of the malignant illness.[76] Paré adds a description of more internal signs, giving a very vivid portrait of the afflicted, then of the dying, person based on his own experience, since Paré was not only a healer but also a patient of the plague, as we will see in the next section. Consider these passages from Paré:

> en la peste, le coeur, auquel gist la vie, est principalement assailly [...] Parquoy les malades frappez de peste ont souvent defaillance de cœur, et tombent comme esvanouis. Le pouls est quelquesfois remis, et par fois trop frequent, et principalement la nuict. Ils sentent des punctions et demangeaison par tout le corps, et principalement aux narines, comme piqueures d'espingles, qui procedent de la vapeur maligne, montant des parties inferieures [...] Ils ont semblablement la poictrine chaude et ardente, avec grande palpitation et battement de cœur, disans sentir grande douleur sous le mammelon du tetin senestre, avec courte haleine, et grande difficulté de respirer [...] Pareillement ils ont toux et douleur d'estomach, enfleure de flancs ou costez: pour-ce qu'à cause de la debilité de la chaleur naturelle, se multiplient beaucoup de ventositez, qui sont cause de ladite extension: voire que le ventre en est quelquesfois si fort enflé, qu'on diroit estre une espece d'hydropisie, nommee *Tympanites*. D'avantage, ils ont nausee, ou appetit de vomir, c'est à dire, que l'estomach leur bondist, qui vient à raison qu'il a connexion avecques les parties nobles, et se ressentent du venin mortel de tout le corps: autres ont grands vomissemens et frequens, jettans une cholere jaune, et aucunefois verde ou noire, correspondante aux selles en varieté de matiere et couleur: et à aucuns sort le sang tout pur en grande abondance, non seulement par le vomissement, mais aussi quelquesfois par le nez, par le siege, et par la verge, et aux femmes par leur matrice [...] la face se monstre hideuse, et est veue de couleur plombee et livide, les yeux ardens, estincelans, rouges, et comme pleins de sang, ou d'autre couleur, et larmoyans. Le tour des paupieres est livide et noir, comme si elles avoyent esté battues et meurdries, et ont la face hideuse à voir, et tout le corps jaunastre, tellement qu'ils ne resemblent point à eux-mesmes, de façon qu'on les decognoist, et telle chose signifie la mort proche.[77]

---

76 Ambroise Paré, 'Livre de la Peste', in Ambroise Paré, *Les oeuvres*, vol. 3, Edition critique par Evelyne Berriot-Salvadore, Jean Céard et Guylaine Pineau, Sous la direction d'Evelyne Berriot-Salvadore (Paris: Classiques Garnier, 2019), Chap. 14 'Des signes de la peste presente', pp. 2315-16.

77 Paré, 'Livre de la Peste', pp. 2316–17. For the English translation, see Ambroise Paré, 'Of the Plague', in *The Workes of that famous Ambrose Parey*, Translated out of Latine and compared with the French by Tho. Johnson (London: Printed by Richard Cotes, and Willi Du-Gard, 1649), Chap. 13 'Of the signs of such as are infected with the Plague', pp. 546–47: 'Wherefore the chiefest and truest signs of this diseas are to bee taken from the heart, beeing the mansion of life [...] Therefore they that are infected with the Pestilence, are vexed with often swoundings and fainting; their puls is feebler and flower then other, but somtimes more frequent, but that is specially in the night-season; they feel prickings over all their bodie, as if it were the pricking of needles; but their nostrils do itch especially by occasion of the malign vapors riseing upwards [...] their breast burneth, their heart beateth with pain under the left dug, difficultie of takeing breath, ptissick, cough, pain of the heart, and such an elation or puffing up of the *Hypocondria*, or sides of the bellie, distended with the abundance of vapors raised by the force of the feverish heat, that

> Les signes mortels, et qui demonstrent le cœur estre saisi, sont fiévres tresardentes et continues, la langue aride et seiche, de couleur noire, et quand les malades ont grande difficulté d'inspirer [...] Autres ont veilles continuelles, dont s'ensuit resverie et alienation d'esprit, et souvent meurent comme furieux et enragez. Aucuns ont une contraction et convulsion de tous les members, defaillances frequentes de cœur, accompagnees de hocquets, et tombent souvent en syncope. [...] et ont appetit continuel de vomir, qui provient de la venenosité de la matiere [...] le vomissement est puant, et de matiere verde, comme jus de porreaux, et quelquesfois de couleur noire ou rouge: aussi aucunesfois est de sang tout pur, comme nous avons dict, et ont sueur froide, la face livide, hideuse et noire, et le regard esgaré.[78]

Ambroise Paré resorts to a rich panoply of images and colours to convey the suffering of the patient, especially the signs which indicate the pain and the decomposition of the body. All the body is affected: the pictures and gravures of the plague cannot produce the same effect, since they cannot express the physical and psychological status of the patient.

In Paré's text, the reader hears the patient vomiting, grasping for breath, suffering from abdominal pain. The body of the patient empties of blood, and the face becomes the portrait of death. What can a physician, a surgeon, or anyone present do to save the patient or at least relieve his or her suffering? According to the texts, one should intervene as soon as possible with surgical operations, such as bloodletting and enemas, and pharmaceutical treatments in order to drive away the poisonous contamination and protect the heart. Moreover, in the case of a bubo, the surgeon should induce suppuration, practice drainage and scarification; in the case of a carbuncle, the treatments include scarification, suction cups, bloodletting and topical applications. These treatments are only some of the medical and surgical therapies, since the patient is also to be submitted to special diets, sweatings, and fastings.[79] Once again, Paré's text provides a colourful description of the procedures, especially when the surgeons have to practice an operation, such as removal of the bubo. Differential

---

the patient will in a manner seem to have the Tympanie. They are molested with a desire to vomit, and oftentimes with much and painful vomiting, wherein green and black matter is seen, and alwaies of divers colors, answering in proportion to the excrements of the lower parts [...] oftentimes blood alone, and that pure, is excluded and cast up in vomiting [...], but also verie often out of the nostrils, fundament; and in women, out of the womb; [...] all the whole face hath an horrid aspect, and as it were the color of lead, the eies are burning red, and as it were swoln, or puffed up with blood, or anie other humor, shed tears; and to conclude, the whole habit of the bodie is somwhat changed, and turned yellow'.

78 Paré, 'Livre de la Peste', Chap. 15 'Des signes mortels de la peste', p. 2320. See Paré, 'Of the Plague', Chap. 14 'What signs in the Plague are mortal', p. 547: 'It is a most deadlie sign in the Pestilence, to have a continual and burning fever, to have the tongue drie, rough, and black, to breathe with difficultie [...] to have phrensie and madness together, with [...] great watching; to have convulsions, the hicket, heart-beating, and to swound verie often and vehemently [...] and dailie vomits of a green, black, and bloodie color; and the face pale, black, of an horrid and cruel aspect, bedewed with a cold sweat, and verie mortal signs'.

79 For a portrayal of the means employed, see Coste, *Représentations et comportements*, pp. 270–307.

diagnosis allows the practitioner to appreciate the nature and dangerousness of the bubo:

> Au commencement que la fluxion de la bosse se fait, les malades disent sentir à l'emunctoire comme une corde tendue, ou un nerf dur, avec douleur poignante: puis la matiere s'assemble comme une glande, et peu à peu, et en brief temps s'engrossit et s'enflamme [...] Si la tumeur est rouge et se grossit peu à peu, c'est bon signe. Celle qui est livide et noire et tardive à venir, est dangereuse. Aussi il en y a qui viennent promptement et d'une grande furie, et ne tiennent la forme commune, c'est à dire, que subitement deviennent enflammees avec grande tumeur et douleur intolerable, et telles sont communément mortelles.[80]

The therapy for treating the bubo is a long and arduous, since it is based on the application of 'cupping-glass', which implies special treatment with unguents, vesicatories, cantharids, cataplasms, fomentations, and cauteries.[81] The everyday life of a medical practitioner consisted of such acts, performed in the context of a general mobilization of the entire community. In fact, because of the recurrent outbreaks of plague during the second pandemic, officials and physicians became involved in the creation of public health boards, health officers, permanent institutions and magistracies. Large and small towns and states in what is now Italy were pioneers in this respect from the arrival of the Black Death in 1348, as Carlo M. Cipolla has pointed out: other countries, including France, Switzerland, and England, followed the Italian examples.[82] Dialogue between officials and physicians was essential in order to establish the diagnosis of plague and activate public health measures. Medical error or under-estimation of the health situation could cause a delay in carrying out the necessary sanitary measures and thereby lead to a high rate of illness and death. During the outbreak of the plague of 1575–76, in Venice, the university professors of medicine Girolamo Mercuriale (1530–1606) and Girolamo Capodivacca (1523–89) argued that the disease was not plague and defended their diagnosis before other colleagues, who did not agree with them, and officials. As reconstructed by Richard Palmer, a medical debate was held in the 'Sala del Maggior Consiglio' in Venice, and the resulting decision was that this disease was not plague. A conflict between the two

80 Paré, 'Livre de la Peste', Chap. 33 'De l'aposteme pestiferee, appellee bubon ou bosse', pp. 2385–86. See Paré, 'Of the Plague', Chap. 30 'Of a pestilent *Bubo*, or Plague-sore', p. 563: 'In the beginning, while the *Bubo* is breeding, it maketh the patient to feel, as it were, a cord or rope stretched out in the place, or a hardned nerv with pricking pain: and shortly after the matter is raised up as it were into knob, and by little and little it groweth bigger, and is inflamed [...] If the tumor be red, and increas by little and little, it is a good and salutarie sign: but if it bee livid or black, and com verie slowly unto his just bigness, it is a deadlie sign; It is also a deadlie sign if it increas suddenly, and com to his just bigness as it were with a swift violence, and as in a moment, have all the symptoms in the highest excess; as pain, swelling and burning'.

81 Paré, 'Livre de la Peste', Chap. 34 'De la cure de l'aposteme pestifieré', pp. 2386–94.

82 Carlo M. Cipolla, 'The origin and development of the Health Boards', in Id., *Public Health and the Medical Profession in the Renaissance* (Cambridge: Cambridge University Press, 1976), pp. 11–66.

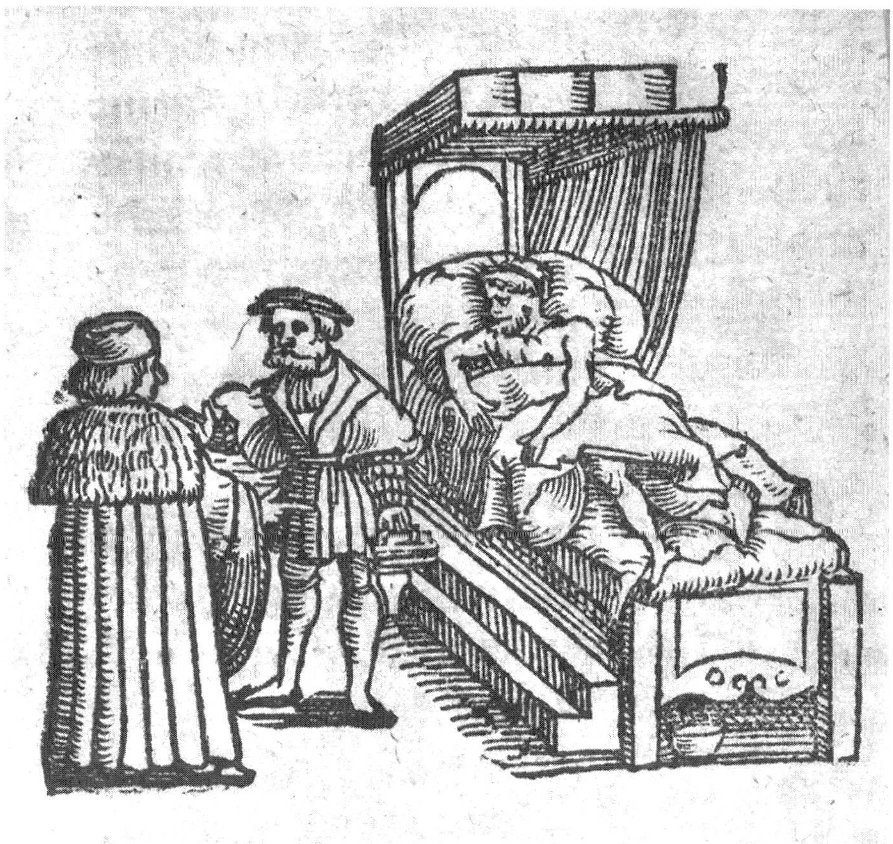

Figure 3. Luys Lobera de Avila, Bancket oder Gastmal der Hofe und Edellent (Francfort: Charles Egen, 1563). © Collection BIU Santé Médecine

physicians and the 'Provveditori alla Sanità' erupted, as well as an increasing number of deaths.[83]

The 'Provveditori alla Sanità', who did not agree with the two physicians, had to take care of the population and prevent the demographic, economic, and social disaster of yet another outbreak of plague. The numerous registers, diaries, and chronicles conserved in the archives and libraries of all Europe describe the fear, even panic, and the misery of daily life.[84] These sources are essential if one wants to understand the impact of the lists of deaths, sick persons, houses marked and shops closed, interruptions of public services, and persons confined in *lazarettos*. In the 'Relatione del contaggio di Goritia' (1682) by Giovanni Maria Marusig (1641–1712),

83 Richard Palmer, 'Girolamo Mercuriale and the Plague of Venice', in *Girolamo Mercuriale. Medicina e cultura nell'Europa del Cinquecento*, ed. by Alessandro Arcangeli and Vivian Nutton (Firenze: Leo S. Olschki, 2008), pp. 51–65. See also Vivian Nutton, 'With Benefit of Hindsight: Girolamo Mercuriale and Simone Simoni on Plague', *Medicina e Storia*, 11 (2006), pp. 5–19.

84 On the fear, see Jean Delumeau, *La peur en Occident* XIVe–XVIIIe *siècle* (Paris: Fayard, 1978), pp. 98–142.

one finds a day-by-day catalogue of dead persons, of houses closed and marked by the sign announcing the presence of sick persons, of ways to find food and remedies, of measures to prevent acts of violence, of religious vigils and prayers to ward off the disease, of ways of providing assistance to poor persons and children. The lists of deaths are not numbers, but persons, identified by name, age, and links with other persons.[85]

4. Preserving People from Plague: The Doctor and the Patient

Given the extremely high rate of mortality during an outbreak of plague, preservation from it was one of the major preoccupations, not only of treatises, but also of medical practice, especially in the relationship between the doctor and the patient. Medical and historical researchers highlight the practical side of Renaissance medicine, showing how attentively the doctor stays at the bedside of the patient, listening to him or to her, working with other professional colleagues, such as surgeons, midwives, and apothecaries.[86] Nevertheless, the nature of the medical visit during a wave of pestilence still needs more investigation. Early modern medical sources are rich in descriptions of the way physicians and their assistants could remain safe from the plague when visiting the patient. In these sources, one can also find many commentaries describing how to take care of sick and dying persons, which show the ethical and charitable commitment of these doctors.

The highly dangerous contamination of plague was a reason either to flee or to be protected, if it was necessary to stay in the towns, as was especially the case for the physicians treating victims of plague. The first medical advice for avoiding contagion was to protect oneself from the infectious breath of the patient, as well as from the contaminated bed sheets, pillows, and clothes. As one can read in Pietro da Tossignano's treatise, the air of the patient's room must be purified in the interest, not only of the sick person, but also of those who stay with him. For this purpose, one could make use of rose-branches dampened with vinegar and sandalwood, as well as perfumes made of myrrh, incense, aloe, and so on. Bed sheets must be immersed in vinegar and changed frequently; the walls of the room must be washed with water and vinegar. A large number of lemons should be placed on the bed.[87] In such a purified room, the physician follows a strict procedure in treating the patient. Pietro

85 Maria Cristina Cergna, *Il diario della peste di Giovanni Maria Marusig (1682), Edizione del testo e delle illustrazioni originali dell'autore*, con un saggio di Rienzo Pellegrini (Mariano del Friuli: Edizioni della Laguna, 2005). For a historical picture of the religious actions undertaken to repel out the plague, see Biraben, *Les hommes et la peste*, vol. 2, pp. 56–84.

86 Jerome Bylebyl, 'The manifest and the hidden in the Renaissance clinic', in *Medicine and the five senses*, ed. by William F. Bynum and Roy Porter (Cambridge: Cambridge University Press, 1993), pp. 40–60; Michael Stolberg, 'Bedside Teaching and the Acquisition of Practical Skills in Mid-Sixteenth-Century Padua', *Journal of the History of Medicine and Allied Sciences*, 69 (2014), pp. 633–64.

87 Pietro da Tossignano, '*Consilium pro peste evitanda*' (1491), Chap. 4, 'De modo curativo', fol. b7r: 'Aer camere sic rectificetur pro illis qui stant in camera sicut pro egro aspergendo cum ramis et frondulis, et rosis madefactis in aceto cum sandalis cum prefumigiis ex mira, ture, silloxaloe, storace, et similibus.

explains that, after the body of the patient has been purified by bloodletting and enema, the surgeon can intervene with scarification of the bubo (*apostema*) or the carbuncle (*anthrax*), a very dangerous operation because of the matter that can flow out of these excrescences.[88] The practitioners have to be very cautious for additional reasons: the heat of both the means of treatment (cauterisation) and the exhalations from the body of the patient is very dangerous. In this situation, the physicians must be particularly careful because of the noxious vapours, and he should avoid physical contact. The matter of these exhalations is so dangerous, so subtle and poisonous, that this explains why physicians fall ill: 'Caveat sibi medicus a malis fumis, et non tangat cum manu, quia una materia distillari subtilis est contagiosa intantum quod medici postea infirmantur'. Thus, Pietro suggests a recipe for a purifying drug.[89]

The very practical medical chapters of Pietro da Tossignano's treatise inspired an illustration of a medical visit to a plague-stricken patient in the 1493 edition of the *Fasciculo di medicina* by Johannes de Ketham; this illustration was not present in the first edition of 1491, but was retained in the following latin editions.[90]

A quite similar explanation of the way the physicians could be protected from the plague when visiting the patient in his house was proposed by the French physician Auger Ferrier (1513–88). Ferrier, born in Toulouse, studied medicine at the University of Montpellier and became a personal physician of Queen Catherine de' Medici (1519–89).[91] During the epidemic of 1548, he wrote a book proposing ways to be preserved from contagion: *Remedes preservatifs et curatifs de peste*. Reading Ferrier's pages on the medical visit allows one to appreciate the precautions physicians had to adopt in order to avoid contagion, as well as their fear, and particularly the meticulous measures advised to prevent contact with the body of the patient, his excrements, and his family:

> Quand vous serez pres de la maison du pestiferé, envoyez quelcun devant, qui face ouvrir toutes les portes de la maison, et les fenestres de la chambre ou gist le patient: et tandis arrestez vous un peu à la rue.
> Et commandez que lon allume bon feu à la chambre du malade.

Ponendo lintheamina madefacta in aceto cum cortinis, et sepe renovando, etiam muri camere aspergantur sepe aqua et aceto. Et sint super lecto et banchis multi citri'.

88 Pietro da Tossignano, '*Consilium pro peste evitanda*' (1491), Chap. 4, 'De corporis evacuatione et de cristeri faciendo', 'De cura apostematis', 'De cura Antracis', fol. b7r.

89 Pietro da Tossignano, '*Consilium pro peste evitanda*' (1491), Chap. 4, 'Cura circa accidentia quae veniunt a pravitate materie', fol. b7v ('The physician has to avoid bad exhalations, and he must not touch. In fact, a single stuff of a thin catarrh is contagious. This is why physicians get sick').

90 Pietro da Tossignano, 'Consiglio per la peste', in Johannes de Ketham, *Fasciculo di medicina* Vulgarizato per Sabastiano Manilio Romano (Venexia: Zuane et Gregorio di Gregorii, 1493), fol. e2r. See, for instance, Pietro da Tossignano, '*Consilium pro peste evitanda*', in Johannes de Ketham, *Fasciculus medicine* (Venetiis: per Joannem et Gregorium de Gregoriis fratres, 1500), fol. c5r.

91 On Auger Ferrier, see Ingrid De Smet, 'Of Doctors, Dreamers and Soothsayers: The Interlinking Worlds of Julius Caesar Scaliger and Auger Ferrier', *Bibliothèque d'Humanisme et Renaissance*, 70, 2, (2008), pp. 351–76; Jean-François Gourdou, *Le professeur Augier Ferrier et la reine Catherine de Médicis* (Paris: Saint Honoré éditions, 2016).

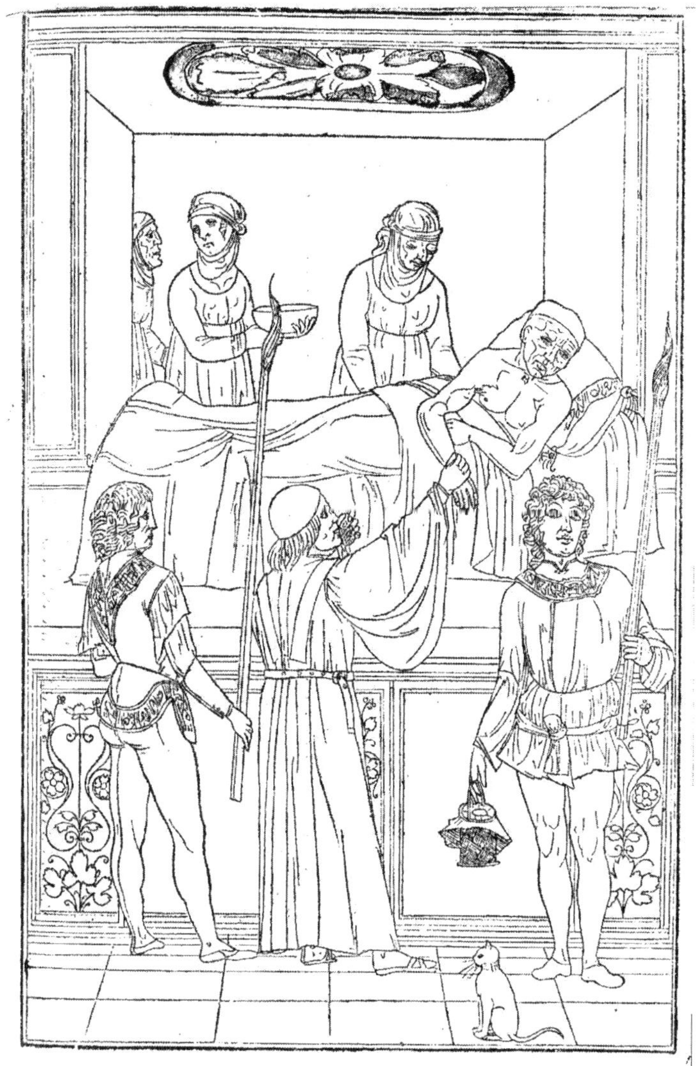

Figure 4. Johannes de Ketham, *Fasciculus medicine* (Venetiis: per Johannes et Gregorium de Gregoriis fratres, 1495). © Wellcome Collection

Puis ferez descendre une eschauffette pleine de charbons ardans, avec l'encens, roses, myrrhe, benioin, ladanum, styrax, cloux de giroffle, et semblables odeurs, pour en faire fumigation.

Et quant et quant faites allumer votre piece de boys de genevrier: et ainsi entrez hardiment, faisant passer devant vous ledit personnage avec ladite fumigation d'encens, myrrhe, etc. et le suyvez, tenant à l'une main ledit boys allumé: et à l'autre vostre pomme de senteur, ou vostre bouquet, ou latide esponge, l'appliquant au nez.

Et en ceste façon marcherez iusques dens la chambre, là ou ferez mettre ladite eschauffette avec ledit encens, à celle fin que l'odeur s'espande par toute la chambre.
Ainsi, tenant dens la bouche quelque chose de vostre massapan, et tenant l'une main au pres du nez avec lesdites odeurs, et ayant en l'autre ladite piece de genevrier allumee: vous regarderez d'un peu loing vostre patient, et l'interroguerez de son mal, et de ses accidens: et s'il ha douleur, ou quelque tumeur en aucune partie, la visiterez.
Puis vous approcherez, et en luy tournant le dos, baillerez vostre piece de boys à quelcun qui la tienne devant vostre face. Et avec vostre main tournee en arriere, toucherez le pouls du malade, et le front, et la region du cœur: tenant tousiours quelque senteur au pres du nez.
Puis visiterez l'urine, et autres excremens, si bon vous semble, et si la condition du malade le merite. Car certainement il est fort dangereux s'approcher des excremens de telz malades.
Parquoy s'il fault que vous les visitez, faites tenir ledit genevrier fumigant et allumé au devant de vostre face, et n'oubliez tenir quelques odeurs au pres du nez.
Ce fait prenant congé de vostre patient, prenez vostre genevrier allumé, et le tenant au devant de vous, sortez hors de la maison.
Incontinent que serez hors, iettez ce que vous aviez dens la bouche, et prenez quelque autre chose dudit massapan. Laquelle macherez tout au long du chemin, et ainsi vous en retournerez à votre logis.
Et notez qu'au lieu dudit boys de genevrier, vous pouvez user de une torche, en la mesme forme et maniere qui ha esté dit du genevrier.[92]

92 Auger Ferrier, *Remedes preservatifs et curatifs de peste* (Lyon: par Iean de Tournes, 1548), 'Quand le medecin, ou autre va voir les malades de peste', pp. 52–56 ('When you are near the house of the plague-afflicted person, send someone ahead to open all the doors of the house and the windows of the room where the patient is lying. During this time, wait a little in the street.
Order a good fire to be lit in the room of the sick person.
Then, you will order a warming-pan to be brought down full of burning coals, with incense, roses, myrrh, benzoin, labdanum, styrax, cloves, and similar herbs, in order to perform fumigations.
At the same time, ask for your piece of juniper-wood to be lit. So, enter boldly, having the person go ahead who is holding the said fumigation of incense, myrrh, and so on. Follow him with, in one hand, the said wood ignited and, in the other, either your pomander or your bouquet or the previously mentioned sponge, applying it to your nose.
In this way, you will proceed to the room, where you ask the warming-pan previously mentioned, with its incense, to be placed, so that the scent spreads through the whole room.
So, keeping some of your marzipan in your mouth and one of your hands near your nose with the previously mentioned aromatics, and in the other hand the lighted juniper previously mentioned, you will look at your patient from a little distance and ask him about his disease and symptoms; and if he feels pain or has a tumour anywhere, you will examine this.
Then, you will approach him and turn your back, giving your piece of wood to someone so that he keeps it before your face. And with the back of your hand, you will touch the wrist of the sick person, his forehead, and the region of the heart, always keeping some scent near your nose.
After this, you will examine the urine and the other excrements, if you think it is important and if the state of the sick person justifies it. For to come close to the excrements of these sick persons is undoubtedly very dangerous.

The physician, as well as any person who is going to visit a person afflicted by the plague, is urged to avoid any direct or indirect contact, since the disease can reach a person through infected air, objects, and the sick body itself. Direct and indirect contacts must to be prevented by purifying the air with perfumed smoke, by keeping oneself distant from the excrements and the body of the sick person, and by turning away one's own face in order not to inhale his poisonous breath. The ordinary act of taking the pulse necessitates a specific manoeuvre, with the physician keeping his back turned to the patient. Moreover, the physician is protected by a kind of pharmacological marzipan, the ingredients of which are chosen from the remedies against poison of galenic medicine.

All the gestures and techniques that one can see in the illustration from Pietro da Tossignano–Ketham and read about the pages of Auger Ferrier are designed to protect the breath of the physician, and his body. In the same period, physicians also proposed other methods of keeping safe from contagion. In his 1566 treatise on the plague, the physician François Valleriole (1504–80) underlines how the lives of those attending the sick person are in danger, since they breathe the same air and are close to the excrements of their bodies. So, according to Valleriole, after praying to God to save him and taking all the possible precautions against contagion, the practitioner turns his face from the sick person in order to avoid his breath and the infection (*infection*). Moreover, the practitioner must wear clean clothes and be scrupulous about his physical hygiene.[93]

In 1567, one year after the publication of Valleriole's book, the Chancellor of the University of Medicine of Montpellier and personal physician of the King of Navarre, Laurent Joubert (1529–83), described the clothes the doctor should wear if he wants to be protected from the plague, since these clothes impede the passage of the poisonous and bad-smelling air coming from the patient. It is very important that the tissue of these clothes should be thick and tightly woven. The best material is animal leather, especially the kind made from goat-skin, called *Marroquina*, as well as

Thus, if you must examine them, have the fumigant and lighted juniper kept before your face, and do not forget to keep some scent near your nose. When this is done, in taking leave of your patient, take with you your lighted juniper, and, holding it in front of you, get out of the house.
As soon as you are outside, throw away what you had in your mouth and take another piece of the previously mentioned marzipan. You will chew this all along the way and in this manner return to your lodging.
Note that you can make use of a torch instead of the juniper-wood mentioned in the same form and manner as has been specified regarding the juniper'.
See Coste, *Représentation et comportements*, pp. 264–65.

93 François Valleriole, *Traicté de la peste* (Lyon: par Antoine Oryphius, 1566), Chap. 16 'De l'ordre et regime que doibvent observer ceux qui assistent aux malades de peste pour le servir', pp. 186–91. On Valleriole and the plague, see Véronique Montagne, 'Le discours didascalique sur la peste dans les traités médicaux de la Renaissance: rationaliser et/ou inquiéter', *Réforme, Humanisme, Renaissance*, 70 (2010), pp. 103–12; Guylaine Pineau, 'Soigner la peste sans défier la colère divine dans les traités médicaux du XVIe siècle', Seizème siècle, 8 (2012), pp. 173–90. Véronique Montagne has also analysed Valleriola's rhetorical language concerning plague in her book: Véronique Montagne, *Médecine et rhétorique à la Renaissance. Le cas du traité de peste en langue vernaculaire* (Paris, Classiques Garnier, 2017).

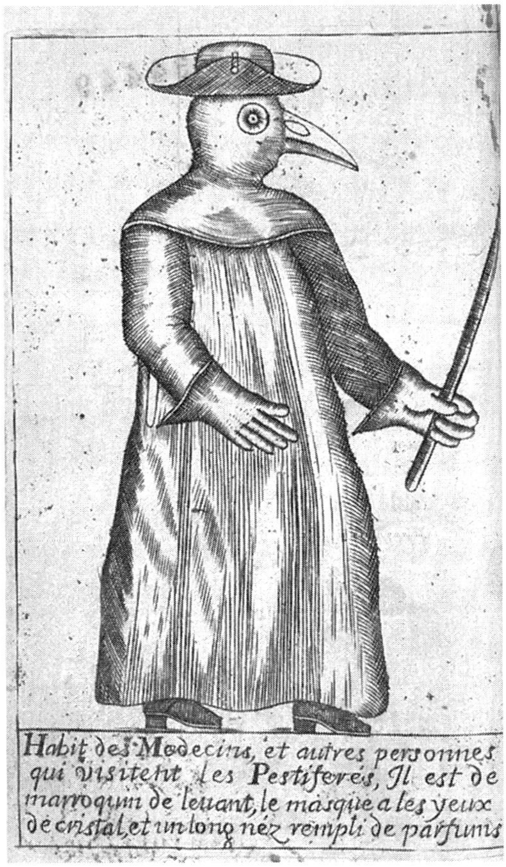
Habit des Medecins, et autres persones
qui visitent les Pestiferés, Il est de
marroquin de leuant, le masque a les yeux
de cristal, et un long néz rempli de parfums

Figure 5. Jean-Jacques Manget, *Traité de la peste* (Genève: chez Philippe Planche, 1721). © Collection BIU Santé Médecine

clothes without fur, such as those made with silk.[94] In the following years, physicians continued to search for garments offering protection from the plague, as Joël Coste explains, citing sources from the seventeenth and eighteenth centuries,[95] until they arrived at the very famous costume of the plague doctor to be seen in one of the last treatises on the pandemic which had started in Europe in the mid-fourteenth century, namely the 1721 *Traité de la peste* by the Genevan physician Jean-Jacques Manget (1652–1742):[96]

94 Laurent Joubert, *De peste liber unus* (Lugduni: apud Ioannem Frellonium, 1567), Chap. 11 'In aere pestilenti quomodo agendum sit: et de illius correctione, quot, quibusque modis fiat', pp. 75–77. Joël Coste quotes the passage from the French edition of 1581: Coste, *Représentations et comportements*, p. 265.

95 Coste, *Représentations et comportements*, pp. 266–267.

96 See Jean-Jacques Manget, *Traité de la peste* (Genève: chez Philippe Planche, 1721), Chap. 12 'L'ordre que les Magistrats doivent tenir pour se conserver en santé en tems de Peste, et se garantir de ce mal contagieux', pp. 170–71.

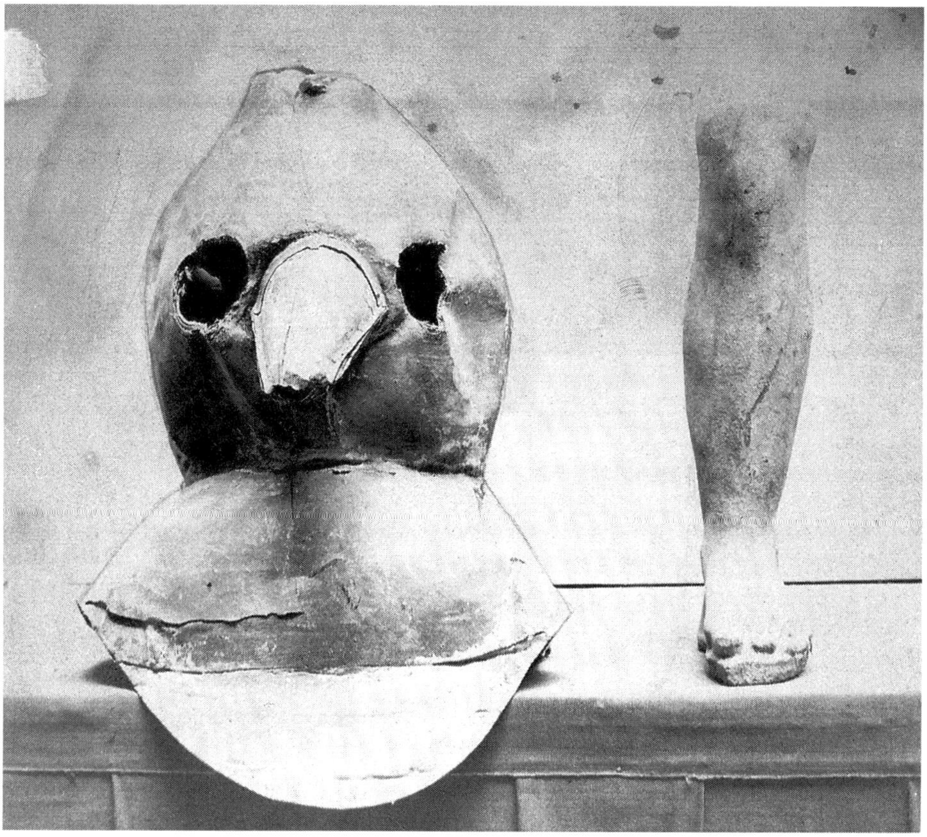

Figure 6. Plague apparatus from a lazaretto in Venice. © Wellcome Collection

This clothing resembles the protective apparel physicians could wear when working in a *lazaretto*, such as is shown in The Wellcome Collection:

The interest of the physicians in protective measure was justified because of the great number of them who contracted the plague. The famous surgeon Ambroise Paré underlines the human and ethical engagement practitioners make when treating plague-stricken patients, and recounts his own activity at their bedsides during three years. As he explains in his treatise on the plague of 1568, he practiced surgery in order to heal such patients. He was asked by the Queen to write the treatise after she saw, in 1564, a great many sick and dying patients in Lyon. Paré accepted, since, according to him, despite the great number of treatises already written on plague, he had to practice Christian charity by healing the miserable victims of the plague ('une infinite de pauvres maladies pestiferez').[97] Paré knew the suffering of the patients not only because he treated them, as we have seen, but also because he had experienced

97 Ambroise Paré, *Traicté de la Peste, de la petite Verolle et Rougeolle: avec une brefve description de la Lepre* (Paris: de l'Imprimerie d'André Wechel, 1568), 'Epistre à Monsieur Castellan', fols *2v–4r.

the disease, with a painful bubo in his right armpit and carbuncle on the belly. He hopes that his experience may encourage young students to engage actively with their patients.[98]

Respect for the patient, compassion for his suffering, and for the entourage at the moment of dying — all these elements are at the core of both the experience and the treatise of the physician Nicolas de Nancel (1539–1610), who practiced medicine in the French town of Tours during the epidemic of the 1580s. This humanist physician is especially known for his former activity as pupil, colleague, and secretary of Pierre de la Ramée (Ramus: 1515–72), of whom he wrote a very interesting biography.[99] Because of the wars of religion, Nancel left Paris in the 1560s and went to Douai, where he studied medicine. In 1570 he settled in Tours, working as a physician in the town, then as the personal physician of Eléonore de Bourbon, the abbess of Fontevraud.[100] In 1581, his treatise *Discours tres ample de la Peste, divisé en trois livres, adressant à Messieurs de Tours*, was published in Paris. The treatise is divided into three large books: the first one is on the definition and causes of the plague; the second is about prophylactic measures against the plague; the last explains the therapies. In his treatise, Nancel makes many references to the nature of Touraine, its food, and the possibility of finding many ingredients for remedies. Moreover, he wants to show how a surgeon in Tours's *lazaretto* operates in treating plague-stricken patients and understanding their illness. At the end of the first book, Nancel copies description by the surgeon Simeon, who was treating patients in the *Sanitat* (Lazaretto) of Tours. This description was written at the request of Nancel, who wanted to know the signs of the plague the surgeon could see in the *Sanitat*. Simeon explains what the signs are, such as headache, stomach pain, vomiting, trembling, cold sweat, palpitation, syncope, and so on. After this list, Simeon describes the pestilential bubo and points out that he dissected dead persons, finding putrefaction in the left ventricle of the heart and alteration of the blood and the liver, which becomes violet and black.[101]

In this work, the reader is immersed in the everyday life of a practitioner, by way of a case-history report intended to inform other physicians, surgeons, and especially public officials. In fact, Nancel explicitly writes for the officials of Tours, *Messieurs de Tours*, who are responsible for the public health of the town and the working conditions of the practitioners. This is why Nancel closes his treatise with another

98 Paré, *Traicté de la Peste*, fol. *4r: 'Davantage, ceste experience a esté faicte en moy mesme ayant esté touché de ce mal et souffert l'aposteme pestilent souz l'aisselle dextre, et le charbon au ventre. [...] Quand ores le tout ne profiteroit que pour donner courage aux ieunes estudiants, qui desirent parvenir à la Chirurgie, cela leur peut donner asseurance de traicter les pauvres malades'.

99 Marie-Dominique Couzinet et Jean-Marc Mandosio, 'Nouveaux éclairages sur les cours de Ramus et de ses collègues au Collège de Presles d'après des notes inédites prises par Nancel', in *Ramus et l'Université* (Paris: Editions rue d'Ulm, 2004), pp. 11–48; Katharine MacDonald, *Biography in Early Modern France, 1540–1630. Forms and Functions* (Leeds: Legenda, 2007), Chap. 4 'Medicine and Method in Nicolas de Nancel's *Petri Rami Vita* (1599)', pp. 61–79.

100 MacDonald, *Biography in Early Modern France*, p. 62.

101 Nicolas de Nancel, *Discours tres ample de la Peste, divisé en trois livres, adressant à Messieurs de Tours* (Paris, Chez Denys du Val, 1581), Book 1, 'S'ensuit un advertissement du Chirurgien du Sanitat de Tours, touchant ce qu'il a trouvé et descouvert en la peste, de l'an present 1580', pp. 106–08.

discourse, written by himself, which provides officials with a procedure for protecting people during a pestilence: *Advertissement particulier à Messeiurs de Tours, touchant la police et reglement qu'on doit garder et tenir en temps de peste.*[102] After the description of the beautiful and wholesome territory of Tours, Nancel explains how to purify the air using fire perfumed by the many medicinal plants of the abbey-gardens. He suggests some measures for avoiding contagion. For instance, when meeting someone, it is sufficient to shake hands instead of kissing; one should also avoid meeting if one is not protected by an antidote; the food markets, especially those with meat, must be placed outside the town; one should avoid selling the goods of the dead, since they can retain the contagious poison of the plague; and of course, to flee is the best way to ensure safety.[103] Nevertheless, the physician must not forget the poor and sick, whose lives are in danger during the outbreak of plague. According to Nancel, nobody must mistreat the plague-afflicted. On the contrary, it is important to treat them with kindness and grace, without either keeping them imprisoned or burying them before they die. In fact, this is the reason why many people conceal their illness, thereby creating great danger for their entourage. Nancel points out that some sick people are prepared to be interred in their gardens because they fear the way they may be treated by physicians and their assistants in the *lazaretto*. So, officials must ensure that sick people are transported to the *Sanitat* in order to be nourished and healed at the expenses of the citizens and the bourgeois. All their bedding must be preserved, cleaned, and given back to them or their heirs:

> Ie seroye d'advis [...] qu'on traittast les povres malades gratieusement et humainement, sans leur barrer, bacler, cadenasser et cheviller leurs portes et fenestres, et les enterrer auparavant qu'ils soient morts. Qui est occasion, que plusieurs celent et dissimulent leur mal, au grand danger de leurs domestiques, parens, voysins et amis : et craignants telle rigueur, endurent leur maladie, sans y prouvoir ; ainsi mourants, craignant de mourir : et quelquefois se faisant enterrer en leurs caves et celiers, ou iardins, s'ils en ont.
> Les povres doivent estre transportés à l'hostel Dieu, ou au Sanitat [...], pour y estre nourris et secourus aux despens des citadins et bourgeois et emportés avec eux, leurs lits et coites, draps et couvertures, ciels et cortines, estants ja infectés de la contagion. et demeurer audit Sanitat ou Hospital, pour l'usage d'eux et des autres malades : pour crainte, que les laissant en leur maison, ou y estant remportés, ils baillent le mal aux autres domestiques ; comme nous en avons veu l'experience. il en sera fait registre et memoire, pour leur rendre, ou à leurs successeurs et heritiers, long temps aprés tout le mal cessé.[104]

102 Nancel, *Discours*, pp. 342–66.
103 Nancel, *Discours*, pp. 342–60.
104 Nancel, *Discours*, p. 362 ('In my opinion [...] one should treat the poor sick persons graciously and humanely, and not bar, close, lock, and bolt their doors and windows, burying them before they are dead. This is why many of them conceal and hide their disease, presenting a great danger to their servants, relatives, neighbours, and friends. And being afraid of this harshness, they put up with their disease and do

These are the last pages of Nancel's treatise, which echoes Ambroise Paré's engagement on behalf of the patient. The experience of the disease — and in Paré's case also as a patient — pushes these practitionners to ask for compassion, respect, and care for the patient, including the dying. What Nancel's pages show is the destiny of a poor patient, who cannot be treated in his own house. In fact, the illustration of the medical visit in the treatises of Pietro da Tossignano and Auger Ferrier concerns a patient who can stay in his own room, able to have a doctor come to him. But what about the others? Nicolas de Nancel et Ambroise Paré describe their condition, especially Nancel in his portrait of the situation in Tours. The plague-afflicted patient is not afraid of death. He is afraid of the conditions of the *Sanitat*. So he prefers to die at home and does not reveal his disease. A physician cannot accept this situation for two reasons: it is a way of propagating of disease; it is an unethical violation of the relationship between the doctor and the patient, contrary to the deontology of the Hippocratic medical oath.[105] Nancel asks the officials to work to safeguard the human dignity of the plague-stricken poor. For his part, the physician must ensure correct diagnosis and have experience of the disease. In this way, he can identify and treat the real sick patient, without committing a fatal error by sending someone to the *Sanitat* who does not have plague:

> Ainsi seroit bon, qu'il y eust quelque Medecin gagé et deputé, qui aiant veu et manié une fois les malades, donnast certain iugement, si c'est peste ou non peste. Car nous avons veu, que par ignorance du mal, et seule souspeçon, plusieurs ont esté portés au Sanitat des pestiferés, qui n'avoient point de peste.[106]

Conclusion

As this short view of the impact of contagion and pandemics in societies and medicine shows, since Antiquity physicians confronted themselves with epidemics they called plague. Independently from the nature of ancient epidemics, the development of a

---

not have it taken care of. So they die, while fearing to die. And sometimes, they have themselves buried in their cellars or gardens, if they have them.
Poor people should be carried to the Hôtel-Dieu or to the Sanitat [...] to be fed and assisted at to the expense of the town-dwellers and wealthier citizens. And with them should be brought their beds, clothes, sheets, blankets, canopies, and bed curtains, which have already been infected by the contagion. These are to remain in the said Sanitat or Hospital to be used by them and other patients, for fear that, if they are left in their house or are taken back to it, they will propagate the disease to the others who live there, as we have already seen happen. A register and list of them will be made so they may be returned, or given to their successors and heirs, well after the disease is over and done').

105 See Thomas Rütten, 'Receptions of the Hippocratic "Oath" in the Renaissance: The Prohibition of Abortion as a Case Study in Reception', *Journal of the History of Medicine and Allied Sciences*, 51 (1996), pp. 456–83.

106 Nancel, *Discours*, p. 364 ('It would be a good thing if there were some physicians employed and empowered, who, having previously seen and handled the sick, would judge with certainty if a disease is plague or not. For we have seen that, because of lack of knowledge of the disease and simple suspicion, many persons have been brought to the Sanitat for the plague-afflicted who had no plague whatever').

theoretical thought in Hippocratic and Galenic medicine about what contagion is and how people react to it, as well as the accumulation of experiences in the fight against transmissible diseases were conveyed to medieval and modern medicine as sources to face the pandemics of the Black Death (1347–1351), which dwelled in Europe until the eighteenth century. During the four centuries the plague, *Yersinia pestis,* lasted in Europe, physicians had the possibility to elaborate theories about its causes, the way of its communication from one person to another, and the reasons way some people could survive to it. During the sixteenth century, a lexicon about contagion was elaborated, which mirrored the epistemological thought about the way natural phenomena communicate, exchange, attire and repel each other. The philosophical substratum to the medical theory, mixed with the clinical experience of the disease, let physicians like Fracastoro question the Galenic notion of the responsibility of the patient in contracting the plague. The survivors were no more the good patients physicians could hope to treat, but they were people whose body was predisposed by its own nature to repel or fight the seeds of the plague.

This deontological switch in medicine echoed the direct experience of the plague by doctors and surgeons, who were involved in the daily treatment of patients. The narrative by a surgeon like Ambroise Paré, who was both a person affected by the disease and a caregiver, allows us to hear the voice of the patients, whose suffering body is decomposed by the disease. Paré listened to his patients ("les malades disent", patients say) in order to understand how the plague acted in their body, in every body. Thus, physicians and surgeons were precious collaborators for the magistrates and officials, who had to create public health boards in order to contain the spread of the epidemics. Being protected from the plague by special clothes and gestures, they could be useful in the fight against the disease. Nevertheless, the preventive measures and the creation of *lazarettos* should not be a discharge for caregivers in their ethical engagement to respect the patient until his or her last breath of life. The local experience of a doctor like Nicolas de Nancel and the surgeon Simeon of Tours becomes an epistemic tool for other physicians and surgeons, who need to develop means to ensure the best treatment for patients suffering from plague. So, one of the major questions for a physician or a caregiver, who wants to preserve the dignity of patients affected by a tremendous disease like plague, becomes how to accompany them and take care of their future life or their unavoidable death.

Bibliography

Aristotle, *On the Soul*, in Aristotle, *On the Soul, Parva naturalia, On Breath* with an English trans. by Walter Stanley Hett (Cambridge, Mass.-London: Harvard University Press-William Heinemann, 1935).

Calepinus (Impressum Rhegii Lingobardiae industria presbyteri Dionysii Berthochi impressoris, 1502).

Calepinus *hoc est Lexicon Latinum* (Patavii: Typis seminarii, 1741).

Compendium de epidimia per Collegium Facultatis medicorum Parisius ordinatum, ed. by H. Emile Rébouis, in Id., *Étude historique et critique sur la peste* (Paris: Alphone Picard–Croville-Morant et Foucart, 1888), pp. 70–145.

d'Holbach, Paul-Henri Thiry, *La contagion sacrée ou Histoire naturelle de la superstition*, ed. by Jean Pierre Jackson (Paris: Coda, 2006).

Dictionarium Latinogallicum (Lutetiae: apud Iacobum Dupuys, excudebat Franciscus Stephanus, 1570).

Ferrier, Auger, *Remedes preservatifs et curatifs de peste* (Lyon: par Iean de Tournes, 1548).

Ficino, Marsilio, *Consilio contro la pestilenza*, ed. Enrico Musacchio et con un saggio introduttivo di Giampaolo Moraglia (Bologna: Cappelli editore, 1983).

Fracastoro, Girolamo, *De sympathia et antipathia rerum liber unus. De contagione, contagiosis morbis et curatione libri tres* (Venetiis: apud heredes Lucaeantonii Iuntae Florentini, 1546).

———, *De contagione et contagiosis morbis et eorum curatione*, Translation and notes by Wilmer Cave Wright (New York–London: G. P. Putnam's Sons, 1930).

———, *De sympathia et antipathia rerum Liber I*, Edizione critica, traduzione e commento a cura di Concetta Pennuto (Roma: Edizioni di Storia e Letteratura, 2008).

Galenus, *De differentiis febrium*, in Galenus, *Opera omnia*, ed. by D. Carolus Gottlob Kühn, vol. 7 (Lipsiae: Prostat in officina libraria Car. Cnoblochii, 1824).

Hippocrates, *Breaths*, in Hippocrates with an English trans. by William Henry Samuel Jones, vol. 2, The Loeb Classical Library, (Cambridge, Mass.-London: Harvard University Press-William Heinemann, 1959).

———, *Nature of man*, in Hippocrates, English trans. by William Henry Samuel Jones, vol. 4, The Loeb Classical Library, (Cambridge, Mass.-London: Harvard University Press-William Heinemann, 1959).

Joubert, Laurent, *De peste liber unus* (Lugduni: apud Ioannem Frellonium, 1567).

Luis Lobera de Avila, *Vanquete de nobles cavalleros e modo de bivir … et trata del regimiento curativo e preservativo de las fiebres Pestilenciales et de la Pestilencia* (Lutetiae Parisiorum: Georgii Iosse, S. D. [Augsburg: H. Steiner, 1530]).

Manget, Jean-Jacques, *Traité de la peste* (Genève: chez Philippe Planche, 1721).

Nicolas de Nancel, *Discours tres ample de la Peste, divisé en trois livres, adressant à Messieurs de Tours* (Paris, Chez Denys du Val, 1581).

Paré, Ambroise, *Traicté de la Peste, de la petite Verolle et Rougeolle: avec une brefve description de la Lepre* (Paris: de l'Imprimerie d'André Wechel, 1568).

———, 'Of the Plague', in *The Workes of that famous Ambrose Parey*, Translated out of Latine and compared with the French by Tho. Johnson (London: Printed by Richard Cotes, and Willi Du-Gard, 1649).

———, 'Livre de la Peste', in Ambroise Paré, *Les oeuvres*, vol. 3, Edition critique par Evelyne Berriot-Salvadore, Jean Céard et Guylaine Pineau, Sous la direction d'Evelyne Berriot-Salvadore (Paris: Classiques Garnier, 2019).

Petrus Aponensis, *Conciliator controversiarum, quae inter philosophos et medicos versantur* (Venetiis: apud Iuntas, 1565).

Pietro da Tossignano, '*Consilium pro peste evitanda*', in Johannes de Ketham, *Fasciculus medicine revisus per Georgium de Monteferrato* (Venetiis: per Joannem et Gregorium fratres de Forlivio, 1491).

———, 'Consiglio per la peste', in Johannes de Ketham, *Fasciculo di medicina* Vulgarizato per Sabastiano Manilio Romano (Venexia: Zuane et Gregorio di Gregorii, 1493).

———, '*Consilium pro peste evitanda*', in Johannes de Ketham, *Fasciculus medicine* (Venetiis: per Joannem et Gregorium de Gregoriis fratres, 1500).

Valleriole, François, *Traicté de la peste* (Lyon: par Antoine Oryphius, 1566).

***

Armstrong, Elizabeth, *Robert Estienne, royal printer* (Cambridge: Cambridge University Press, 1954).

Barry, Stéphane, and Gualde, Nobert, 'La Peste noire dans l'Occident chrétien et musulman 1346/1347–1352/1353', in *Epidémies et crises de mortalité du passé*, ed. by Dominique Castex and Isabelle Cartron (Pessac: Ausonius, 2007) pp. 193–227.

Beecher, Donald, 'Windows on Contagion', in *Imagining Contagion in Early Modern Europe*, ed. by Claire L. Carlin (Houndmills: Palgrave, 2005), pp. 32–46.

Bériac, Françoise, 'A propos de la fin de la lèpre: XIIIe-XVe siècles', in *The Regulation of Evil. Social and Cultural Attitudes to Epidemics in the Late Middle Ages*, ed. by Agostino Paravicini Bagliani and Francesco Santi (Firenze: Sismel-Edizioni del Galluzzo, 1998), pp. 159–73.

Bertrand, Dominique, 'Contagious Laughter and the Burlesque: From the Literal to the Metaphorical', in *Imagining Contagion in Early Modern Europe*, ed. by Claire L. Carlin (Houndmills: Palgrave, 2005), pp. 177–194.

Biraben, Jean-Noël, *Les hommes et la peste en France et dans les pays européens et méditerranéens*, 2 vols (Paris-La Haye: Mouton, 1975–76).

Bos, Kirsten I., and , 'A draft genome of *Yersinia pestis* from victims of the Black Death', *Nature*, 478 (2011), pp. 506–10.

———, and , 'Eighteenth century *Yersinia pestis* genomes reveal the long-term persistence of an historical plague focus', *eLife* (2016), https://www.ncbi.nlm.nih.gov/pmc/articles/PMC4798955/

Brancher, Dominique, 'Du poème à la chair: La contagion érotique des traités médicaux (XVIe–XVIIe siècles), in *La contagion. Enjeux croisés des discours médicaux et littéraires (XVIe–XIXe siècle)*, ed. by Ariane Bayle (Dijon: Editions Universitaires de Dijon, 2013), pp. 25–40.

Bylebyl, Jerome, 'The manifest and the hidden in the Renaissance clinic', in *Medicine and the five senses*, ed. by William F. Bynum and Roy Porter (Cambridge: Cambridge University Press, 1993), pp. 40–60.

Carmichael, Ann G., 'Universal and Particular: The Langage of Plague, 1348–1500', in *Pestilential Complexities: Understanding Medieval Plague*, ed. by Vivian Nutton (London: The Wellcome Trust Centre for the History of Medicine, 2008), pp. 17–52.

———, 'Plague Persistence in Western Europe: A Hypothesis', in *Pandemic Disease in The Medieval World. Rethinking The Black Death*, ed. by Monica H. Green (Kalamazoo-Bradford: ArC Medieval Press, 2015), pp. 157–91.

Cergna, Maria Cristina, *Il diario della peste di Giovanni Maria Marusig (1682), Edizione del testo e delle illustrazioni originali dell'autore*, con un saggio di Rienzo Pellegrini (Mariano del Friuli: Edizioni della Laguna, 2005).

Cipolla, Carlo M., 'The origin and development of the Health Boards', in Id., *Public Health and the Medical Profession in the Renaissance* (Cambridge: Cambridge University Press, 1976), pp. 11–66.

———, *Contro un nemico invisibile. Epidemie e strutture sanitarie nell'Italia del Rinascimento* (Bologna: Il Mulino, 1985).

Colet, Anna, and , 'The Black Death and Its Consequences for the Jewish Community in Tàrrega: Lessons from History and Archeology', in *Pandemic Disease in The Medieval World. Rethinking The Black Death*, ed. by Monica H. Green (Kalamazoo-Bradford: ArC Medieval Press, 2015) pp. 63–96.

Comba, Rinaldo, 'Il rilevamento demografico : prima e dopo la peste nera', in *La peste nera: dati di una realtà ed elementi di una interpretazione* (Spoleto: Centro Italiano di Studi sull'Alto Medioevo, 1994), pp. 155–73.

Cook, Harold J., 'Policing the Health of London: the College of Physicians and the Early Stuart Monarchy', *The Society for the Social History of Medicine*, 2 (1989), pp. 1–33.

Coste, Joël, *Représentations et comportements en temps d'épidémie dans la literature imprimée de peste (1490–1725). Contribution à l'histoire Culturelle de la peste en France à l'époque moderne.* Préface du professeur Yves-Marie Bercé (Paris: Honoré Champion Editeur, 2007).

Couzinet, Marie-Dominique, and Mandosio, Jean-Marc, 'Nouveaux éclairages sur les cours de Ramus et de ses collègues au Collège de Presles d'après des notes inédites prises par Nancel', in *Ramus et l'Université* (Paris: Editions rue d'Ulm, 2004), pp. 11–48.

Day, Matthew, 'The Sacred Contagion: John Trenchard, Natural History, and the Effluvial Politics of Religion', *History of Religions*, 50 (2010), pp. 144–161.

De Ferrari, Augusto, 'Curialti, Pietro', in *Dizionario Biografico degli Italiani*, 31 (Roma: Istituto *della Enciclopedia italiana*, 1985) https://www.treccani.it/enciclopedia/pietro-curialti_(Dizionario-Biografico)/

De Smet, Ingrid, 'Of Doctors, Dreamers and Soothsayers: The Interlinking Worlds of Julius Caesar Scaliger and Auger Ferrier', *Bibliothèque d'Humanisme et Renaissance*, 70, 2, (2008), pp. 351–76.

Delumeau, Jean, *La peur en Occident* XIVe–XVIIIe *siècle* (Paris: Fayard, 1978), pp. 98–142.

Demaitre, Luke, *Leprosy in Premodern Medicine. A Malady of the Whole Body* (Baltimore: The Johns Hopkins University Press, 2007).

Demeure, Christian E., and , '*Yersinia pestis* and the plague: an updated view on evolution, virulence determinants, immune subversion, vaccination, and diagnostics', *Genes & Immunity*, 20 (2019), pp. 357–70.

Demont, Paul, 'Notes sur le récit de la pestilence athénienne chez Thucydide et sur ses rapports avec la médecine grecque de l'époque classique', in *Formes de pensée dans la Collection hippocratique*. Actes du IV Colloque International Hippocratique, Lausanne 21–26 septembre 1981, ed. by François Lasserre and Philippe Mudry (Genève: Librairie Droz, 1983), pp. 341–353.

Deutscher, Thomas B., 'Ambrogio Calepino', in *Contemporaries of Erasmus*, vol. 1, ed. by Peter G. Bietenholz and Thomas B. Deutscher (Toronto-Buffalo-London: University of Toronto Press, 1985) p. 244.

Drancourt, Michel, 'Plague in the genomic area', *Clinical Microbiology and Infection*, 18 (2012), pp. 224–30.

Duncan-Jones, R. P., 'The Antonine Plague Revisited', *Arctos*, 52 (2018), pp. 41–72.

Eckert, Edward A., *The Structure of Plagues and Pestilences in Early Modern Europe. Central Europe, 1560–1640* (Basel: Karger, 1996).

Fortuna, Stefania, De differentiis febrium *tradotto da Burgundio da Pisa*, in 'Galeno Latino. Catalogo della tradizione latina di Galeno: manoscritti ed edizioni', https://www.galenolatino.com/traduzioni.php?id = 1

Glatter, Kathryn A., and Finkelman, Paul, 'History of the Plague: An Ancient Pandemic for the Age of Covid-19', *The American Journal of Medicine*, 134 (2021), pp. 176–81.

Gourdou, Jean-François, *Le professeur Augier Ferrier et la reine Catherine de Médicis* (Paris: Saint Honoré éditions, 2016).

Gourevitch, Danielle, 'Peut-on employer le mot d'*Infection* dans les traductions françaises de textes latin?', in *Mémoires V, Textes Médicaux Latins Antiques*, ed. by Guy Sabbah (Saint-Etienne: Publications de l'Université de Saint-Etienne, 1984), pp. 49–52.

Grmek, Mirko D., 'Les vicissitudes des notions d'infection, de contagion et de germe dans la médecine antique', in *Mémoires V, Textes Médicaux Latins Antiques*, ed. by Guy Sabbah (Saint-Etienne: Publications de l'Université de Saint-Etienne, 1984), pp. 53–70.

Guellil, Meriam, and , 'A genomic and historical synthesis of plague in 18th century Eurasia', *Proceedings of the National Academy of Sciences of the United States of America*, 117 (2020), pp. 28328–35.

Holladay, A. J., and Poole, J. C., 'Thucydides and the Plague of Athens', *The Classical Quarterly*, 29 (1979), pp. 282–300.

Jarcho, Saul, *The Concept of Contagion in Medicine, Literature, and Religion* (Malabar: Krieger Publishing Company, 2000).

Jouanna, Jacques, 'Air, miasme et contagion à l'époque d'Hippocrate et survivance des miasmes dans la médecine posthippocratique', in *Air, miasmes et contagion. Les épidémies dans l'Antiquité et au Moyen Age*, ed. by Sylvie Bazin-Tacchella and others (Langres: Dominique Guéniot, 2001), pp. 9–11.

Kallet, Lisa, 'Thucydides, Apollo, the Plague, and the War', *The American Journal of Philology*, 134 (2013), pp. 355–82.

Katinis, Teodoro, 'A Humanist Confronts the Plague: Ficino's *Consilio contro la Pestilentia*', *Modern Language Notes*, 125 (2010), pp. 72–83.

———, 'Per la fortuna di Ficino nel Cinquecento: il caso dei *Dialoghi sopra le cause della peste universale* di Alessandro Puccinelli', *Bruniana et Campanelliana*, 26 (2020), pp. 453–66.

Lieber, Elinor, 'Old Testament "Leprosy", Contagion and Sin', in *Contagion. Perspectives from Pre-Modern Societies*, ed. by Lawrence I. Conrad and Dominik Wujastyk (Aldeshot: Ashgate, 2000), pp. 97–136.

Little, Lester K., 'Life and Afterlife of the First Plague Pandemic', in *Plague and the End of Antiquity. The Pandemic of 541–750*, ed. by Lester K. Little (Cambridge: Cambridge University Press, 2007), pp. 3–32.

Longrigg, James, 'Epidemic, ideas and classical Athenian society', in *Epidemics and ideas. Essays on the historical perception of pestilence*, ed. by Terence Ranger and Paul Slack (Cambridge: Cambridge University Press, 1992), pp. 21–44.

MacDonald, Katharine, *Biography in Early Modern France, 1540–1630. Forms and Functions* (Leeds: Legenda, 2007).

McGough, Laura J., 'Quarantining Beauty: The French Disease in Early Modern Venice', in *Sins of the Flesh. Responding to Sexual Disease in Early Modern Europe*, ed. by Kevin Siena (Toronto: Centre for Reformation and Renaissance Studies, 2005), pp. 211–237.

Mc Gough, Laura J., *Gender, Sexuality, and Syphilis in Early Modern Venice* (New York: Palgrave Macmillan, 2011).

Monneret, Philippe, 'Epilogue linguistique. La contagion comme métaphore', in *La contagion. Enjeux croisés des discours médicaux et littéraires (XVIe–XIXe siècle)*, ed. by Ariane Bayle (Dijon: Editions Universitaires de Dijon, 2013), pp. 161–75.

Montagne, Véronique, 'Le discours didascalique sur la peste dans les traités médicaux de la Renaissance: rationaliser et/ou inquiéter', *Réforme, Humanisme, Renaissance*, 70 (2010), pp. 103–12.

———, *Médecine et rhétorique à la Renaissance. Le cas du traité de peste en langue vernaculaire* (Paris, Classiques Garnier, 2017).

Naphy, William, and Spicer, Andrew, *Plague. Black Death and Pestilence in Europe* (Wiltshire: Tempus, 2004).

Nutton, Vivian, 'The Seeds of Disease: An Explanation of Contagion and Infection from the Greeks to the Renaissance', *Medical History*, 27 (1983), pp. 1–34.

———, 'The Reception of Fracastoro's Theory of Contagion: The Seed That Fell among Thorns?', *Osiris*, 6 (1990), pp. 196–234.

———, 'Did the Greeks Have a Word for It? Contagion and Contagion Theory in Classical Antiquity', in *Contagion. Perspectives from Pre-Modern Societies*, ed. by Lawrence I. Conrad and Dominik Wujastyk (Aldeshot: Ashgate, 2000), pp. 137–62.

———, 'With Benefit of Hindsight: Girolamo Mercuriale and Simone Simoni on Plague', *Medicina e Storia*, 11 (2006), pp. 5–19.

Palmer, Richard, 'Girolamo Mercuriale and the Plague of Venice', in *Girolamo Mercuriale. Medicina e cultura nell'Europa del Cinquecento*, ed. by Alessandro Arcangeli and Vivian Nutton (Firenze: Leo S. Olschki, 2008), pp. 51–65.

Pastore, Alessandro, and Peruzzi, Enrico (eds.), *Girolamo Fracastoro fra medicina, filosofia e scienze della natura* (Firenze: Leo S. Olschki, 2006).

Perfetti, Amalia, 'La *Syphilis sive de morbo gallico* de Jérôme Fracastor: exemple de la diffusion de Lucrèce en Italie dans la première moitié du XVIe siècle', *Revue d'histoire des sciences*, 55 (2002), pp. 263–72.

Peruzzi, Enrico, 'Antioccultismo e filosofia naturale nel *De sympathia et antipathia rerum* di Girolamo Fracastoro', *Atti e memorie dell'Accademia Toscana di Scienze e Lettere* La colombaria, 45 (1980), pp. 41–131.

Pesenti, Tiziana, *Il* Fasciculus medicinae, *ovvero le metamorfosi del libro umanistico* (Treviso: Antilia, 2001).

Pineau, Guylaine, 'Soigner la peste sans défier la colère divine dans les traités médicaux du XVIe siècle', Seizème siècle, 8 (2012), pp. 173–90.

Price-Smith, Andrew T., *Contagion and Chaos. Disease, Ecology, and National Security in the Era of Globalization* (Cambridge, Mass.–London, England: The MIT Press, 2009), pp. 16–18.

Rébouis, H. Emile, *Étude historique et critique sur la peste* (Paris: Alphone Picard–Croville-Morant et Foucart, 1888).

Rütten, Thomas, 'Receptions of the Hippocratic "Oath" in the Renaissance: The Prohibition of Abortion as a Case Study in Reception', *Journal of the History of Medicine and Allied Sciences*, 51 (1996), pp. 456–83.

Samama, Evelyne, 'Thucydide et Procope: Le regard des historiens sur les épidémies', in *Air, miasmes et contagion. Les épidémies dans l'Antiquité et au Moyen Age*, ed. by Sylvie Bazin-Tacchella and others (Langres: Dominique Guéniot, 2001), pp. 55–74.

Sánchez, Carlos José Hernando, 'El banquete de damas y caballeros, la corte galante de Carlos V en Nápoles', *Bulletin hispanique*, 119 (2017), pp. 427–58.

Schuenemann, Verena J., and , 'Targeted enrichment of ancient pathogens yielding the pPCP1 plasmid of *Yersinia pestis* from victims of the Black Death', *Proceedings of the National Academy of Sciences of the United States*, 108 (2011), pp. 746–52.

Singer, Charles, and Singer, Dorothea, 'The Scientific Position of Girolamo Fracastoro (1478?-1553) with Especial Reference to the Source, Character and Influence of his Theory of Infection', *Annals of Medical History*, I (1917), pp. 1–34.

Stolberg, Michael, 'Bedside Teaching and the Acquisition of Practical Skills in Mid-Sixteenth-Century Padua', *Journal of the History of Medicine and Allied Sciences*, 69 (2014), pp. 633–64.

Teyssou, Roger, *La thérapeutique de Fracastor. Lexique des médicaments* (Paris: L'Harmattan, 2017).

Touati, François-Olivier, 'Contagion and Leprosy: Myth, Ideas and Evolution in Medieval Minds and Societies', in *Contagion. Perspectives from Pre-Modern Societies*, ed. by Lawrence I. Conrad and Dominik Wujastyk (Aldeshot: Ashgate, 2000), pp. 179–201.

Wajeman, Lise, 'La contagion pétrifiante ou des dangers de l'agalmatophilie', in *La contagion. Enjeux croisés des discours médicaux et littéraires (XVIe–XIXe siècle)*, ed. by Ariane Bayle (Dijon: Editions Universitaires de Dijon, 2013), pp. 41–55.

MARIANGELA PRIAROLO

6. New Sciences and Old Diseases

Seventeenth-Century Readings of the Causes of the Plague

▼ **ABSTRACT** As Carlo Cipolla remarked in one of his memorable inquiries into Italian plague epidemics, the endurance over time of the miasmatic paradigm of explanation for the plague should be considered a sort of historical mystery. Indeed, from a reading of the entry that Louis de Jancourt devoted to the plague in the eighteenth-century *Encyclopédie*, we get the impression that the 'Scientific Revolution' hardly affected the standard analysis of the 'Black Death'. In this regard, the early modern criticisms of Galenism, especially those coming from mechanist philosophers, would appear to have concerned more the notion of natural faculties — which was perceived as an outgrowth of the already discredited philosophy of Scholastic-Aristotelianism, and, in general, of Galen's philosophical principles — than the concrete descriptions which he had provided of specific diseases, like the plague. The thesis of this chapter — which aims to propose a (partial) solution to Cipolla's 'mystery' — is that one of the reasons for the persistence of the Galenic model of explanation of the plague until the nineteenth century is that, instead of being challenged by mechanism, the new dominant scientific paradigm in the seventeenth century, this model was reinforced by it. As we will see, this seems due to the fact that the seventeenth-century corpuscular version of mechanism, through a re-interpretation of Fracastoro's notion of seeds of contagion, made it possible to interpret the Galenic (putrid) exhalations, or 'effluvia', as (very tiny) parts of matter in motion that could be described, analysed and quantified, and hence rightfully be included within the new view of the world.

Epidemics and Pandemics, ed. by Michele Nicoletti and Alessandro Palazzo (Turnhout: Brepols, 2024), pp. 167–188
BREPOLS PUBLISHERS 10.1484/M.STPH-EB.5.136410

> [A]s he listened to the cries of joy rising from the town, Rieux remembered that such joy is always imperiled. He knew what those jubilant crowds did not know but could have learned from books: that the plague bacillus never dies or disappears for good; that it can lie dormant for years and years in furniture and linen-chests; that it bides its time in bedrooms, cellars, trunks, and bookshelves; and that perhaps the day would come when, for the bane and the enlightening of men, it would rouse up its rats again and send them forth to die in a happy city.
>
> *Albert Camus,* The Plague, *chap. 30, Engl. transl. by Stuart Gilbert (New York: Vintage Books, 1991 [ebook])*

Introduction

In the 1769, at the end of the article that, in the *Encylopédie*, he had devoted to the plague, Louis de Jancourt (1704–1780), the 'soldier of the Enlightenment',[1] wrote these sorrowful words:

> From what has been said about the plague, we must conclude that such a disease is completely unknown to us with regard to its causes and its treatment, and that only experience has taught us its tragic effects.[2]

In truth, in his entry Jancourt had presented several hypotheses on the causes of the plague. He had explained that the plague

> is an epidemic, contagious, very acute disease, which is caused by a subtle venom, diffused in the air, which penetrates into our bodies, and produces buboes, anthrax, exanthemas, and other very annoying symptoms.[3]

Jancourt's definition clearly reveals the medical background of his conception of the plague: the long-lasting miasmatic interpretation stemming from the Galenic medical tradition.[4] The Galenic approach is also attested by the lexicon used by

1 Such definition comes from Thomas Ferenczi's 'The Chevalier de Jancourt, a Soldier for the Enlightenment', *Le philosophoire*, 47. 1 (2017), pp. 77–133.

2 *Encyclopédie, ou dictionnaire raisonné des sciences, des arts et des métiers, etc.*, ed. by Denis Diderot and Jean-Baptiste Le Rond D'Alembert, 17 vols (Lucques: Giuntini, 2nd edition, 1758–71), vol. 13, art. 'Peste', p. 367, 'On doit conclure de tout ce qui a été dit sur la *peste*, que cette maladie nous est totalement inconnue quant à ses causes et son traitement; que la seule expérience ne nous a que trop instruit de ses funestes effets'.

3 *Encyclopédie*, vol. 13, art. 'Peste', p. 364: '[c]'est une maladie épidemique, contagieuse, très-aiguë, causée par un venin subtil, répandue dans l'air, qui pénetre dans nos corps et y produit les bubons, des charbons, des exanthemes, et d'autres symptome très-fâcheux'.

4 As is widely known, Galen borrowed this doctrine from Hippocrates. See Jacques Jouanna, 'Air, miasme et contagion à l'époque d'Hippocrate et survivance de miasmes dans la médecine posthippocratique (Rufus d'Éphèse, Galien et Palladios)', in *Air, miasmes et contagion, Les épidémies dans l'Antiquité et au Moyen Âge*, ed. by *Sylvie Bazin-Tacchella and others* (Langres: Dominique Guéniot, 2001), pp. 9–28. Engl. trans. in

Jancourt in presenting the different causes of the plague, a lexicon abounding in terms like 'humours', 'putridity', and 'humidity', all related to the Galenian doctrine of humours.[5] According to Jancourt, for example, the internal causes, which are connected to the individual condition of the subject considered, include 'le vice des parties' ('the vices of the parts'), and 'la corruption du sang et des autres humeurs' ('the corruption of the blood and other humours'), but also passions like sadness or fear, a bad diet, and excesses.[6] The external causes, on the other hand, concern meteorological conditions such as 'les vents du midi' ('southern winds'), 'un hiver trop doux' ('an overly mild winter'), 'les froid violens et les chaleurs excessives' ('violent cold or excessive heat'), and 'l'air fort sec ou fort humide' ('very dry or very humid air').[7] These causes are, then, summarized by invoking the 'cause véritable' ('true cause') of the plague, namely 'la reception d'exhalaisons putrides dans l'air qui viennent des pays chauds' ('putrid exhalations in the air that come from hot countries'), usually identified with the Middle East or Asia, and which is 'aidée et fomentée par la disposition de nos corps ('aided and fueled by the disposition of our body').[8] If we consider that an almost identical description of the causes of the plague can be found in the treatise *De peste* published two centuries before, more precisely in 1554, by the Galenist physician Georgius Agricola[9] — whose reputation is actually due more to his mineralogical research than to his work as a doctor[10] —,

Jacques Jouanna, *Greek Medicine from Hippocrates to Galen. Selected Papers* (Leiden-Boston: Brill, 2012), pp. 121–36.

5 The doctrine of humours was, again, a legacy of Hippocrates, but Galen had expanded and defended it against its critics. See on this, Keith Andrew Stewart, *Galen's Theory of Black Bile. Hippocratic Tradition, Manipulation, Innovation* (Leiden-Boston: Brill, 2018), esp. pp. 55–58.

6 *Encyclopédie*, vol. 13, art. 'Peste', p. 365.

7 *Encyclopédie*, vol. 13, art. 'Peste', p. 365.

8 *Encyclopédie*, vol. 13, art. 'Peste', p. 365.

9 See for instance: Georgii Agricolae *De Peste. Libri tres* (s.l. [but Basel]: Hyeronimus Froben, 1554), pp. 8, 11: 'Nemo autem dubitare potest, quin pestis ex aere pestilente vel ex eiusdem diuturna intemperantia orta morbus sit communis [...] pestis saepius oritur ex aere gravi et pestilente, minus saepe ex diuturna aeris intemperie, rarius ex malis cibis et potionibus, quae gignunt corporis succos ad putrescendum aptos' ('Nobody can doubt that the plague is a common disease which arises from pestilential air or enduring bad weather [...] The plague more often arises from heavy and pestilential air, less often from enduring bad weather, seldom from bad food and drugs, which produce bodily juices that are able to cause putrefaction').

10 Georgius Agricola (1494–1555), the Latin name of Georg Pawer or Bauer, was widely known in the sixteenth and seventeenth centuries for his treatise *De re metallica*, published posthumously (1556). However, between 1524 and 1526, he studied medicine in Italy, namely in Padua and Bologna. Eventually, he moved to Venice, where he became acquainted with the editor of the works of Hippocrates and Galen, Andrea Torresano (also known as Asolano from his birthplace Asola in Lombardy). Despite his interests in the domain of mineralogy and his commitment with the emergent mining industry, to which he provided an essential contribution, Agricola mostly earned his living as a physician. A portrait of Agricola can be found in Hans Prescher, 'Georgius Agricola. Ein sächsischer Humanist ond Naturforscher von europäischer Bedeutung', in *Georgius Agricola. 500 Jahre. Wisseschaftliche Konferenz vom 25.-27.März 1994 in Chemnitz, Freistaat Sachsen*, ed. by Friedrich Naumann (Basel–Boston–Berlin: Birkhäuser Verlag, 1994), pp. 11–34.

we get the impression that the seventeenth-century 'Scientific Revolution'[11] hardly affected the standard analysis of the 'Black Death'. In this regard, the early modern criticisms of Galenism, especially those coming from mechanism, would appear to have concerned more the notion of natural faculties — which was perceived as an outgrowth of the already discredited philosophy of Scholastic-Aristotelianism, and, in general, of Galen's philosophical principles — than the concrete descriptions which he had provided of specific diseases, like the plague.[12] The thesis of this chapter is that one of the reasons for the persistence of the Galenic model of explanation of the plague until the nineteenth century is that, instead of being challenged by mechanist philosophers, the new dominant scientific paradigm in the seventeenth century, this model was reinforced by it. As we will see, this is due to the fact that the corpuscular version of mechanism, which had become particularly widespread across the Channel after the famous London plague of 1665, made it possible to interpret the Galenic (putrid) exhalations, or 'effluvia', as (very tiny) parts of matter in motion that could be described, analysed and quantified, and hence rightfully be included within the new view of the world.

In the following pages, therefore, I will first present the common way in which the causes of the plague are described in some early modern English texts and then examine some passages that one of the most important seventeenth-century exponents of the new science, Robert Boyle, devoted to the notion of effluvia. Through this inquiry I would like to suggest that although it is certainly difficult to maintain the traditional interpretation of the 'Scientific Revolution' as an event that completely overturned the vision of the world, since changing the framework of one's knowledge does not (necessarily) mean abandoning old beliefs overnight, nevertheless when a new explanatory model — like mechanism[13] — appears, it radically transforms the way in which long-standing convictions are interpreted. As a consequence, only those ideas that are able to adapt to such a new model can survive. In this sense, as Thomas

11 It is well known that the existence of a unitary phenomenon called 'Scientific Revolution' has been a source of endless discussion among scholars. See Daniel Garber's considerations in Daniel Garber, 'Why the Scientific Revolution Wasn't a Scientific Revolution, and Why It Matters', in *Kuhn's Structure of Scientific Revolutions at Fifty. Reflections on a Science Classic*, ed. by Robert J. Richards and Lorraine Daston (Chicago-London: University of Chicago Press, 2016), pp. 133–48.

12 A useful overall presentation of Galenism in early modern philosophy is Matteo Favaretti Camposampiero, 'Galenism in Early Modern Philosophy and Medicine', in *Encyclopedia of Early Modern Philosophy and Science*, ed. by Dana Jalobeau and Charles T. Wolfe, (Cham: Springer, 2018). On the reception of Galenism between the seventeenth and the nineteenth century, see Maria Pia Donato, 'Galen in an Age of Change (1650–1820)', in *Brill's Companion to the Reception of Galen*, ed. by Petros Bouras-Vallianatos and Barbara Zipser, (Leiden-Boston: Brill 2019), pp. 487–507.

13 However, it must be said that Boyle's status as a mechanical philosopher is not unanimously shared by scholars. Antonio Clericuzio, for instance, has stated that Boyle's corpuscular philosophy cannot be conceived of a purely mechanical theory of matter (see Antonio Clericuzio, 'A Redefinition of Boyle's Chemistry and Corpuscular Philosophy', *Annals of Science*, 6. 47 (1990), pp. 561–89, and, more recently, *Elements, Principles and Corpuscles. A Study of Atomism and Chemistry in the Seventeenth Century* (Dordrecht: Springer, 2000), esp. pp. 103–48. Clericuzio's position has been disputed by William R. Newman, *Atoms and Alchemy: Chymistry and the Experimental Origins of the Scientific Revolution* (Chicago-London: University of Chicago Press, 2006).

Kuhn claimed, the notion of progress should not be expelled from the history of science along the traditional historicism that entails it, but rather re-interpreted in an evolutionary sense.[14]

1. A Contagious Disease

The early modern interest in the plague is hardly surprising, considering how many waves of such a disease affected European countries up to the end of the eighteenth century.[15] Carlo Cipolla has devoted several studies to the diffusion of the plague in Italy, which, between 1348 and 1700, had 'una struttura d'avanguardia in Europa nel settore della prevenzione sanitaria e dell'igiene pubblica' ('a pioneering structure in Europe in the field of health prevention and public hygiene'), subsequently adopted by other countries.[16] In Cipolla's view, despite the dominant medical interpretation of the plague as caused by certain noxious elements of the air, the public authorities used to manage epidemics of this kind as though they were contagious diseases. In this regard, quarantines, lockdowns, and lazarettos could be seen as a means for fighting the plague not because of the medical conceptions of the time but *notwithstanding* them for, according to Cipolla's account, the humoral-miasmatic theory of the plague should be considered as opposed to the contagious one. However, after having disputed the thesis that the Italian physician Girolamo Fracastoro (*c.* 1478–1553) — the author of a treatise on contagion to which we will return[17] — was neglected until

14 I am referring, in particular, to the famous, and much discussed, remark by which Kuhn closed his *The Structure of the Scientific Revolution* (1962): 'The analogy that relates the evolution of organisms to the evolution of scientific ideas can easily be pushed too far. But with respect to the issues of this closing section it is very nearly perfect. The process described in Section XII as the resolution of revolutions is the selection by conflict within the scientific community of the fittest way to practice future science. The net result of a sequence of such revolutionary selections, separated by periods of normal research, is the wonderfully adapted set of instruments we call modern scientific knowledge. Successive stages in that developmental process are marked by an increase in articulation and specialization. And the entire process may have occurred, as we now suppose biological evolution did, without benefit of a set goal, a permanent fixed scientific truth, of which each stage in the development of scientific knowledge is a better exemplar' (Thomas Kuhn, *The Structure of the Scientific Revolution* [Chicago: University of Chicago Press, 1970], p. 172). As I have mentioned, the relation between Kuhn's thesis and the notion of evolution is much discussed. See, for instance, Barbara Gabriella Renzi, 'Kuhn's Evolutionary Epistemology and Its Being Undermined by Inadequate Biological Concepts', *Philosophy of Science*, 76. 2, (2009), pp. 143–59.

15 See the classic work Jean-Noël Biraben, *Les hommes et la peste en France et dans les pays Europeéens et Méditerranées* (Paris-La Haye: Mouton, 1975). Biraben's conclusions on the difference between the consequences of the plague in northern and southern Europe has been disputed by Guido Alfani, who has proposed a different reading of the data presented by Biraben. See Guido Alfani, 'Plague in Seventeenth-Century Europe and the Decline of Italy: an Epidemiological Hypothesis', *European Review of Economic History*, 17 (2013), pp. 408–30.

16 Carlo M. Cipolla, *Miasmi ed umori. Ecologia e condizioni sanitarie in Toscana nel Seicento* (Bologna: Il Mulino, 1989) p. 11. See also *Public Health and the Medical Profession in the Renaissance* (Cambridge: Cambridge University Press, 1973). I would like to thank Daniela Brogi for her precious help in checking Cipolla's references.

17 See Girolamo Fracastoro, *De contagione et contagiosis morbis et curatione, libri tres* (Venetiis: Lucaeantonii Iuntae, 1546). According to an enduring reading, Fracastoro's *De contagione* foreshadowed the modern

the nineteenth century because his doctrine of contagion rejected the traditional view of the plague, the historian of medicine Vivian Nutton concludes that

> [t]he word contagion, especially if defined as involving indirect as well as direct transmission of harmful material, was far from incompatible with a theory of noxious air.[18]

In support of Nutton's claim one could adduce the definition of contagion present in Antoine Furetière's *Dictionnaire universel*, which widely circulated in Europe and was also promoted by Pierre Bayle:

> Contagion — Furetière writes — Mal qui se gagne par communication. [...] se dit par excellence et absolument de la peste ('Contagion. Disease that one obtains through communication [...] It is said par excellence and absolutely of the plague').[19]

The plague, then, appears to have been commonly — and wrongly — considered a contagious disease whose propagation, as already mentioned, mostly depended on the condition of the air.[20] This reading is apparent in the countless pamphlets written by medical officers in England during the seventeenth century. Let us turn, for instance, to the pamphlet authored by Francis Hering, a fellow of the London College of Physicians during the terrible plague of 1625–26 poetically described by John Milton.[21] After having recalled that the first and fundamental cause of the plague is 'God's wrath', for which the only 'appropriate and special antidote is *seria poenitentia, et conversio ad Deum*', Hering stressed the importance of burying the dead at 'some good distance from the city and the suburbs',

> for all men that have the least insight in philosophy know that from the dead corps, by force of the sun, certain vapours or exhalations are elevated, which

germ theory. However, this thesis has been widely reappraised. See Vivian Nutton's observations in 'The Reception of Fracastoro's Theory of Contagion: The Seed That Fell among Thorns?', *Osiris*, 6 (1990), pp. 196–234 (pp. 196–97). For more on Fracastoro, see also section 3 of chapter 5 of this volume.

18 Nutton, 'The Reception of Fracastoro's Theory of Contagion', p. 198.

19 *Dictionaire universel, contenant généralement tous les mots françois tant vieux que modernes et les termes de toutes les sciences et des arts* (La Haye-Rotterdam: Arnout et Reinier Leers, 1690), vol. 1, ad vocem.

20 It may be useful to recall the 'true' cause of the plague — which was discovered only at the end of the nineteenth century by Alexandre Yersin (1863–1943) and, at the same time, by Shibasáburo Kitasato (1852–1931), i.e. the bacillus now known as 'Yersinia pestis', usually present in parasites borne by rats. The diffusion of the plague is due to the fact that, after exhausting their preferred resources (rats), fleas would attack human beings. Strictly speaking, therefore, the plague cannot be considered a contagious disease, for the infection mostly follows from the direct contact between the parasite and its host, be it a rat or human. The idea that the plague is contracted via contagion may derive from the observation of a particular set of sick people, those affected by a pulmonary form of plague. In this case, the infection is spread by the diseased people's droplets, which therefore act as a (possible) source of infection.

21 John Milton, *On the Death of Bishop of Winchester*, in Id., *The Latin Poems*, ed. by W. Mackellar (New Haven: Yale University Press, 1930), pp. 74–75: 'Moestus eram, et tacitus, nullo comitante, sedebam/ Haerebantque animo tristia plura meo,/ Protinus en subiit funestae cladis imago/ Fecit in Anglico quam Libitina solo' (Silent and alone I sat in sorrowful mood, and many griefs laid hold upon my soul, when suddenly arose the phantom of the deadly plague which Libitina sent upon England).

> partake of the nature of those bodies, and do undoubtedly taint, corrupt and poison the air with their ill quality.[22]

To preserve the air from infection, the place of burial 'should be on the south side of the city', where 'the sun may draw the vapours from it',[23] the streets must be free from the 'carcasses of horses, dogs, cats, etc.',[24] the river must be enabled to flush out the gutters,[25] and fires must be lit to purge the air.[26] In private houses, the air must be purified with herbs like thyme, rosemary, fennel, marjoram, and cinnamon, and the interior must be cleaned with vinegar. Feasts, plays, and dances must be banned, first because they dishonour God, and therefore increase his rage, and second because, by providing an occasion for 'drunkness, and other riots and excesses', they predispose bodies to infection. People must avoid those foods which 'corrupt and putrify in the stomach' and particular attention must be given to eschew 'all perturbations of mind, especially anger and fear'. Beer is allowed, or indeed recommended, but not spirits or Rosa-solis, the Italian Rosolio, which can increase the heat in the stomach and the process of putrefaction that, as already mentioned, is considered to lie at the basis of the disease.

The humoral-miasmatic approach to the plague can be detected in another significant text, namely the (partial) English version of the famous *Traicté de la peste* by Ambrosius Paré (1510–90), published in 1568.[27] It circulated widely across Europe, especially during the recurrent plague epidemics of those years.[28] After a description of the plague, which is presented as 'a cruell and contagious Disease' depending on 'a certaine poysonous and venenate malignitie, the force whereof exceeds the condition

---

22 Francis Hering, *Certaine Rules, Directions, or Advertisments for This Time of Pestilentiall Contagion with a Caveat to Those That Weare about Their Neckes Impoisoned Amulets as a Preservative from the Plague* (London: William Iones, 1625), without page numbers, point 2 (I have modernized the spelling of the passages quoted in the main text).

23 Hering, *Certaine Rules*, point 3.

24 Hering, *Certaine Rules*, point 4.

25 Hering, *Certaine Rules*, point 5–6.

26 Hering, *Certaine Rules*, point 7.

27 *Traicté de la peste, de la petite Verolle et Rougeolle. Avec une brefue description de la Lepre par Ambroise Paré premier Chirurgien du Roy et Iuré à Paris* (Paris: André Wechel, 1568). The English version, which appeared in 1630, four years after the aforementioned 1625–25 episode, presented the chapters with the same layout as the original, but in a very abridged form, so this publication is best regarded as a summary of Paré's arguments than as a translation of his book — as the English subtitle actually already suggests. See *A Treatise of the Plague contayining Causes, Signes, Symptomes, Prognosticksm and Cure thereof. Together with sundry other remarkable passages (for the prevention of, and preservation from the Pestilence) never yet published by anie man. Collected out of the Workes of the no lesse learned than experimented and renowned Chirurgian Ambrose Parey* (London: Michael Parke, 1630).

28 The Italian translation, for instance, was published in the same year of the tragic Marseilles epidemic: *Trattato della peste di Ambrosio Pare de Laval al Mene … diviso in LII. capitoli ne' quali tra le altre cose si leggono i presaggi, le cause divine o umane, e le sementi generali della peste … Tradotto dal francese nell'italiano da Gio. Michele Du' Bois e dato in luce … con l'aggionta di alcune ricette…* (Bologna: Benacci's heirs, 1720). Notice the use of the word 'sementi' (seeds).

of common putrefaction',[29] the *Treatise of Plague* sets out — along traditional lines — by establishing God's will as the first cause:

> It is a confirmed, constant, and received opinion in all Ages amongst Christians, that the Plague and other Diseases which violently assaile the life of Man, are often sent by the iust anger of God punishing our offenses.[30]

The analysis of the scriptural passages in support of this belief — to which the original text devoted nine pages and the English version only two — gives way to an explanation of the natural causes of disease, which from the beginning invokes Galen's analysis:

> The generall and naturall causes of the Plague are absolutely two, that is, the infection of corrupt Aire, and a preparation and fitnesse of corrupt humours to take that infection; for it is noted before out the Doctrine of Galen, that our humours may be corrupted, and degenerate into such an alienation which may equall the malignitie of Poyson.[31]

The air becomes putrid because seasons have not 'their seasonableness', for winter is too warm or spring too cold, autumn 'ominous by Fires [...], with Starres shooting, and as it were falling downe, or terrible Comets, never seene without some disaster', and summer 'cloudy and moist, and without Winds'[32] — all elements that, as Paré recalls, had already been noted by Hippocrates in his book on epidemics. Here the French version and the English one slightly differ, since the latter — and only the latter — ascribes the responsibility for the modifications of humours which give rise to plague to some 'seeds':

> the Aire from hence [i.e. the unusual features of seasons] draws the Seeds of Corruption and the Pestilence, which at the lenght, the like excesse of qualities being brought in, it sends into the humours of our Bodyes, chiefly such as are thin and serous.[33]

The notion of 'seeds of contagion', which in Paré's inspired treatise is of secondary importance, is instead pivotal in one of the several inquiries written during the Great Plague of London (1665), namely the brief report by Gideon Harvey, who worked as a physician to Charles II. This text is particularly significant, for, although it newly presents the standard view, it shows that some relevant changes have occurred in the medical domain. The first thing to be noted is the disappearance of God among the causes of the plague. Indeed, in his *Discours on the plague*, a sort of 'instant book'

29 *A Treatise of the Plague*, p. 1.

30 *A Treatise of the Plague*, p. 3.

31 *A Treatise of the Plague*, p. 4.

32 *A Treatise of the Plague*, pp. 4–5.

33 *A Treatise of the Plague*, p. 5. In the French version one reads: "Telles constitutions de saisons sont escrites par Hippocrates au libre des Epidemies: et veritablement elles rendent l'air du tout pestiferé: car alors par son intemperature il dispose à pourriture les humeurs sereux de nostre corps, et par sa chaleur non naturelle les brule et enflamme", *Traicté de la peste*, p. 10.

published in 1665, Harvey starts by providing a definition of the plague, which — once again — is traditionally seen as 'a most malignant and contagious feaver, caused through pestilential *miasms*, insinuating into the humoral and consistent parts of body'.[34] According to Harvey, the miasmas activate a process of putrefaction which leads to 'a great ebullition or fermentation' of the 'vital spirits'.[35] This activation depends on the peculiar nature of pestilential miasm, which are made of 'arsenical fumes'[36] that are produced by 'stinking or putrid bodies'[37] whose evaporation gives rise to rains that fall onto the earth. Here the polluted water forms gutters, pools, and ponds that diffused the venomous fumes. When these miasmas are inhaled, they gradually corrupt the blood and poison the entire body, which will eventually die.[38] Although he adopts the traditional humoral framework, in describing the structure of the miasmas Harvey speaks of 'flaming atoms', 'pestilential atoms'[39] and 'pestilent seminaries',[40] a notion which he explicitly draws from Fracastoro. In answering the question concerning the means by which the plague spreads, Harvey states that contagion occurs in two ways:

> immediately, by conversing with infected persons; or mediately, by pestilent seminaries, propagated through the air by continuation; or by those dense bodies, that easily incarcerate infected air, as wollen cloaths, beds, furniture, in which the contagion may be preserved several years, as *Fracastorius* relates.[41]

Harvey's reference reproduces the first two of the three ways in which contagion occurs according to Fracastoro: 1) directly; 2) by means of an agent, the so-called *fomites*; 3) from a distance.[42] The second and the third manner are — and have been for scholars — particularly relevant because it is in discussing them that Fracastoro specifically uses the notion of 'seeds of contagion'.[43] In defining *fomites*, for instance, Fracastoro states that they are those objects, like 'clothes or wood or similar things', which can 'conserve [...] the seeds of contagion (*contagionis seminaria*)'[44] and then propagate the infection. The same term appears in Fracastoro's analysis of the contagion from a distance. Here Fracastoro explains that the seeds of contagion cannot be conceived of as occult properties, but are most likely corporeal qualities.[45] This

34 Gideon Harvey, *Discourse of the Plague containing the Nature, Causes, Signs, and Presages of the Pestilence in general. Together with the state of the present Contagion. Also most rational Preservatives for Families, and choiche Curative Medicines both for Rich and Poor. With several waies for purifying the air in houses, streets, etc.* (London: Angel, 1665), p. 2 (Harvey's emphasis).

35 Harvey, *Discourse of the Plague*, p. 2.

36 Harvey, *Discourse of the Plague*, p. 5.

37 Harvey, *Discourse of the Plague*, p. 5.

38 See Harvey, *Discourse of the Plague*, p. 7.

39 Harvey, *Discourse of the Plague*, pp. 6, 8.

40 See Harvey, *Discourse of the Plague*, p. 9.

41 Harvey, *Discourse of the Plague*, p. 9.

42 Fracastoro, *De Contagione*, Book 1, Chap. 2, p. 29.

43 See on this Vivian Nutton, 'The Seeds of Disease. An Explanation of Contagion and Infection from the Greeks to the Renaissance', *Medical History*, 27 (1983), pp. 1–34.

44 Fracastoro, *De Contagione*, Book 1, Chap. 2, p. 29, my emphasis.

45 Fracastoro, *De Contagione*, Book 1, Chap. 6, pp. 31–33.

thesis would appear to be inspired by Lucretius' atomism[46] and could be supported by some passages of the chapter that Fracastoro devotes to clarifying the way in which infection from a distance occurs. As we read in one passage, these seeds

> ab iis [...] igitur quae solo contactu afficiunt differre videtur, quod haec in forti mistione constituta videtur et lentore quodam, illae vero non. Ab iis vero quae fomite solo et contactu inficiunt, differunt eae quae ad distans protenduntur, quod validior adhuc mistio iis inesse videtur, et subtilitas maior, propter quod et penetrant magis, et maiorem actionem habent.[47]

The diversity in terms of viscosity, strength, and subtlety, which appear to be the material properties of these particles, is also responsible for the varying levels of virulence of diseases, an aspect that is stressed by Harvey too:

> The differences of Plagues are specified by the degree, qualification, or *modus substantia* of the Pestilent Seminaries, which according to their grosseness or subtility, activity, or hebetude, cause more or less truculent plagues.[48]

However, as Isabelle Pantin has shown, Fracastoro modified Lucretius' notion of *pestifera semina* 'by giving them all the properties of the *species spirituales*, and as well, those of the *spiritus* that lived in animated bodies'.[49] It is because of these features that, according to Fracastoro, the seeds of contagion can act at a distance, because, inasmuch as they also possess the properties of the spiritual world, they have the power to modify the nature of things, and therefore to produce new infections in (hitherto) healthy bodies. In this regard, Fracastoro's theory of contagion could be seen as a synthesis of ancient and medieval doctrines whose 'result was assuredly new, but it would be hazardous to assert that it was decidedly 'modern'',[50] for not only is the framework of his medical notions still the traditional Aristotelian world of substances composed by both spiritual and material elements but the source of

---

46 Fracastoro was well acquainted with Lucretius' work. See Charlotte Goddard, 'Lucretius and Lucretian Science in the Works of Fracastoro', *Res Publica Litterarum*, 16 (1993), pp. 185–92 and Andrea Ceccarelli, '*Neve Lucretius a me indefensus maneat*: Girolamo Mercuriale, il *De rerum natura* e la medicina nel Rinascimento', *Lexicon philosophicon. International Journal for the History of Ideas*, 5 (2017) pp. 161–88 (pp. 166–67).

47 Fracastoro, *De Contagione*, Book 1, Chap. 7, p. 33: '[the seeds] seem to differ from those which infect only by contact, for the former seem to be made of a strong and viscous mixture and the latter not. The seeds which extend from a distance also differ from those which infect through a sole fomite or by contact, because it seems that their composition is stronger and their subtlety higher, and this is the reason why they penetrate more easily and exercise a broader action'.

48 Harvey, *Discourse of the Plague*, p. 10.

49 Isabelle Pantin, 'Fracastoro's *De Contagione* and Medieval Reflection on 'Action at a Distance': Old and New Trends in Renaissance Discourse on the Plague', in *Imagining Contagion in Early Modern Europe*, ed. by Claire Carlin (New York: Palgrave, 2005), pp. 3–15 (p. 9).

50 Pantin, 'Fracastoro's *De Contagione* and Medieval Reflection on 'Action at a Distance'', p. 10. A similar reading in Concetta Pennuto, 'La natura dei contagi in Fracastoro', in *Girolamo Fracastoro. Fra medicina, filosofia e scienze della natura*, ed. by Alessandro Pastore and Enrico Peruzzi (Florence: Leo Olschki, 2006) pp. 57–71.

any activity on the part of these substances is the spiritual element.[51] In other words, Fracastoro's seeds of contagion cannot be completely reduced to corporeal elements, but owe their power to spread to properties that, although not occult, belong to a non-material domain. It is not an aim of this chapter to discuss the true meaning or the possible novelty of Fracastoro's notion of seeds of contagion, or even its divergence from the Galenic description of the causes of the plague.[52] What I would like to show is rather that seventeenth-century thinkers, who read Fracastoro through the lens of a doctrine that actually reduced all properties of bodies to matter and motion, i.e. mechanism, did not draw upon his theories in order to abandon the old approach to the plague, but, on the contrary, to support it. This is the case for instance with Robert Boyle, who devoted a lot of pages to defining effluvia, a term which is widely present in Fracastoro too.[53]

2. The Effluvia and the Plague: Robert Boyle

As Silvia Parigi has highlighted,[54] Boyle's interest in effluvia dates back to the mid-1650s, although probably the most systematic writings on this subject are those collected in the *Essays of the Subtilty, Efficacy, Determinate Nature of Effluviums* (1673). Boyle begins his inquiry by stating that the hypothesis of effluvia could work both within an atomistic framework, such as the one proposed by Gassendi, and within a Cartesian or even Aristotelian one, according to which matter is 'indefinitely, if not infinitely divisible'.[55] The reason for this is that Boyle conceives of effluvia as 'emanations [...] subtil enough to get through the pores, even of the closest bodies'.[56] Consequently, it is not necessary to regard them as the ultimate constituents of a portion of matter. These emanations can explain many natural phenomena, such as, for instance, the attractive power of loadstones — whose effluvia are responsible for the turning of compass needles — or the emetic virtue of certain substances.[57] In this

---

51 With this in view, Peter Anstey has warned, for instance, against the mistake of confusing the Scholastic notion of first and second qualities adopted by Fracastoro with Locke's distinction between first and secondary qualities. See Peter Anstey, *The Philosophy of Robert Boyle* (London-New York: Routledge, 2000), note 17, pp. 33–34. The continuity of Fracastoro's doctrine with the previous tradition could also explain why his doctrine was not perceived as revolutionary in the medical discussion of his time. See Nutton, 'The Reception of Fracastoro's Theory of Contagion', pp. 229–34.

52 Still useful in this respect the aforementioned Nutton, 'The Seeds of Disease'. A rich historical analysis of the notion of *semina rerum* is provided by Hiro Hirai, *Le concept de semence dans les théories de la matière à la Renaissance. De Marsile Ficin à Pierre Gassendi* (Turnhout: Brepols, 2005).

53 See especially Girolamo Fracastoro, *De sympatia et antipathia rerum liber unus. De contagione, contagiosis morbis et curatione libri tres* (Venetiis: apud heredes Lucaeantonii Iuntae Florentini, 1546), which precedes his treatise on contagion. On this work, see Concetta Pennuto, *Simpatia, fantasia e contagio. Il pensiero medico e il pensiero filosofico de Girolamo Fracastoro* (Roma: Edizioni di storia e letteratura, 2008).

54 See Silvia Parigi, 'Effluvia, Action at a Distance, and the Challenge of the Third Causal Model', *International Studies in the Philosophy of Science*, 29. 4 (2005), pp. 351–68.

55 I quote from *The Works of the Honourable Robert Boyle*, edited by Thomas Birch, 6 vols, vol. 3, p. 661.

56 Robert Boyle, *Essay on the Great Efficacy of Effluviums*, in, *The Works of Boyle*, vol. 3, p. 669.

57 See Boyle, *Essay on the Great Efficacy of Effluviums*, pp. 670–72.

regard, Boyle grounds — or believes to be grounding — all his statements in specific observations, which he describes in great detail. One of these, namely the observation of dogs' ability to follow a track will become a sort of *topos* in the discussion on effluvia. In Boyle's account, the reason why many dogs are able to find their prey in the woods lies in the fact that a partridge or a hare 'probably communicate to the grass, or ground, but some of those effluxions that transpire out of his feet'.[58] Such 'effluxions', which can be considered as '*fomes*' of 'steams'[59] are transported by wind or fresh air and eventually perceived by dogs, and since they fill the atmosphere, they can last a long-time. As Boyle puts it,

> you may take notice, that the effluvia, mentioned to have been smelt by animals, are, though invisible, yet big enough to be the objects of sense; so that it is not improbable, that among the steams that no sense can immediately perceive, there should be some far more subtil than these and consequently capable of furnishing an atmosphere much longer, without quite exhausting the effluviating matter that afforded them.[60]

It is precisely for this reason that according to Boyle — who supported his claim by referring to what several authors have stated (in his opinion) — the plague can break out at intervals.[61] 'The learned *Sennertus*', i.e. the famous German doctor Daniel Sennert (1572–1637), for instance, had observed

> that in the year one thousand five hundred and forty-two, there did in the city of *Uratislavia*, [*sic*], vulgarly *Breslaw*, when he afterwards practised physick, die of the plague, in less than six months, little less of six thousand men, and that from that time the pestilential contagion was kept folded up a linen cloth about fourteen years, and at the end of that time being displayed in another city, it began a plague there, which infected also the neighbouring towns, and other places.[62]

The wind, the air, and in general particular meteorological conditions reactivate the motion and the power of those effluvia, which, however, are nothing but material corpuscles. In this regard, as we read in the second essay devoted to 'the great efficacy of Effluviums', Boyle does not attribute their capacity to any spiritual property — as

58 Boyle, *Essay on the Great Efficacy of Effluviums*, p. 675.

59 See Boyle, *Essay on the Great Efficacy of Effluviums*, p. 675. As we have seen in the previous paragraph the term 'fomes' belongs to Fracastoro's lexicon. This is one of the hints that may support to the thesis that Boyle knew Fracastoro's doctrine of contagion. On the source of Boyle's acquaintance with Fracastoro see below note 62.

60 Boyle, *Essay on the Great Efficacy of Effluviums*, pp. 675–76.

61 Among others, Boyle refers to 'Forestus' (probably the Dutch physician Pieter van Foreest 1521–1597), 'Alexander Benedictus' (Alessandro Benedetti, *c.* 1420–1512, the author of two writings on the plague, *De pestilenti febre liber*, 1490, and *De observatione pestilentia*, 1493), and 'Trincavella' (most likely Vittore Trincavelli, 1496–1568, the great Humanist, who was Professor of Practical Medicine at Padua).

62 Robert Boyle, *On the Strange Subtlity of Effluviums*, in *The Works of Boyle*, vol. 3, p. 676. According to Thorndike, Sennert is one of the probable sources of Boyle's acquaintance with Fracastoro's thought (see Lynn Thorndike, *A History of Magic and Experimental Science*, vols 8, *The Seventeenth Century* (New York: Columbia University Press, 1958) p. 174.

Fracastoro instead did, if Pantin is right — but rather to merely quantitative features, namely 'the shape, size, situation, and texture both of the agent and of the patient'.[63] Basically, the effluvia of a body can operate upon another because of 'the great number of emitted corpuscles', 'the congruity and incongruity of their bulk and shape with the pores of the bodies they are to act upon' and their motion.[64] Being material corpuscles, therefore, effluvia behave accordingly to the same mechanical principles which in Boyle's view govern nature.

This idea was already present in another interesting essay, Boyle's *Cosmical Suspicions*, an appendix to his treatise *Of the Systematical or Cosmical Qualities of Things* (1671), in which he mostly presented examples of phenomena related to gravity and magnetism. Similar phenomena, according to Boyle, could be explained by certain qualities whose existence, while only suspected,[65] would also appear to be governed by the laws of nature, even if at present such laws are still unknown:

> And whereas, *Pyrophilus*, I have in the former discourse taken in the structure and established laws of the universe, as an help toward the giving an account of the cosmical attributes of things, I shall here also ingeniously confess to you, that I much fear, whether we have yet attentively enough taken notice either of the number, or the kinds of those Laws. For as I am by some notions and observations inclined to think, that there may be a greater number even of the more general Laws than have been yet distinctly enumerated.[66]

Some laws, therefore, must also govern those effluvia, or 'pestilential steams', which — as Boyle explains in a later text, *An Experimental Discourse on Some Unheeded Causes of the Insalubrity and Salubrity of the Air* (1690) — originate from some 'expirations from subterraneal bodies'.[67] Not only are these exhalations responsible for the presence of endemical diseases in different countries — such as, for instance, 'an odd kind of colick in one part of France' or 'fluxes of the belly in Ireland'[68] — but they might also lie at the root of the spread of epidemic diseases such as the plague. As Boyle claims,

63 Boyle, *Essay on the Great Efficacy of Effluviums*, p. 678.

64 Boyle, *Essay on the Great Efficacy of Effluviums*, p. 678.

65 As Boyle writes, 'it may now, therefore, be not unreasonable to confess to you that I have had some faint suspicion that [...] there may possibly be some other kind of corpuscles fitted to have considerable operations, when they find congrouous bodies to be wrought on by them [...] there may be, as I was beginning to say, peculiar sorts of corpuscles that have yet no distinct name, which may discover peculiar faculties, and ways of working, when they meet with bodies of such a texture as disposes them to admit, or to concur with the efficacy of these unknown agents' (Robert Boyle, *Cosmical Suspicions [Subjoyned as an Appendix to the Discourse of the Cosmical Qualities of Things]*, in *The Works of Robert Boyle*, vol. 3, p. 316).

66 *Cosmical Suspicions*, in *The Works of Robert Boyle*, vol. 3, p. 318.

67 Robert Boyle, *An Experimental Discourse on Some Unheeded Causes of the Insalubrity and Salubrity of the Air*, in *The Works of Robert Boyle*, vol. 5, p. 42. The importance of this text for understanding the early modern attention toward problems that now fall within the discussion on climate change is stressed by Claire Crignon. See Claire Crignon, 'Peut-on faire une histoire naturelle de l'air? Francis Bacon et Robert Boyle', *Archives de Philosophie*, 84. 1 (2021), pp. 93–113.

68 Boyle, *An Experimental Discourse*, in *The Works of Robert Boyle*, vol. 5, p. 43.

> The changes of the air, that produces epidemical diseases, are sometimes so great and sudden, that they cannot, in my opinion, with probability be imputed to the action of the sun or of the moon (which are causes that act in too general, and too uniform a way, to have those particular and anomalous effects attributed to them) as probably as they may to subterraneal bodies, that often act with more suddenness and impetuosity without any regularity, at least that is known to us.[69]

Such 'noxious effluvia' can explain why epidemics affect certain towns more than others: for instance, a town may lie on particular kinds of minerals which damage the quality of the air. However, since effluvia are exhalations of minerals, and hence 'steams', they could be either carried by winds and therefore reach places that are distant from their original source or, on the contrary, have no effect at all. The reason for this is that

> by being diffused through a greater tract of air, they are more and more dispersed in their passage, and thereby so diluted (if I may so speak) and weakened, as not to be able to do any notorious mischief.[70]

The interaction between the subterraneal effluvia and the air is also essential for the diffusion of the plague for another reason; even when these effluvia are 'in their own nature either innocent enough, or at least not considerably hurtful', the presence in the air of 'certain corpuscles' that are not dangerous in themselves can nevertheless produce a combination which gives rise to 'corpuscles of a new and very morbifick nature'.[71] The combination of these different kinds of corpuscles, i.e. effluvia and those corpuscles present in the air, is also evoked by Boyle to account for some facts that the traditional miasmatic theory of the plague had trouble justifying. This is the case, for instance, with the question 'why in some epidemical diseases some persons may escape much better than others' — a situation which, according to Boyle, derives from the fact that corpuscles can be 'unequally dispersed through the air'.[72] It is also the case with the varying duration of epidemics — depending on the greater or smaller concentration of harmful corpuscles in the air —, or even the varying number of victims,[73] which depends on the presence in human bodies of corpuscles that can react in a bad way to the harmful effluvia.[74] Boyle's corpuscular definition of effluvia, therefore, allowed him not only to provide a unitary explanation for several phenomena, but also to abandon all those spiritual elements which in Fracastoro — as we have seen — were considered necessary to solve the problems posed by the idea of contagion from a distance. In this regard, as Marina Paola Banchetti-Robino has shown, Boyle's analysis of the properties of air and of 'cosmical qualities' — which include the 'subterraneal effluvia' discussed above — can be seen as a response to the

---

69 Boyle, *An Experimental Discourse*, in *The Works of Robert Boyle*, vol. 5, p. 51.
70 Boyle, *An Experimental Discourse*, in *The Works of Robert Boyle*, vol. 5, p. 53.
71 Boyle, *An Experimental Discourse*, in *The Works of Robert Boyle*, vol. 5, p. 53.
72 Boyle, *An Experimental Discourse*, in *The Works of Robert Boyle*, vol. 5, p. 53.
73 Boyle, *An Experimental Discourse*, in *The Works of Robert Boyle*, vol. 5, p. 54.
74 Boyle, *An Experimental Discourse*, in *The Works of Robert Boyle*, vol. 5, p. 55.

use of 'non-material principles prevalent in the natural philosophies of Paracelsians and spagyrists'.[75] However, this new focus on the ultimate nature of the elements responsible for contagion does not entail a rejection of the explanation of the causes of the plague, but, on the contrary, an effort to provide a more solid foundation for what we have defined as the 'standard view of the plague'.

Conclusion

In one of his memorable inquiries into Italian plague epidemics, Carlo Cipolla remarks that the endurance over time of the miasmatic paradigm of explanation for the plague should be considered a sort of historical mystery.[76] In the previous sections I have tried to show one of the possible reasons for such persistence, namely the adaptability of the miasmatic theory of the plague to the new mechanical philosophy. However, one could reasonably object that not all forms of seventeenth-century mechanisms can be reduced to Boyle's corpuscularism, which I have taken as the main example of a new approach to old doctrines. Nevertheless, it should be noted that almost in the same years we find a use of effluvia very similar to Boyle's even in the country that preferred a Cartesian version of mechanism to his, namely France. I am referring in particular to the debate that focused several thinkers' attention on a mysterious murder which had taken place in Lyons in 1692 and had, apparently, been solved by a local farmer, Jacques Aymar, by means of a divining rod.[77] In the late summer of 1692, the French intellectual scene was divided between those who ascribed Aymar's ability to supernatural causes — God or, most likely, the devil — and those — the majority — who thought there were natural reasons for it.[78] Among

75 Marina Paola Banchetti-Robino refers in particular to Boyle's statement in *Relations betwixt Flame and Air* (1672) that cosmical qualities must be interpreted in a mechanical sense. See M. Paola Banchetti-Robino, *The Chemical Philosophy of Robert Boyle: Mechanicism, Chymical Atoms, and Emergence* (Oxford: Oxford University Press, 2020) p. 142. According to Banchetti-Robino Boyle's target here is Henry More, who had developed a vitalistic interpretation of Boyle's experiments with the air-pump.

76 See Cipolla, *Miasmi ed umori*, pp. 14–15.

77 On this subject there is a wide literature. See especially Stanis Pérez, 'La République des Lettres menée à la baguette? L'affaire Jacques Aymar', *xviie siècle*, 226 (2005), pp. 145–64.

78 Proof of this is, for instance, the verdict we find in *Mercure Galant*, August 1692, pp. 126–27, one of the most widely read journals of that time: 'on ne croit pas que le mouvement excité sur le passage du Criminel et sur le lieu du Crime, soit plus surnaturel et plus difficile à expliquer, que celuy qu'on apperçoit en suivant les rameaux d'une source, qui quelquefois a plus de sept ou huit toises de profondeur, ou sur les veines d'une mine, ou sur de l'argent monnoyé et caché, lequel estant separé de la mine, semble devoir bien moins exciter l'agitation au dehors, que le metal qui est encore dans la terre, et dont les emissions sont incessamment attirées par la chaleur du Soleil' ('We do not believe that the movement excited on the passage of the criminal and on the place of the crime is more supernatural and more difficult to explain than that which we see by following the branches of a spring, which is sometimes more than seven or eight toises deep, or on the veins of a mine, or on silver coined and hidden, which, being separated from the mine, seems to excite much less agitation outside than the metal which is still in the earth, and whose emissions are incessantly attracted by the heat of the Sun'). On the French debate see Mariangela Priarolo, 'Demoni o corpuscoli? La bacchetta divinatoria e la nuova scienza alla fine del XVII secolo', *Intersezioni*, 3 (2020), pp. 333–58.

the latter, an important role was played by a Lyons physician, Pierre Chauvin, the first author to suggest a mechanical explanation for the powers of the divining rod. In his *Letter to the Marquise de Senozan,*[79] which opened with a 'declaration of faith' in Descartes' method,[80] Chauvin stated that Aymar's reactions to the discovery of the traces of the murder, namely palpitations, sweat, nausea, and an increased heartbeat, depended on some 'little particular corpuscles, distinct and different from the subtle matter, and more subtle than air, and whose configuration let this subtle matter pass through their pores'.[81] These corpuscles had been released by the murderers through the transpiration caused by the agitation of their blood, a consequence of the strong passions that they experienced because of their crime.[82] According to Chauvin, then, the motion of the divining rod resulted from the interaction between the corpuscles emitted by the criminals (the agents) and their reception by Aymar (the patient). In Chauvin's opinion, the objection that considerable time passed before Aymar's discovery, and that the corpuscles thus ought have 'evaporated', so to speak, was not a good argument because the same experience is common during hunting. Recovering an argument that we have already found in Boyle, Chauvin observed that hunting dogs can follow the traces of a deer even 'une heure aprés qu'il a traversé une riviere'

---

79 *Lettre de M. Chauvin, à Madame la Marquise de Senozan, sur les moyens dont on s'est servy pour découvrir les Complices d'un assassinat commis à Lyon, le 5eme de Juillet 1692* (Lyon: chez Jean Baptiste et Nicolas De Ville, 1692).

80 See Chauvin, *Lettre à la Marquise*, pp. 24–25.

81 Chauvin, *Lettre à la Marquise*, p. 29: 'little particular corpuscles […], distinct and different from the pure air and the subtle matter, which I can imagine more subtle than the first, and which can dispose the pores in a manner that make freely pass the latter'.

82 Chauvin explicitly refers here to Santorio Santorio's (1561–1636) experiments on transpiration. See Simone Mannola, *La ragione e l'incertezza. Filosofia e medicina nella prima età moderna* (Milano: Franco Angeli, 2012), pp. 266–71. A follower and friend of Chauvin's, Pierre Garnier, a Lyons physician who supported his view with similar arguments, was to add that the behaviour of a murderer's corpuscles is analogous to that of magnets: 'il faut penser que cet amas de corpuscules sortis du corps du meurtrier dont il a êté tant parlé, et que j'appellerai ici, par allegorie à la matière magnetique, la matière meurtriere, fait des la premiere fois qu'elle touche le corps de Jaques [*sic*] Aymar dans le tissu de sa peau, et peut-étre aussi dans les parties de son sang, de certaines moulures, et de certaines traces, à raison desquelles elle se conserve toûjours un passage et une entrée libre dans le corps, et dans le sang de cet homme disposé à les recevoir plutôt qu'un autre homme; de même que la matiere magnetique sortant de l'ayman fait ces traces ou ces moulures en écroües dans le pores du fer, et non pas dans les pores des autres corps qu'elle peut toucher, à cause qu'elle trouve les pores du fer disposés à laisser passer les petites écroües, et que les pores des autres corps ne sont pas disposés de la méme façon' ('It must be thought that this mass of corpuscles which came out of the body of the murderer of whom so much has been said, and which I shall call here, by allegory to the magnetic matter, the murderous matter, makes from the first time it touches the body of Jaques [*sic*] Aymar in the tissue of his skin, and perhaps also in the parts of his blood, certain mouldings, and certain traces, by reason of which it always preserves for itself a passage and a free entrance into the body, and into the blood of this man disposed to receive them rather than another man; just as the magnetic matter coming out of the magnet makes these traces or mouldings in the pores of the iron, and not in the pores of the other bodies which it can touch, because it finds the pores of the iron so disposed to let the little particles pass through, and the pores of the other bodies are not disposed in the same way'), (Pierre Garnier, *Dissertation physique en forme de lettre à Monsieur de Seve… dans laquelle il est prouvé que les talens extraordinaires qu'à Jacques Aymar de suivre avece une Baguette les Meurtries et les Voleurs à la piste, de trouver de l'eau, l'argent chaché, les bornes transplantées, etc. dépendent d'une cause tres-naturelle et tres ordinaire* [Lyon: chez Jean-Baptiste de Ville, 1692], pp. 45–46).

('one hour after it has crossed a river'),[83] a clear demonstration of the fact that corpuscles can survive in the air for a long-time. The reason why only Aymar, and not other people, could sense the murderers' corpuscles is the same as why only certain dog breeds are able to smell animal traces, namely the peculiar dimension of their pores, which can let in corpuscles that other individuals cannot receive.[84]

It is worth noting that a similar reference to the 'porousness of bodies' as a reason for hunting dogs' skills is present in another text written by Boyle, *Essay on the Porousness of Animal Bodies*.[85] This work is particular interesting because it testifies to Boyle's absolute confidence in the explanatory powers of effluvia. Indeed, to Boyle's eyes, effluvia account even for those phenomena which apparently resist from natural explanation and which in the Renaissance were usually regarded as examples of the activity of occult qualities, i.e. amulets.[86] As we read in the aforementioned *Essays of Effluviums*, the positive effect of objects like 'blood-stones, cornelian, nephritick stones, lapis Malacensis, and some other substances, applied by physicians outwardly to our bodies',[87] although occurring 'not often, much less always', indeed derives

> from the subtle emanations that pass thorough the pores of the skin to the inward parts of the body, as is evident in those, who by holding cantharides in their hands, or having them applied to some remote external part, have grievous pains produced in their urinary pars, as it has happened to me, as well as to many others.[88]

In the *Essay on the Porousness of Animal Bodies* Boyle resumes these statements and invokes his own experience as a further proof of them:

> that some of them [i.e. amulets], especially on some patients, may have considerable, not to say admirable, operations, I confess, myself, by other motives, as well as authority, to be persuaded. Having been one summer frequently subject to bleed at the nose, and reduced to employ several remedies to check that distemper; that, which I found the most effectual to stanch the blood, was some moss of a dead man's skull (sent for a present out of Ireland, where it is far less rare than in most other countries) though it did but touch my skin, till the herb was a little warmed by it. And, though I remember not, that I have known any

83 Chauvin, *Lettre à la Marquise*, p. 87.

84 Chauvin, *Lettre à la Marquise*, p. 54 : 'Il y a donc des hommes, dont les pores peuvent être disposez de la maniere dont il s'agit; come il y a des hommes dont toutes les inclinations, et tous les traits exterieurs sont tres divers; ce qui ne peut arriver que par un arrangement et une configuration de la matiere differente dans châque individu' ('There are people, therefore, whose pores may be arranged in such manner; as there are people whose inclinations, and all their external features, are very diverse; which can only happen by a different arrangement and configuration of matter in each individual').

85 This essay was the first part of *Experiments and Considerations about Porosity in Two Essays* (1684). The second one was devoted to the porousness of solid bodies. See *The Works of Robert Boyle*, vol. 4, pp. 759–93.

86 On the seventeenth-century interpretation of amulets, see Martha Baldwin, 'Toads and Plague: Amulet Therapy in Seventeenth-Century Medicine', *Bulletin of the History of Medicine*, 67. 2 (1993), pp. 227–47.

87 Boyle, *Essay on the Great Efficacy of Effluviums*, p. 688.

88 Boyle, *Essay on the Great Efficacy of Effluviums*, p. 688.

> greater matter done to stop haemorrhages by the bare outward application of other blood-stones; yet, of one, that looked almost like an agate, I admired the effects, especially upon a young and extraordinary sanguine person.[89]

Boyle's personal experience, then, supports an idea which — as already mentioned — is widespread in his writings on effluvia, namely the thesis that the passage of effluvia from one body to another depends on the particular configuration of both bodies, and hence on mechanical properties. In this regard, the rhapsodical effects of specific remedies like amulets is taken not to disprove validity of the thesis adopted but, on the contrary, to prove that the mechanical properties of effluvia (size, shape, and texture) are what influences their behaviour. As we have seen, a similar argument is present in Chauvin's discussion of Aymar's peculiar divinatory powers: far from being considered a 'red flag', the exceptionality of these powers was regarded as a further element supporting a natural explanation of his striking discovery. Both these points, in my opinion, attest to the validity of those interpretations of the Scientific Revolution — evoked at the beginning of this chapter — according to which, when a new view of the world is developed, old beliefs do not immediately disappear, but, in a sense, struggle to survive within the current ones. At the same time, as the treatment of judicial astrology by Boyle and other seventeenth-century thinkers shows,[90] not all opinions endure over the centuries, but only those which possess features that are compatible with the new frameworks. The miasmatic interpretation of the plague appears to be one of them.

89 Boyle, *Essay on the Porousness of Animal Bodies*, in *The Works of Robert Boyle*, vol. 4, p. 767.

90 On this topic see H. Darrel Rutkin, 'How to Accurately Account for Astrology's Marginalization in the History of Science and Culture: The Essential Importance of an Interpretive Framework', *Early Science and Medicine*, 23 (2018), pp. 217–43.

Bibliography

Agricola, Georg, *De Peste. Libri tres* (s.l. [but Basel]: Hyeronimus Froben, 1554).

Boyle, Robert, *Cosmical Suspicions [Subjoyned as an Appendix to the Discourse of the Cosmical Qualities of Things]*, in *The Works of the Honourable Robert Boyle*, edited by Thomas Birch, 6 vols (London: 1744), vol. 3.

———, *Essay on the Great Efficacy of Effluviums*, in, *The Works of the Honourable Robert Boyle*, edited by Thomas Birch, 6 vols (London: 1744), vol. 3.

———, *On the Strange Subtlity of Effluviums*, in *The Works of the Honourable Robert Boyle*, edited by Thomas Birch, 6 vols (London: 1744), vol. 3.

———, *Essay on the Porousness of Animal Bodies*, in *The Works of the Honourable Robert Boyle*, edited by Thomas Birch, 6 vols (London: 1744), vol. 4.

———, *An Experimental Discourse on Some Unheeded Causes of the Insalubrity and Salubrity of the Air*, in *The Works of the Honourable Robert Boyle*, edited by Thomas Birch, 6 vols (London: 1744), vol. 5.

Chauvin, *Lettre à Madame la Marquise de Senozan, sur les moyens dont on s'est servy pour découvrir les Complices d'un assassinat commis à Lyon, le 5eme de Juillet 1692* (Lyon: chez Jean Baptiste et Nicolas De Ville, 1692).

Diderot, Denis, and D'Alembert, Jean-Baptiste Le Rond (ed.), *Encyclopédie, ou dictionnaire raisonné des sciences, des arts et des métiers, etc.*, 17 vols (Lucques: Giuntini, 2nd edition, 1758–71), vol. 13.

Fracastoro, Girolamo, *De sympatia et antipathia rerum liber unus. De contagione, contagiosis morbis et curatione libri tres* (Venetiis: apud heredes Lucaeantonii Iuntae Florentini, 1546).

Furètiere, Antoine, *Dictionaire universel, contenant généralement tous les mots françois tant vieux que modernes et les termes de toutes les sciences et des arts* (La Haye-Rotterdam: Arnout et Reinier Leers, 1690), vol. 1.

Garnier, Pierre, *Dissertation physique en forme de lettre à Monsieur de Seve… dans laquelle il est prouvé que les talens extraordinaires qu'à Jacques Aymar de suivre avece une Baguette les Meurtries et les Voleurs à la piste, de trouver de l'eau, l'argent chaché, les bornes transplantées, etc. dépendent d'une cause tres-naturelle et tres ordinaire* [Lyon: chez Jean-Baptiste de Ville, 1692].

Harvey, Gideon, *Discourse of the Plague containing the Nature, Causes, Signs, and Presages of the Pestilence in general. Together with the state of the present Contagion. Also most rational Preservatives for Families, and choiche Curative Medicines both for Rich and Poor. With several waies for purifying the air in houses, streets, etc.* (London: Angel, 1665).

Hering, Francis, *Certaine Rules, Directions, or Advertisments for This Time of Pestilentiall Contagion with a Caveat to Those That Weare about Their Neckes Impoisoned Amulets as a Preservative from the Plague* (London: William Iones, 1625).

Milton, John, *The Latin Poems*, ed. by W. Mackellar (New Haven: Yale University Press, 1930).

Traicté de la peste, de la petite Verolle et Rougeolle. Avec une brefue description de la Lepre par Ambroise Paré premier Chirurgien du Roy et Iuré à Paris (Paris: André Wechel, 1568).

Trattato della peste di Ambrosio Pare de Laval al Mene … diviso in LII. capitoli ne' quali tra le altre cose si leggono i presaggi, le cause divine o umane, e le sementi generali della peste … Tradotto dal francese nell'italiano da Gio. Michele Du' Bois e dato in luce … con l'aggionta di alcune ricette… (Bologna: Benacci's heirs, 1720).

A Treatise of the Plague contayining Causes, Signes, Symptomes, Prognosticksm and Cure thereof. Together with sundry other remarkable passages (for the prevention of, and preservation from the Pestilence) never yet published by anie man. Collected out of the Workes of the no lesse learned than experimented and renowned Chirurgian Ambrose Parey (London: Michael Parke, 1630).

***

Alfani, Guido, 'Plague in Seventeenth-Century Europe and the Decline of Italy: an Epidemiological Hypothesis', *European Review of Economic History*, 17 (2013), pp. 408–30.

Anstey, Peter, *The Philosophy of Robert Boyle* (London-New York: Routledge, 2000).

Baldwin, Martha, 'Toads and Plague: Amulet Therapy in Seventeenth-Century Medicine', *Bulletin of the History of Medicine*, 67. 2 (1993), pp. 227–47.

Banchetti-Robino, M. Paola, *The Chemical Philosophy of Robert Boyle: Mechanicism, Chymical Atoms, and Emergence* (Oxford: Oxford University Press, 2020).

Biraben, Jean-Noël, *Les hommes et la peste en France et dans les pays Europeéens et Méditerranées* (Paris-La Haye: Mouton, 1975).

Ceccarelli, Andrea, '*Neve Lucretius a me indefensus maneat*: Girolamo Mercuriale, il *De rerum natura* e la medicina nel Rinascimento', *Lexicon philosophicon. International Journal for the History of Ideas*, 5 (2017) pp. 161–88.

Cipolla, Carlo M., *Public Health and the Medical Profession in the Renaissance* (Cambridge: Cambridge University Press, 1973).

———, *Miasmi ed umori. Ecologia e condizioni sanitarie in Toscana nel Seicento* (Bologna: Il Mulino, 1989).

Clericuzio, Antonio, 'A Redefinition of Boyle's Chemistry and Corpuscular Philosophy', *Annals of Science*, 6. 47 (1990), pp. 561–89.

———, *Elements, Principles and Corpuscles. A Study of Atomism and Chemistry in the Seventeenth Century* (Dordrecht: Springer, 2000).

Crignon, Claire, 'Peut-on faire une histoire naturelle de l'air? Francis Bacon et Robert Boyle', *Archives de Philosophie*, 84. 1 (2021), pp. 93–113.

Donato, Maria Pia, 'Galen in an Age of Change (1650–1820)', in *Brill's Companion to the Reception of Galen*, ed. by Petros Bouras-Vallianatos and Barbara Zipser, (Leiden-Boston: Brill 2019), pp. 487–507.

Favaretti Camposampiero, Matteo, 'Galenism in Early Modern Philosophy and Medicine', in *Encyclopedia of Early Modern Philosophy and Science*, ed. by Dana Jalobeau and Charles T. Wolfe, (Cham: Springer, 2018).

Ferenczi, Thomas, 'The Chevalier de Jancourt, a Soldier for the Enlightenment', *Le philosophoire*, 47. 1 (2017), pp. 77–133.

Garber, Daniel, 'Why the Scientific Revolution Wasn't a Scientific Revolution, and Why It Matters', in *Kuhn's Structure of Scientific Revolutions at Fifty. Reflections on a Science Classic*, ed. by Robert J. Richards and Lorraine Daston (Chicago-London: University of Chicago Press, 2016).

Goddard, Charlotte, 'Lucretius and Lucretian Science in the Works of Fracastoro', *Res Publica Litterarum*, 16 (1993), pp. 185–92.

Hirai, Hiro, *Le concept de semence dans les théories de la matière à la Renaissance. De Marsile Ficin à Pierre Gassendi* (Turnhout: Brepols, 2005).

Jouanna, Jacques, 'Air, miasme et contagion à l'époque d'Hippocrate et survivance de miasmes dans la médecine posthippocratique (Rufus d'Éphèse, Galien et Palladios)', in *Air, miasmes et contagion, Les épidémies dans l'Antiquité et au Moyen Âge*, ed. by Sylvie Bazin-Tacchella and others (Langres: Dominique Guéniot, 2001), pp. 9–28.

———, *Greek Medicine from Hippocrates to Galen. Selected Papers* (Leiden-Boston: Brill, 2012).

Kuhn, Thomas, *The Structure of the Scientific Revolution* (Chicago: University of Chicago Press, 1970).

Mammola, Simone, *La ragione e l'incertezza. Filosofia e medicina nella prima età moderna* (Milano: Franco Angeli, 2012), pp. 266–71.

Newman, William R., *Atoms and Alchemy: Chymistry and the Experimental Origins of the Scientific Revolution* (Chicago-London: University of Chicago Press, 2006).

Nutton, Vivian, 'The Seeds of Disease. An Explanation of Contagion and Infection from the Greeks to the Renaissance', *Medical History*, 27 (1983), pp. 1–34.

———, 'The Reception of Fracastoro's Theory of Contagion: The Seed That Fell among Thorns?', *Osiris*, 6 (1990), pp. 196–234.

Pantin, Isabelle, 'Fracastoro's *De Contagione* and Medieval Reflection on 'Action at a Distance': Old and New Trends in Renaissance Discourse on the Plague', in *Imagining Contagion in Early Modern Europe*, ed. by Claire Carlin (New York: Palgrave, 2005), pp. 3–15.

Parigi, Silvia, 'Effluvia, Action at a Distance, and the Challenge of the Third Causal Model', *International Studies in the Philosophy of Science*, 29. 4 (2005), pp. 351–68.

Pennuto, Concetta, 'La natura dei contagi in Fracastoro', in *Girolamo Fracastoro. Fra medicina, filosofia e scienze della natura*, ed. by Alessandro Pastore and Enrico Peruzzi (Florence: Leo Olschki, 2006) pp. 57–71.

———, *Simpatia, fantasia e contagio. Il pensiero medico e il pensiero filosofico de Girolamo Fracastoro* (Roma: Edizioni di storia e letteratura, 2008).

Pérez, Stanis, La République des Lettres menée à la baguette? L'affaire Jacques Aymar', *XVIIe siècle*, 226 (2005), pp. 145–64.

Prescher, Hans, 'Georgius Agricola. Ein sächsischer Humanist ond Naturforscher von europäischer Bedeutung', in *Georgius Agricola. 500 Jahre. Wisseschaftliche Konferenz vom 25.-27.März 1994 in Chemnitz, Freistaat Sachsen*, ed. by Friedrich Naumann (Basel–Boston–Berlin: Birkhäuser Verlag, 1994), pp. 11–34.

Priarolo, Mariangela, 'Demoni o corpuscoli? La bacchetta divinatoria e la nuova scienza alla fine del XVII secolo', *Intersezioni*, 3 (2020), pp. 333–58.

Renzi, Barbara Gabriella, 'Kuhn's Evolutionary Epistemology and Its Being Undermined by Inadequate Biological Concepts', *Philosophy of Science*, 76. 2, (2009), pp. 143–59.

Rutkin, H. Darrel, 'How to Accurately Account for Astrology's Marginalization in the History of Science and Culture: The Essential Importance of an Interpretive Framework', *Early Science and Medicine*, 23 (2018), pp. 217–43.

Stewart, Keith Andrew, *Galen's Theory of Black Bile. Hippocratic Tradition, Manipulation, Innovation* (Leiden-Boston: Brill, 2018).

Thorndike, Lynn, *A History of Magic and Experimental Science*, vols 8, *The Seventeenth Century* (New York: Columbia University Press, 1958).

FABRIZIO MEROI

7. Contagion and Epidemics in Twentieth-Century Thought

A Hypothesis about Bergson

▼ **ABSTRACT** In the twentieth century, as in previous centuries, there was also much talk, at various levels and in the most diverse cultural fields, of epidemics and, more generally, of contagion. After some references to authors and works dealing with epidemics and contagion in the literary, philosophical, and human sciences fields, the essay focuses specifically on the theme of contagion and on one of the greatest thinkers of the early twentieth century, Henri Bergson, in whose works this theme is very present, albeit in a very peculiar form. Bergson often resorts to terms and concepts such as those of influence, diffusion, propagation, and transmission, when dealing with: psychological and gnoseological issues, the central theme of the evolution of life, and anthropological, ethical, and religious themes. In conclusion, it is hypothesized that in Bergson there is not simply a metaphorical use of the idea of contagion, but the presence of an original theoretical model of interpretation of reality consisting of a dynamic of interaction and transfer, which constitutes a conceptual structure characteristic of his thought.

1. Literature, Philosophy, and the Human Sciences

Since ancient times, the topic of epidemics and, more generally, contagion has been very present in the cultural production of Western civilization. The twentieth century, in this sense, is certainly no exception: epidemics, pandemics, and infectious diseases in general, real or fictional, have been the subject of various descriptions, representations, treatments, and interpretations; and the idea of contagion, extrapolated from its medical context, has been widely used in the most diverse fields to indicate and

Epidemics and Pandemics, ed. by Michele Nicoletti and Alessandro Palazzo (Turnhout: Brepols, 2024), pp. 189–214
BREPOLS PUBLISHERS 10.1484/M.STPH-EB.5.136411

define dynamics similar to those of the diffusion and transmission of a pathological phenomenon in the strict sense.[1]

In a literary context, the most famous example in terms of contagious diseases is certainly the novel *La peste* (1947) by Albert Camus, in which the epidemic at the centre of the narrative is, on the one hand, the metaphor of the World War and of the Nazi horror that had haunted Europe for years; on the other hand, it is an opportunity for a series of broader reflections on the problem of evil and on the absurdity and incomprehensibility of the human condition.[2] But an infectious disease plays a far from marginal role in two other twentieth-century literary masterpieces: *Der Tod in Venedig* (1912) and *Der Zauberberg* (1924) by Thomas Mann. In the former, the cholera epidemic that is spreading in Venice is the background — and counterpart — to the protagonist's insane amorous passion and the last days of his life;[3] in the latter, the scenario in which the narrated event takes place is a tuberculosis sanatorium where the protagonist himself has been hospitalized.[4] The dating of Mann's two above-mentioned novels is reflected in that of two other works: *The Scarlet Plague* (1912), a short apocalyptic novel in which Jack London foreshadows a distant future in which humanity is almost entirely wiped out by a pandemic of colossal proportions;[5] and *Semmelweis* (1924), the dissertation in Medicine in which a young Louis-Ferdinand Céline retraces the biography of the brilliant but unheeded discoverer of the true causes of puerperal infection.[6] Two years after *La peste* by Camus, Curzio Malaparte's *La Pelle* (1949) was published, a raw and shocking portrait of the city of Naples freed by the Allies and overwhelmed by a plague epidemic that does not corrupt the body but the spirit.[7] And in the second half of the last century other important narrative works appeared that revolve around epidemics of various kinds, whether they had actually occurred or were imaginary: from *Le hussard sur le toit* (1951) by Jean Giono to Marcel Pagnol's *Les Pestiférés* (1977, published

1 For a recent and comprehensive historical-social framework of the phenomenon of epidemics, see Frank M. Snowden, *Epidemics and Society: From the Black Death to the Present* (New Haven: Yale University Press, 2019); see also *Epidemics and Ideas: Essays on the Historical Perception of Pestilence*, ed. by Terence Ranger and Paul Slack (Cambridge: Cambridge University Press, 1992). Regarding the idea of contagion in particular, see *Contagion: Perspectives from Pre-Modern Societies*, ed. by Lawrence I. Conrad and Dominik Wujastyk (Aldershot: Ashgate, 2000); Saul Jarcho, *The Concept of Contagion in Medicine, Literature, and Religion* (Malabar: Krieger, 2000); *Contagion: Historical and Cultural Studies*, ed. by Alison Bashford and Claire Hooker (London and New York: Routledge, 2001); *Imagining Contagion in Early Modern Europe*, ed. by Claire L. Carlin (New York: Palgrave Macmillan, 2005); Antonio Lucci, 'Ansteckung. Plädoyer für eine Ethik der Kontingenz', in *Die Corona-Gesellschaft. Analysen zur Lage und Perspektiven für die Zukunft*, ed. by Michael Volkmer and Karin Werner (Bielefeld: transcript Verlag, 2020), pp. 357–67.

2 Albert Camus, *La peste* (Paris: Gallimard, 2021).

3 Thomas Mann, *Der Tod in Venedig* (Frankfurt a. M.: Fischer, 1992).

4 Thomas Mann, *Der Zauberberg* (Frankfurt a. M.: Fischer, 2003).

5 Jack London, *The Scarlet Plague* (New York: Macmillan, 1915).

6 Louis-Ferdinand Céline, *Semmelweis* (Paris: Gallimard, 1999).

7 Curzio Malaparte, *La pelle* (Milano: Adelphi, 2010).

posthumously), from *El amor en los tiempos del cólera* by Gabriel García Márquez (1985) to *Ensaio sobre a Cegueira* by José Saramago (1995).[8]

There have been quite a few philosophers who have spoken, in various senses, of contagion and contagious diseases. Just a few examples, among the many possible. At the beginning of the century, Otto Weininger, in a part of the concluding section of *Über die letzten Dinge* (1903), the collection of writings published immediately after his death, sees malaria as the symbol of an 'innerer Versumpfung' ('interior swamping'), that is, of an unhealthy condition in which the current of life can flow: in fact, 'die Gefahr des Flusses ist die Versumpfung. Dort sind die Mücken und das Fieber' ('the risk for the river is to end up in the swamps, where there are mosquitoes and fever'); and a little further on he still uses the image of the insect carrier par excellence of malaria to allude to the sense of persecution of those who have committed a crime: 'der Verbrecher halluziniert die giftige Mücke und stirbt an falscher Furcht durch Herzschlag' ('the criminal has the hallucination of the poisonous mosquito and dies of a broken heart from an unfounded fear').[9] In a chapter of *Histoire et utopie* (1960) Emil Cioran identifies the reason for Russia's superiority over the West in its being immune from the contagion of the 'virus de la liberté' ('virus of freedom') and argues that, by virtue of its rampant imperialist ideology, it extends beyond its own borders like 'une épidémie, salutaire parfois, souvent nuisible, toujours fulgurante' ('an epidemic, sometimes healthy, often harmful, always meteoric'); while, in another chapter of the same work, he lashes out against the act of procreation and against the cult of the human species: 'la chair se propage avec l'impudeur d'un fléau' ('the flesh spreads with the impudence of a scourge') and all our thoughts appear 'contaminées par la présence de l'humain' ('contaminated by the presence of the human'), as well as unable to grasp any truth since 'cette pestilence asphyxie l'esprit et le rend impropre à considérer autre chose que l'animal pernicieux et fétide dont il subit les émanations' ('this pestilence suffocates the spirit and makes it unfit to consider anything other than the pernicious and fetid animal whose emanations it suffers').[10] And in the introduction to *Mille plateaux* (1980), the sequel to the better known *L'anti-Œdipe*, Gilles Deleuze and Félix Guattari refer, among other things, to viruses to explain the nature of the rhizome (one of the key notions of the work) and, more precisely, its characteristic of linking together very heterogeneous elements or beings: since through a virus genetic information of an organism can be transferred to another organism even of a completely different species, across the board with respect to lines of biological evolution, then it can be said that 'nous faisons rhizome avec nos virus,

8 Jean Giono, *Le hussard sur le toit* (Paris: Gallimard, 1995); Marcel Pagnol, *Les Pestiférés* (Paris: Éditions de Fallois, 2020); Gabriel García Márquez, *El amor en los tiempos del cólera* (Barcelona: Bruguera, 1985); José Saramago, *Ensaio sobre a Cegueira* (Lisbon: Caminho, 1995).

9 Otto Weininger, *Über die letzten Dinge* (Munich: Matthes & Seitz Verlag, 1997), pp. 186–87.

10 Emil M. Cioran, *Histoire et utopie*, in *Œuvres* (Paris: Gallimard, 1995), pp. 979–1061 (pp. 1001, 1004, 1020–21). And note that, to define the scope of politics and history as it appears in Cioran's vision, the author of the afterword to the Italian translation of *Histoire et utopie* uses the expression 'universe of total contamination': Mario A. Rigoni, 'Contaminazione totale', in Emil M. Cioran, *Storia e utopia* (Milan: Adelphi, 1982), pp. 147–59 (p. 153).

ou plutôt nos virus nous font faire rhizome avec d'autres bêtes' ('we make rhizomes with our viruses, in fact our viruses make us make rhizomes with other beasts'); and they conclude: 'nous évoluons et nous mourons de nos grippes polymorphes et rhizomatiques, plus que de nos maladies de descendance ou qui ont elles-mêmes leur descendance' ('we evolve and die because of our polymorphic and rhizomatic fevers, rather than from our diseases transmitted by descent or which have their own descent').[11]

Michel Foucault, who dealt with epidemics and contagion in some of his most important works, deserves a special mention. 'À la fin du Moyen Âge, la lèpre disparaît du monde occidental' ('At the end of the Middle Ages, leprosy disappeared from the Western world'): this is the opening sentence of the first chapter of the first part of the *Histoire de la folie à l'âge classique* (1961).[12] The thesis that Foucault argues in the subsequent pages is that this terrible infectious disease disappeared from the European scenario in the fifteenth century and that its place was first taken (in the sixteenth century) by venereal diseases, but only in a, so to speak, provisional form and in the sense that those who were affected by them were housed, at least initially, in leper hospitals by then devoid of lepers; and later (in the seventeenth century) by madness, which can be considered the heir of leprosy in a much deeper sense. In fact, according to Foucault, during the period of its 'grand renfermement' ('great confinement'), that is, in the heart of the modern age, madness was the object of the same exclusion mechanism to which leprosy had previously been subjected during the Middle Ages. This is a mechanism for which the act of exclusion, of forced separation from the community, entails at the same time a purification, a form of salvation: just as once the removal of the leper left him alone with his disease, which was a punishment for his sins and, as such, brought him closer to the grace of God, so now the imprisonment of the madman is what, in addition to preserving the world of reason from the risk of being confused with madness, offers him an opportunity for the redemption from a mental disorder which is considered a moral guilt.[13] But madness also inherited something else from leprosy: the contagion dimension. Foucault dedicates the first chapter of the third part of the work to the 'grande peur' ('great fear'): towards the mid-eighteenth century people began to fear that, from the places of the confinement of madness, the contagion of a disease, both physical (the so-called 'fièvres des prisons', 'fevers of prisons') and moral (the depravity of inmates), that infects the body and the spirit and causes the decomposition of the flesh and the corruption of morals, could spread.[14] In the second chapter of *Naissance de la clinique* (1963), several pages deal with the eighteenth-century medical study

11 Gilles Deleuze and Félix Guattari, *Mille plateaux. Capitalisme et schizophrénie 2* (Paris: Les Éditions de Minuit, 1980), p. 18.

12 Michel Foucault, *Histoire de la folie à l'âge classique* (Paris: Gallimard, 2017), p. 15.

13 Foucault, *Histoire de la folie*, pp. 15–21, 76–80, 112, 120–21, 179–85.

14 Foucault, *Histoire de la folie*, pp. 445–53 (but also pp. 153–54). Of this work we should also remember, among others, the pages in which Foucault deals with syphilis, which is mixed with madness in the places of the 'great confinement' (pp. 116–21), and the relationship between 'sympathy' — that is the ability of the internal organs of the human body to interact and receive stimuli — and nerve diseases (pp. 366–74).

of epidemics. In the context of the analysis of the progressive overcoming of a classification-based medicine, Foucault outlines, in this regard, a very precise picture. The epidemic differs from individual disease not by its nature or typology, but because it affects many people at the same time, that is, it is distinguished on the basis of a perception — writes Foucault — not 'essentielle et ordinale' ('essential and ordinal'), but 'quantitative et cardinale' ('quantitative and cardinal'); it is therefore a question of identifying not the general form of the disease, but the variable and singular element that unites all those affected by it. In this perspective, the contagion factor is of little importance: it can certainly be one of the causes of the epidemic, but it is only one of the many aspects of the issue. In any case, as epidemics have their own historical specificity and are collective phenomena, they require a detailed description on the one hand and a multiple point of view on the other hand, but also constant and constricting intervention, that is, a policing action. This experience of epidemics is thus at the origin of the definition of a political statute for medicine and the establishment of a medical awareness with both information and monitoring tasks.[15] This last point is taken up and developed in *Surveiller et punir* (1975), where the phenomenon of epidemics is examined in relation to the development, especially between the seventeenth and eighteenth centuries, of the techniques for applying the discipline. In particular, the inspection, recording and surveillance practices that medical and political powers adopt to combat the plague are seen by Foucault as the answer to the real and imaginary disorder that the latter embodies; and the disciplinary schemes generated by the plague are also compared — and here Foucault's discourse is linked not to the *Naissance de la clinique* but to the *Histoire de la folie* — with the rituals of exclusion to which, at the time, leprosy had been subject.[16]

Moreover, the idea of contagion enjoyed a widespread currency, especially between the end of the nineteenth century and the beginning of the twentieth century, in the context of studies on magic and the sacred in ancient or primitive societies. Suffice it to mention James Frazer, who, in his famous *The Golden Bough* (published in several volumes and in subsequent editions between 1890 and 1915, but also in a reduced version of great circulation in 1922), studies, on the one hand, the principles and the manifestations of 'contagious magic', which is based on the assumption that things that have once come into contact continue to interact at a distance, even when the contact has ceased; on the other hand, religious practices by means of which it is believed to be able to free an individual from the misfortunes or diseases (often of an epidemic nature) that afflict him, transferring them (almost always through physical contact, direct or indirect) on to inanimate objects, animals or other individuals.[17] Or consider Émile Durkheim, who, in *Les formes élémentaires de la vie religieuse* (1912), to explain the system of religious prohibitions, uses the principle (which had already

15 Michel Foucault, *Naissance de la clinique. Une archéologie du regard médical* (Paris: Presses Universitaires de France, 2007), pp. 21–26.

16 Michel Foucault, *Surveiller et punir. Naissance de la prison* (Paris: Gallimard, 2020), pp. 228–33.

17 James Frazer, *The Golden Bough: A Study in Magic and Religion* (London: Palgrave Macmillan, 1990), esp. Chapters 3 and 55.

been studied in previous years by other authors, including Frazer himself) of the 'contagiosité du sacré' ('contagiousness of the sacred'): both in totemic religions and in the more advanced ones, the need to keep the profane and the sacred worlds strictly separate depends on the exceptional tendency of the latter to spread and be transmitted, even through superficial and mediated contact, to everything that surrounds it; and this contagiousness, this capacity of the sacred to pass from one body to another, is in turn made possible by the fact that the forces that are at stake here, that is, the religious forces, are conceived as something external and independent of the person in whom they act and, therefore, as something extremely mobile that can easily transfer itself to another person, contaminating him.[18] Nor can we forget René Girard, who in much more recent years, while investigating the phenomenon of ritual sacrifice in *La violence et le sacré* (1972), identifies in the contagious character of violence the cause of religious impurity, also contagious: the objective of sacrificial practices is to take precautions to prevent violence from spreading and to protect, as far as possible, those who have already been contaminated by it and are therefore impure; and the fact that these precautions (which essentially consist in avoiding any form of contact) appear very similar to those adopted by modern medicine to combat epidemics is the reason why many scholars have seen in them a sort of anticipation of scientific empiricism.[19]

But there was also talk, again during the twentieth century, of 'emotional contagion' (to indicate the passive and involuntary forms, that is, without cognitive mediation, of affective sharing) in the context of psychology studies in general;[20] more specifically, there was talk — but also in this case, as in that of studies on magic and the sacred, as early as the nineteenth century — of 'psychic contagion' (or 'mental', 'moral', 'social') in the field of the psychology and sociology of the masses (an aspect which will be discussed later); Max Weber spoke of 'methodologische Pestilenz' ('methodological pestilence') with regard to the risks of over-reflecting on the method to be adopted in the field of historical-social research;[21] Victor Klemperer spoke of a deviated form of the German language as a pathogen, not only as a symptom, but also a vehicle of contagion of that Hitlerian rhetoric in particular and of

---

18 Émile Durkheim, *Les formes élémentaires de la vie religieuse. Le système totémique en Australie* (Paris: Presses Universitaires de France, 1990), pp. 453–64.

19 René Girard, *La violence et le sacré* (Paris: Grasset, 1972), pp. 47–55. By Girard see also 'The Plague in Literature and Myth', *Texas Studies in Literature and Language*, 15 (1974), pp. 833–50. Regarding contagion in Girard, see Ann W. Astell, 'Saintly Mimesis, Contagion, and Empathy in the Thought of René Girard, Edith Stein, and Simone Weil', *Shofar*, 22 (2004), no. 2, pp. 116–31.

20 On the subject, see first of all Elaine Hatfield and others, *Emotional Contagion. Studies in Emotion and Social Interaction* (Cambridge: Cambridge University Press, 1994).

21 Weber uses the above expression in a work of 1913: Max Weber, 'Beitrag zur Werturteildiskussion im Ausschuß des Vereins für Sozialpolitik', in *Max Weber-Gesamtausgabe*, I/12: *Verstehende Soziologie und Werturteilsfreiheit. Schriften und Reden 1908–1917*, ed. by J. Weiß und S. Frommer (Tübingen: Mohr, 2018), pp. 329–82. See Christopher Adair-Toteff, '"Methodological Pestilence": Max Weber's Devastating Critique of Stammler', *Max Weber Studies*, 14 (2014), no. 2, pp. 245–68; Edoardo Massimilla, 'La "pestilenza metodologica" e la "maledizione del rospo": Max Weber lettore di Gustav Meyrink', *Archivio di storia della cultura*, 31 (2018), pp. 263–72.

that Nazi ideology in general that spread in Germany in the 1930s with the virulence of an epidemic...[22] Therefore, in the face of such a complex topic and such a vast panorama, I intend to focus on the idea of contagion, on the early decades of the century in question (but, at least in part, also on the last ones of the previous century), and on a single thinker, Henri Bergson, in whose works the theme of contagion is present in various ways, at different levels and probably — as I will hypothesize in conclusion — in an overall very peculiar form.

2. The Young Bergson and the Plague of Lucretius

It can be said that Bergson is among the authors who inaugurated the thought of the twentieth century: there was the successful *Le rire. Essai sur la signification du comique* (1900);[23] the 1901 essay 'Le rêve', which appeared shortly after Freud's *Traumdeutung*;[24] then there was in 1903 the 'Introduction à la métaphysique', a synthetic but very detailed manifesto of his philosophical method;[25] above all, from 1907 is the very famous *Évolution créatrice*, one of the pre-eminent books of the twentieth century, destined to exert an enormous influence in the most diverse fields of culture and knowledge.[26] However, it is also true that Bergson's activity had already begun in the last years of the previous century, with fundamental works such as the *Essai sur les données immediates de la conscience* (1889) and *Matière et mémoire* (1896), in which the main presuppositions of his philosophical reflections are already fixed.[27] And also dating from the nineteenth century is what can be considered his first significant encounter with the theme of contagion (and epidemics): in fact, in 1883 there appeared the *Extraits de Lucrèce avec commentaire, études et notes*, a commentated anthology of *De rerum natura* for use in schools (Bergson was at that time a high-school teacher) in which the French philosopher also dwells on the plague of Athens described, following in the footsteps of Thucydides, by the Latin poet.[28]

As is well known, in Lucretius's vision (having a Democritean and Epicurean imprint), epidemics, as well as other events that are considered calamities such as earthquakes, volcanic eruptions or floods, should not be attributed to divine anger (this was the prevailing explanation in the previous tradition), but have purely natural

22 Victor Klemperer, *LTI. Notizbuch eines Philologen* (Berlin: Aufbau-Verlag, 1947), esp. pp. 91–92. See Sergio Givone, 'Quando contagioso è il linguaggio', in *Metafisica della peste. Colpa e destino* (Torino: Einaudi, 2012), pp. 50–65.

23 Henri Bergson, *Le rire. Essai sur la signification du comique*, in *Œuvres* (Paris: Presses Universitaires de France, 1959; seconde édition 1963), pp. 381–485.

24 Henri Bergson, 'Le rêve', in *L'énergie spirituelle. Essais et conférences*, in *Œuvres*, pp. 811–977 (pp. 878–97).

25 Henri Bergson, 'Introduction à la métaphysique', in *La pensée et le mouvant. Essais et conférences*, in *Œuvres*, pp. 1249–1482 (pp. 1392–1432).

26 Henri Bergson, *L'évolution créatrice*, in *Œuvres*, pp. 487–809.

27 Henri Bergson, *Essai sur les données immediates de la conscience*, in *Œuvres*, pp. 1–157; *Matière et mémoire*, in *Œuvres*, pp. 159–379.

28 On the Athenian plague, see chapter 1 of this volume.

causes, which ultimately depend on the modalities of aggregation and disgregation of the atoms, that is, of those tiny and invisible entities that form all existing bodies. In the specific case of epidemics, things are simply like this: 'Primum multarum semina rerum | esse supra docui quae sint vitalia nobis, | et contra quae sint morbo mortique necessest | multa volare. Ea cum casu sunt forte coorta | et perturbarunt caelum, fit morbidus aer' ('First of all I explained earlier that there are germs of many substances which are vital for us, and on the contrary, many must be swirling around which bring disease and death. When by chance the latter rise compactly and cloud the sky, the air becomes infected').[29] The distress that assails men in the face of such phenomena is therefore completely unjustified, just as the attribution of responsibility to the gods is unjustified: in order not to incur such errors, it would be sufficient to follow the atomistic conception of reality, thus learning really to know nature and to free oneself from any kind of superstition.

In his commentary on the Lucretian poem, Bergson refers to the verses concerning the plague on three separate occasions. First of all, in the short but important preface, he programmatically declares that he does not want to limit himself to extrapolating, from the text, the 'descriptions à effet' ('striking descriptions'), in order not to run the risk of making the reader of the anthology believe that Lucretius is 'un poète qui a decrit la vie des premiers hommes, ou les effets de la foudre, ou la peste d'Athènes, pour le plaisir de les décrire' ('a poet who described the life of the first men, or the effects of lightning, or the plague of Athens, for the pleasure of describing them'). Lucretius, on the contrary, 'n'a jamais décrit que pour prouver; ses peintures les plus saisissantes sont uniquement destinées à nous faire comprendre, à nous faire accepter quelque grand principe philosophique' ('has always used descriptions to prove something; his most successful representations are only destined to make us understand, to make us accept some great philosophical principle').[30] On this first occasion, therefore, the example of the Athens plague, alongside others, is useful to Bergson to corroborate his idea that the numerous descriptions which embellish the Lucretian work are never ends in themselves, but are always directed at demonstrating a philosophical assumption (which, in the case of the Athenian epidemic, is the completely natural origin of the disease).

Then, at the end of the substantial introduction, concentrating on Lucretius's originality as a philosopher and as a poet, the reference to the plague of Athens is functional to underlining the profound difference which, according to Bergson, exists, beyond the many similarities, between the vision of Lucretius and that of Epicurus. If the doctrine of the latter aims at achieving a serenity, a form of happiness that derives from the elimination of melancholy and disturbances of the soul, superstition and all fear, Lucretius draws instead from the atomism of a Democritean matrix — from which Epicurus himself also draws inspiration — a very different conclusion:

29 Lucretius, *De rerum natura*, ed. by Cyril Bailey (Oxford: Oxford University Press, 1978), VI. 1093–97.
30 Henri Bergson, *Extraits de Lucrèce*, dixième édition (Paris: Delagrave, undated), p. v.

> Comme la fatalité des lois naturelles est ce qui l'a surtout frappé dans la doctrine des atomes, le poète a été pris, malgré la sérénité qu'il affecte, d'une pitié douloureuse pour cette humanité qui s'agite sans résultat, qui lutte sans profit, et que les lois inflexibles de la nature entraînent, malgré elle, dans l'immense tourbillonnement des choses. Pourquoi travailler, prendre de la peine? Pourquoi lutter, pourquoi se plaindre? Nous subissons la loi commune, et la nature se soucie peu de nous. Qu'un vent chargé de germes empoisonnés souffle sur la terre, une épidémie naîtra, les hommes mourront, les dieux n'y pourront rien faire. Et c'est sur l'épouvantable description de la peste d'Athènes que le poème se termine. Lucrèce a voulu nous montrer l'impuissance des hommes et des dieux en présence des lois de la nature; il a voulu que le tableau fût effrayant, que la tristesse envahît notre âme, et que ce fût notre dernière impression.[31]

In short, the prevailing sentiment in Lucretian philosophy would not be that of a serenity that is within man's reach, but that of compassion for a humanity completely at the mercy of events and irremediably subjected to immutable natural laws; and it is no coincidence that *De rerum natura* ends — argues Bergson, who does not believe that the poem is unfinished — with the dramatic image of a humanity more suffering and helpless than ever, which the description of the plague in Athens conveys in a striking and irrefutable way.

Finally, in the anthological part, Bergson introduces the long passage of the poem concerning epidemics in general and the plague of Athens in particular, pointing out that, if the ancients explained the 'maladies épidémiques' ('epidemic diseases') by attributing them to the wrath of the gods, Lucretius, instead, traces them back to absolutely natural causes; recalling that the author of *De rerum natura*, in dealing with the Athenian disease, constantly keeps in mind the model represented by Thucydides; noting the fact that the Lucretian hypothesis on the origin of epidemics (according to which germs first spread in the atmosphere and then develop in the human body) has found a first confirmation in recent scientific observations.[32] And again, in the footnotes that refer to individual verses, he dwells on a series of specific issues: Lucretius's exclusive use of the term *pestilitas* (instead of the more common *pestilentia*); the relationship between certain epidemics and the characteristics of certain places, more favourable than others to the multiplication of germs; the difficulty of establishing with certainty which was the infectious disease that really

31 Bergson, *Extraits de Lucrèce*, p. xxii: 'Since it is above all the fatality of natural laws that struck him in the doctrine of atoms, the poet [Lucretius] is seized, despite the serenity he flaunts, by a painful compassion for this humanity that gets agitated without result, that struggles without profit, and that the inflexible laws of nature drag by force into the immense vortex of things. Why work, why bother? Why fight, why complain? We undergo the common law and nature pays us little attention. It is sufficient for a wind loaded with poisonous germs to blow on the earth and an epidemic will be born, men will die, the gods will not be able to do anything about it. And it is regarding the frightening description of the Athens plague that the poem ends. Lucretius wanted to show us the powerlessness of men and gods in the presence of the laws of nature; he wanted the picture to be terrifying, that sadness should invade our souls, and that this should be our last impression'.

32 Bergson, *Extraits de Lucrèce*, p. 147.

struck Athens (and which scholars have from time to time identified as scarlet fever, yellow fever, smallpox, etc.); the possibility of comparing these pages of Lucretius with those of other classical authors on a similar subject (from Virgil to Ovid, from Lucan to Silius Italicus); Lucretius's intention to demonstrate the gods' disregard for men through the description of 'le plus terrible de tous les fléaux' ('the most terrible of all scourges').[33]

3. From the *Essai* to *La pensée et le mouvant*

If, in the *Extraits de Lucrèce*, Bergson considers the idea of contagion understood in its proper sense, that is relative to the specific field of infections and epidemics, in many other places in his work, that is, those in which he deals with various phenomena of interaction, propagation, and transmission, this same idea reappears, although extrapolated from its original context and formulated more or less explicitly. This can be accounted for through a selection of particularly significant passages, taken from some of the French philosopher's most important texts.

As regards the nineteenth century, both the *Essai sur les données immediates de la conscience* and *Matière et memoire* should be mentioned. In the first chapter of the *Essai*, in the context of the discussion on the intensity of psychological states, Bergson talks about the way in which 'un obscur désir' ('an obscure desire') is gradually transformed into 'une passion profonde' ('a deep passion') by penetrating an ever increasing number of psychic elements and 'les teignant pour ainsi dire de sa propre couleur' ('dyeing them, as it were, with its own colour'); in treating in general the aesthetic feelings and the way in which they develop, he repeatedly resorts to the concepts of sympathy, influence, suggestion, and imitation, as well as the comparison with the effects of hypnosis; and, referring in particular to the plastic arts, he writes that they 'obtiennent un effet du même genre par la fixité qu'ils imposent soudain à la vie, et qu'une contagion physique communique à l'attention du spectateur' ('obtain an effect of the same kind [as that caused by poetry] through that fixity that they suddenly impose on life and which a physical contagion communicates to the spectator's attention').[34] In the second chapter, which concentrates on the multiplicity of the states of consciousness, in order to convey the idea of the reciprocal influence between the perception of the 'extériorité sans succession' ('exteriority without succession') of spatialized time on the one hand and the reality of the 'succession sans extériorité' ('succession without exteriority') of our interior duration on the

33 Bergson, *Extraits de Lucrèce*, pp. 147–49, 156. On the success of Lucretius in nineteenth-century France and, in particular, on Bergson's interpretation, see Salvatore Grandone, *Lucrezio e Bergson. La ricezione del 'De rerum natura' in Francia nel XIX secolo* (Rome: Aracne, 2018); see also Marie Cariou, *L'atomisme. Gassendi, Leibniz, Bergson et Lucrèce* (Paris: Aubier Montaigne, 1978); Patrick Healy, 'The Birthing of Things: Bergson as a Reader of Lucretius', *Footprint*, 8 (2014), pp. 29–39. On the Lucretian theory of epidemics, see Vivian Nutton, 'The Seeds of Disease: An Explanation of Contagion and Infection from the Greeks to the Renaissance', *Medical History*, 27 (1983), pp. 1–34 (pp. 9–11).

34 Henri Bergson, *Essai sur les données immediates de la conscience*, in *Œuvres*, pp. 1–157 (pp. 9, 11–16).

other hand, Bergson brings into play, by analogy, 'ce que les physiciens appellent un phénomène d'endosmose' ('what physicists call a phenomenon of endosmosis'), that is the diffusion of a solvent in a solution.[35] Finally, in the third chapter, in which the philosophical and psychological problem of freedom is directly addressed (on the basis of the theoretical acquisitions of the two previous chapters), the example of hypnotic suggestion is used here once again, to demonstrate that sometimes we can indeed undergo the influence of someone else's will, but this does not in any way mean that our will cannot function freely; moreover, in the final pages, we read that the idea of force, which within our consciousness we perceive as free spontaneity, when instead it is transposed into the external world and overlaps with the idea of necessity, it is 'imprégnée' ('impregnated') with the latter, and, therefore, conceived by us as if it necessarily determined the effects that derive from it.[36]

But let's consider *Matière et mémoire*. In the first chapter, dedicated to the selection of images for representation, it is the act of perception and that of remembering which, according to Bergson, in a sort of mutual contagion, 'se pénètrent donc toujours, échangent toujours quelque chose de leurs substances par un phénomène d'endosmose' ('always interpenetrate each other and always exchange something of their substances through a phenomenon of endosmosis').[37] At the beginning of the second chapter, dealing with the recognition of images, the ideas of influence, conduction, and transmission refer, in a paragraph summarizing what was previously said, to the body: 'le corps, interposé entre les objets qui agissent sur lui et ceux qu'il influence, n'est qu'un conducteur, chargé de recueillir les mouvements, et de les transmettre, quand il ne les arrête pas, à certains mécanismes moteurs, déterminés si l'action est réflexe, choisis si l'action est volontaire' ('the body, interposed between the objects that act on it and those that it influences, is only a conductor, charged with collecting the movements and, in the event that it does not block them, transmitting them to certain motor mechanisms, determined if the action is reflected, chosen if the action is voluntary').[38] In a passage in the third chapter, dealing with the survival of images, Bergson hypothesizes that, in some cases, the memory of a sensation acts, in relation to a sensation in its nascent state, like the hypnotist who exercises a suggestion; while, in another passage, he takes it for granted that 'maladies infectieuses' ('infectious diseases') often provoke madness.[39] Finally, in the fourth chapter, concerned with the delimiting and fixation of images, we find the passage in which we read that our spirit 'a contracté l'habitude utile de substituer à la durée vraie, vécue par la conscience, un temps homogène et indépendant' ('has contracted the practical habit of replacing true duration, experienced by consciousness, with a homogeneous and independent time');[40] but it should also be noted that, in many of

35 Bergson, *Essai*, p. 73. Other references to endosmosis appear on pp. 75, 143, 149.

36 Bergson, *Essai*, pp. 104, 142.

37 Henri Bergson, *Matière et mémoire*, in *Œuvres*, pp. 159–379 (p. 214).

38 Bergson, *Matière et mémoire*, p. 223.

39 Bergson, *Matière et mémoire*, pp. 278–79, 313.

40 Bergson, *Matière et mémoire*, p. 342.

his writings, Bergson refers several times to the act of contracting a habit[41] (as well as, after all, to the ideas of influence, transmission, and propagation themselves, also in *Matière et mémoire* itself).[42]

To move on to the twentieth century, we can first of all state that in *Le rire* the principle — which is also, as we know, a commonplace — of the contagiousness of laughter is not explicitly theorized; but, also in this text better known than others to the general public, Bergson does not fail to use, in various ways and in different contexts, ideas such as those of suggestion, infiltration, propagation, communication, fascination, and imitation: all ideas which — it is easy to understand — are very close to that of contagion.[43] In the first decade of the century, however, what we find in the *Évolution créatrice* is much more important. In this work that is almost unanimously considered Bergson's masterpiece, in fact, the idea of transmission, in all its significance, plays an absolutely fundamental role in defining what is probably the culminating concept — certainly the most famous — of his philosophy: the *élan vital* ('vital impetus'). Bergson first reviews the main evolutionary theories of his time, from neo-Darwinism to neo-Lamarckism, subjecting them to close scrutiny; he then outlines the contours of a new and original evolutionism, of a theory of evolution that is truly capable of explaining — and, we can certainly add, of adequately celebrating — the powerful creative charge of novelty that accompanies and characterizes life. In this perspective, he rejects the principle, dogmatically understood, of the hereditary transmissibility of acquired characteristics as well as of contracted habits, but he does not at all dismiss the idea of transmission in itself, on the contrary: in fact, it is precisely the *élan vital*, life itself, which passes from one generation of germs to the next, through the highly-developed organisms that are like its carriers. Bergson speaks specifically of a 'courant de vie' ('current of life') which is also a 'courant de conscience' ('current of consciousness') and a 'courant d'existence' ('current of existence'): 'ce courant de vie, traversant les corps qu'il a organisés tour à tour, passant de génération en génération, s'est divisé entre les espèces et éparpillé entre les individus sans rien perdre de sa force, s'intensifiant plutôt à mesure qu'il avançait' ('this current of life, passing through the bodies that it has gradually organized, passing from generation to generation, has divided itself among the species and scattered itself among the individuals, without losing any of its strength, in fact becoming more intense as it advanced').[44] Finally, life is 'un fluide bienfaisant [qui] nous baigne' ('a beneficial fluid [that] bathes us'), 'une onde immense qui se propage' ('an immense wave that spreads'), something — we can conclude — that, just like the virus of a colossal epidemic, or rather of an unstoppable pandemic, spreads everywhere, vivifying and contaminating all beings.[45]

41 See e.g. Bergson, *Essai*, pp. 73 and 141.

42 See Bergson, *Matière et mémoire*, passim.

43 See Henri Bergson, *Le rire*, passim.

44 Henri Bergson, *L'évolution créatrice*, in *Œuvres*, pp. 487–809 (pp. 516, 649, 652).

45 Bergson, *L'évolution créatrice*, pp. 657, 720.

Particular mention should be made of the lecture entitled '"Fantômes de vivants" et "recherche psychique"', which Bergson gave on 28 May 1913 at the Society for Psychical Research in London. In this lecture, the text of which would be published six years later in the collection of essays and lectures *L'energie spirituelle*, Bergson aims, on the one hand, at unmasking the metaphysical prejudice that generates the diffidence, derision, and objections encountered by investigations that deal with psychic phenomena — such as telepathy and the so-called true hallucinations, that is the apparitions of sick or dying people to relatives or friends who are at a great distance — whose actual existence is in fact questioned by many; on the other hand, he argues that these phenomena are in reality of the same kind as those which constitute the object of the natural sciences and that 'recherche psychique' ('psychic research') simply studies them following a method which, compared to that adopted by the natural sciences, is very different. Well, in this real apologia for parapsychology — an apologia which, among other things and as is well known, provoked a lot of criticism of Bergson — there is talk of influence, diffusion, and similar dynamics at different points and at different levels. First of all, in general, the phenomenon of true hallucinations is connected with telepathy, that is to the action that a certain consciousness can exercise on another consciousness, communicating with it without a visible intermediary; and telepathy is compared to electricity: 'Nous produisons de l'électricité à tout moment, l'atmosphère est constamment électrisée, nous circulons parmi des courants magnétiques; pourtant des millions d'hommes ont vécu pendant des milliers d'années sans soupçonner l'existence de l'électricité. Nous avons aussi bien pu passer, sans l'apercevoir, à côté de la télépathie' ('We produce electricity at all times, the atmosphere is constantly electrified, we circulate in the midst of magnetic currents; and yet millions of men have lived for thousands of years without suspecting the existence of electricity. Similarly, we could have passed close to telepathy without noticing it').[46] Then, more specifically, the legitimacy of 'psychic research' would also be justified by the fact that memories which are defined 'de rêve' ('as dreams'), as well as perceptions that are defined as 'inconscientes' ('unconscious'), could creep into consciousness.[47] Once again, the 'empiètement réciproque' ('mutual interpenetration') of our consciousnesses is traced back to the 'échanges' ('exchanges') and 'intercommunication' ('intercommunication') which characterize the aforementioned phenomena of endosmosis.[48] And, lastly, mention is made of 'la thérapeutique par suggestion, ou plus généralement par influence de l'esprit sur l'esprit' ('therapy through suggestion or, more generally, through the influence of the spirit on the spirit').[49] But it can also be added that at the beginning of his lecture, while speaking of the mistrust of official science towards 'psychic research', Bergson notes: 'Rien n'est plus désagréable au savant de profession que de voir

46 Henri Bergson, '"Fantômes de vivants" et "recherche psychique"', in *L'energie spirituelle. Essais et conférences*, in *Œuvres*, pp. 811–977, 860–78 (p. 863).

47 Bergson, '"Fantômes de vivants"', p. 874.

48 Bergson, '"Fantômes de vivants"', p. 874.

49 Bergson, '"Fantômes de vivants"', p. 876.

introduire, dans une science de même ordre que la sienne, des procédés de recherche et de vérification dont il s'est toujours soigneusement abstenu' ('There is nothing more unpleasant for the professional scientist than seeing research and verification procedures — introduced in a science of the same order as his own — from which he has always carefully abstained'); and he concludes, in a succinct way: 'Il craint la contagion' ('He fears contagion').[50] And another passage that may be interesting is found towards the end, when Bergson states that, in the history of science, it is thanks to mathematics that 'le besoin de la preuve s'est propagé d'intelligence à intelligence' ('the need for proof has spread from intelligence to intelligence').[51]

As regards the rest of Bergson's corpus, this work confines itself for the moment to a crucial passage from 'La signification de la guerre', the lecture given by Bergson on 12 December 1914 at the Académie des Sciences morales et politiques in Paris; and to some passages from *La pensée et le mouvant*, a collection of essays and lectures published in 1934 (especially from the substantial second part of the introduction, entitled 'De la position des problèmes' and dated January 1922). The text of the Académie lecture is undoubtedly the most famous of Bergson's so-called *écrits de guerre* ('war writings'): in it, the ongoing conflict between France and Germany is presented as a momentous, almost metaphysical, clash between civilization and barbarism, moral strength and material strength, spirit and mechanics. At a certain point, in trying to imagine what the questions that Germany had posed on the threshold of the declaration of war must have been, Bergson — through a pressing series of rhetorical questions — envisages the looming extension of German materialism from its homeland to the whole of humanity in terms which, at least in part, do not seem very different from those that could be used to talk about the spread of a disastrous pandemic:

> Qu'arriverait-il si les forces mécaniques, que la science venait d'amener sur un point pour les mettre au service de l'homme, s'emparaient de l'homme pour le convertir à leur propre matérialité? Que deviendrait le monde si ce mécanisme se saisissait de l'humanité entière et si les peuples, au lieu de se hausser librement à une diversité plus riche et plus harmonieuse, comme des personnes, tombaient dans l'uniformité comme des choses? Que serait une société qui obéirait automatiquement à un mot d'ordre mécaniquement transmis, qui réglerait sur lui sa science et sa conscience, et qui aurait perdu, avec le sens de la justice, la notion de la vérité?[52]

---

50 Bergson, '"Fantômes de vivants"', p. 862.

51 Bergson, '"Fantômes de vivants"', p. 877. On Bergson and 'psychic research', see Camille Pernot, 'Spiritualisme et spiritisme chez Bergson', *Revue de l'enseignement philosophique*, 15 (1964), no. 3, pp. 1–23; Thibaud Trochu, 'Bergson et Freud: la "recherche psychique" et l'"exploration de l'inconscient"', in *Bergson et Freud*, ed. by Brigitte Sitbon (Paris: Presses Universitaires de France, 2014), pp. 197–215.

52 Henri Bergson, 'Discours en séance publique de l'Académie des Sciences Morales et Politiques' ('La signification de la guerre'), in *Mélanges* (Paris: Presses Universitaires de France, 1972), pp. 1107–29 (p. 1115): 'What would happen if the mechanical forces, which science had brought to a point to place them at the service of man, took possession of man to convert him to their own materiality? What would the world become if this mechanism took over all of humanity and if peoples, instead of rising freely to

In *La pensée et le mouvant*, on the other hand, the idea of transmission is certainly present in its various aspects. In the first part of the introduction to the book, entitled 'Croissance de la vérité. Mouvement rétrograde du vrai' and undated, Bergson writes: 'Nous transmettons aux générations futures ce qui nous intéresse, ce que notre attention considère et même dessine à la lumière de notre évolution passée' ('We pass on to future generations what interests us, what our attention considers and also shapes in the light of our past evolution').[53] In the above-mentioned second part of the introduction, we find a reference to the 'transmission héréditaire' ('hereditary transmission') of what is innate; we are warned that 'il ne faut pas croire que la vie sociale soit une habitude acquise et transmise' ('we must not believe that social life is an acquired and transmitted habit'); we read that 'le langage transmet des ordres ou des avertissements' ('language transmits orders or warnings').[54] While, at the beginning of 'La perception du changement' (a text that brings together two lectures held at the University of Oxford between 26 and 27 May 1911), Bergson expresses his gratitude towards the institution that has invited him, describing it as 'un des rares sanctuaires où se conservent, pieusement entretenues, transmises par chaque génération à la suivante, la chaleur et la lumière de la pensée antique' ('one of the rare sanctuaries in which the warmth and light of ancient thought are preserved, maintained with devotion, transmitted from one generation to the next').[55] But in the second part of the introduction there are still two points that are worth dwelling on. In the first place, the phenomenon of endosmosis — which, as we have seen, is the object of frequent references when Bergson wants to allude to the interaction between consciousnesses — is even, so to speak, removed from the sphere of relevance of physical chemistry and delivered without mincing words to that of psychology: 'La sympathie et l'antipathie irréfléchies, qui sont si souvent divinatrices, témoignent d'une interpénétration possible des consciences humaines. Il y aurait donc des phénomènes d'endosmose psychologique' ('The unreflective sympathy and antipathy, which are often diviners, testify to a possible interpenetration of human consciousnesses. There would therefore be phenomena of psychological endosmosis').[56] And, in the second place, to respond to the criticism made by Julien Benda, who had accused his philosophy of being a 'justification de l'instabilité' ('justification of instability') inasmuch as it saw in the 'permanence de la substance' ('permanence

a richer and more harmonious diversity, like people, fell back into uniformity like things? What would a society be that automatically obeyed a mechanically transmitted watchword, that regulated its science and conscience on that watchword, and that had lost, together with the sense of justice, the notion of truth?'. Among the studies worth citing, which deal with Bergson's *écrits de guerre*, apart from the fundamental Philippe Soulez, *Bergson politique* (Paris: Presses Universitaires de France, 1989), there are also the more recent ones: Vincenza Petyx, *Bergson e le streghe di Macbeth. Dagli 'écrits de guerre' a 'Les deux sources de la morale et de la religion'* (Alessandria: Edizioni dell'Orso, 2006); Florence Caeymaex, 'Les discours de guerre (1914–1918). Propagande et philosophie', in *Annales bergsoniennes VII* (Paris: Presses Universitaires de France, 2014), pp. 143–66.

53 Henri Bergson, *La pensée et le mouvant. Essais et conférences*, in *Œuvres*, pp. 1249–1482 (p. 1266).

54 Bergson, *La pensée et le mouvant*, pp. 1298, 1320, 1321.

55 Henri Bergson, 'La perception du changement', in *La pensée et le mouvant*, pp. 1365–92 (p. 1366).

56 Bergson, *La pensée et le mouvant*, p. 1273.

of substance') nothing other than a 'continuité de changement' ('continuity of change'), Bergson formulates the following paradox: 'Autant vaudrait s'imaginer que le bactériologiste nous recommande les maladies microbiennes quand il nous montre partout des microbes' ('We might as well imagine that the bacteriologist is recommending diseases deriving from microbes when he shows us microbes everywhere').[57]

4. Between 'Psychic Contagion' and Moral Imitation

This, albeit partial and concise, reconnaissance of Bergson's corpus may perhaps be sufficient to be able to say that in it, due to the recurring use of terms and concepts such as those — among others — of influence, diffusion, and transmission (but also because of some, more or less occasional, references to infectious pathologies), the idea of contagion — although understood in a rather broad sense — is markedly present (and is on several occasions strictly functional to the development of reflection). But there is more. In some ways, in fact, it can be said that Bergson is included, with his originality, in the line of studies on 'psychic contagion' — in the social sphere — which has already been mentioned in the opening section.

There are several authors who, at the end of the nineteenth century, gave an impetus to this line of studies.[58] Let's just consider a few of them. In *Les lois de l'imitation* (1890), his best known work, Gabriel Tarde argues that all human societies are based on the principle of imitation, which consists in a phenomenon of suggestion, in an assimilation of innovations that is the fruit of the action at a distance exerted by one mind on another, in a repetition which is simultaneously a multiplication, in a real contagion that spreads following a geometric progression (and, to further clarify its nature, he also speaks — as well as, in fact, of contagion — of hypnotism, sympathy, fascination, magnetization, polarization...).[59] It is in *Folla delinquente* (1891) that the Italian Scipio Sighele identifies in imitation, understood as a natural instinct, the origin of what can be called the 'anima della folla' ('soul of the crowd'); and specifies that, if this imitation occurs at an unconscious level, it can certainly be explained — as others have already done — with the notion of 'contagio morale' ('moral contagion'), provided that — however — it is recognized that the latter has a physical basis in the reflective receptivity of the psyche, that is, in a form of suggestion that recalls fascination and hypnotism and which, if it concerns not one but many individuals, generates real epidemics.[60] And Gustave Le Bon, in a widely-read work, *Psychologie des foules* (1895), writes that, when a person wants to sway the crowd and induce it to perform certain actions, if there are favourable circumstances and if he has sufficient prestige, he only has to rely on example; but, otherwise, he must resort to

57 Bergson, *La pensée et le mouvant*, p. 1328. Bergson is referring to Julien Benda, *Une philosophie pathétique* (Paris: Cahiers de la quinzaine, 1913), pp. 80–81.

58 For further discussion of links between crowd psychology and contagion in the late nineteenth century, see section 3 of chapter 10 of this volume.

59 Gabriel Tarde, *Les lois de l'imitation. Étude sociologique* (Paris: Alcan, 1890), esp. pp. 82–98.

60 Scipio Sighele, *La folla delinquente* (Milan: La Vita Felice, 2015), esp. pp. 27–54.

the obsessive repetition of particular and peremptory statements, thus triggering the unnatural mechanism of contagion, which reduces the individual to the condition of the hypnotized person in the hands of the hypnotist: in fact, ideas, emotions, and beliefs are, if spread among crowds, as contagious as microbes.[61] It is then hardly necessary to say that Freud, in *Massenpsychologie und Ich-Analyse* (1921) also dealt with 'psychic contagion' in the social sphere: starting from the text of Le Bon, the founder of psychoanalysis refutes that in order to explain the behaviour of the individual in a throng it is necessary to hypothesize the existence of a psychic entity free from the drives studied by individual psychology; and in particular, considering the conceptual categories of suggestion, imitation, and contagion unsatisfactory, he prefers to resort instead to the notion of *libido*, in the belief that both the essence of the subjective psyche and that of the so-called collective psyche must be sought in love relationships and in emotional ties.[62]

Bergson was well acquainted with and appreciated the theories of social imitation of Tarde, whom he succeeded as holder of the chair of Modern Philosophy at the Collège de France. In fact, he stated in the speech he gave on 12 September 1909, on the occasion of the inauguration of a monument dedicated to him: 'Sans doute, les sociétés humaines sont traversées par des courants; mais à l'origine de chaque courant il y a une impulsion, et l'impulsion vient d'un homme' ('Without a doubt, human societies are crossed by currents; but at the origin of each current there is an impulse, and the impulse comes from a man'); he then added, along the lines of the analogy between the subjective and collective levels: 'Comme l'histoire de chacun de nous s'explique par les initiatives qu'il a prises et par les habitudes qu'il a contractées, ainsi la vie des sociétés est faite des inventions qui ont surgi ça et là et des modifications durables que ces inventions ont amenées en se faisant adopter' ('Just as the story of each of us is expressed through the initiatives he has taken and through the habits he has contracted, so the life of societies is made up of the inventions that have arisen here and there and of the lasting changes that these inventions have brought about by being adopted'); and finally he exclaims: 'Grande et importante idée!' ('A great and important idea!').[63] He also wrote in the preface to a French anthology of selected pages of Tarde published in the same year: 'L'imitation ne manifeste en effet ni une impulsion mécanique ni même, à proprement parler, une attraction morale. C'est une certaine action *sui generis* qui s'exerce d'esprit à esprit. C'est une certaine contagion psychologique se propageant dans une certaine direction déterminée' ('Actually, imitation does not reveal a mechanical impulse or,

---

61 Gustave Le Bon, *Psychologie des foules* (Paris: Presses Universitaires de France, 2020), pp. 72–76.

62 Sigmund Freud, *Massenpsychologie und Ich-Analyse / Die Zukunft einer Illusion* (Frankfurt a. M.: Fischer, 1993), Chapters 2 and 4. What can be considered an updated version of the line of studies on 'psychic contagion' established itself in the last decades of the twentieth century: see in particular Richard Dawkins, *The Selfish Gene* (Oxford: Oxford University Press, 1976; second edition 1989); Daniel C. Dennett, *Consciousness Explained* (Boston: Little, Brown & Co., 1991); Richard Brodie, *Virus of the Mind: The New Science of the Meme* (Seattle: Integral Press, 1996); Aaron Lynch, *Thought Contagion: How Belief Spreads through Society* (New York: Basic Books, 1996).

63 Henri Bergson, 'Discours sur Gabriel Tarde', in *Mélanges*, pp. 799–801 (p. 800).

properly speaking, a moral attraction. It is a kind of *sui generis* action that is exercised from spirit to spirit. It is a kind of psychological contagion that spreads in a certain determined direction').[64]

But, above all, it is worth remembering here the research on great personalities conducted by William James in the essays 'Great Men, Great Thoughts, and the Environment' (1880) and 'The Importance of Individuals' (1890); as well as the pages dealing with the influence exerted on other men by saints and mystics in the work entitled *The Varieties of Religious Experience* (1902).[65] Bergson refers to the content of this latter work both in the preface to the French translation (1911) of the famous *Pragmatism* of his American friend and correspondent: 'Nous baignons, d'après James, dans une atmosphère que traversent de grands courants spirituels. Si beaucoup d'entre nous se raidissent, d'autres se laissent porter. Et il est des âmes qui s'ouvrent toutes grandes au souffle bienfaisant. Celles-là sont les âmes mystiques' ('We are immersed, according to James, in an atmosphere crossed by great spiritual currents. While many of us stiffen, others let themselves be carried away. And there are souls who are totally open to the beneficial breath. These are the mystical souls');[66] and in the preface to the French translation (1924) of a collection of extracts from the New York philosopher's correspondence: 'Il ne voulait rien sacrifier de l'expérience; et comme il croyait à des courants de réalité multiples, plus ou moins indépendants les uns des autres, se juxtaposant et s'entrecroisant pour faire un "univers pluralistique", il allait les chercher dans les consciences individuelles qui en subissaient l'influence et qui les manifestaient' ('He did not want to sacrifice anything to experience; and since he believed in multiple currents of reality, more or less mutually independent, that became juxtaposed and intersected to create a "pluralistic universe", he went to look for them in the individual consciousnesses that were influenced by them and manifested them').[67]

Now, also on the basis of suggestions like these, Bergson develops his own precise conception of moral exemplarity and the action it exercises on humanity. This conception emerges at various times and in various writings.[68] For example, in the text

64 Henri Bergson, 'Préface', in *Pages choisies* de Gabriel Tarde, in *Mélanges*, pp. 811–13 (p. 812).

65 See William James, 'Great Men, Great Thoughts, and the Environment', *The Atlantic Monthly*, 46 (1880), no. 276, pp. 441–59; Id., 'The Importance of Individuals', *Open Court*, 4 (1890), pp. 2437–40; Id., *The Varieties of Religious Experience. A Study in Human Nature* (Cambridge: Cambridge University Press, 2011), Lectures 14 and 15.

66 Henri Bergson, 'Sur le pragmatisme de William James. Vérité et réalité', in *Œuvres*, pp. 1440–50 (p. 1443).

67 Henri Bergson, 'Préface', in William James, *Extraits de sa correspondance*, in *Sur le pragmatisme de William James* (Paris: Presses Universitaires de France, 2011), pp. 37–43 (pp. 40–41). On Bergson and James, see at the very least Frédéric Worms, 'Bergson et James, lectures croisées', *Philosophie*, 64 (1999), pp. 54–68; *Bergson et James. Cent ans après*, ed. by Stéphane Madelrieux (Paris: Presses Universitaires de France, 2011).

68 On this conception of Bergson, see in particular Maria Teresa Russo, *Esperienza ed esemplarità morale. Rileggere 'Le due fonti della morale e della religione' di Henri Bergson* (Pisa: ETS, 2017); see this book also for its thorough comparison between Bergson's position and that of Tarde, James, and other authors: Chapters 5 and 6.

of the conference 'La conscience et la vie', held at the University of Birmingham on 29 May 1911, he states:

> Supérieur est le point de vue du moraliste. Chez l'homme seulement, chez les meilleurs d'entre nous surtout, le mouvement vital se poursuit sans obstacle, lançant à travers cette œuvre d'art qu'est le corps humain, et qu'il a créée au passage, le courant indéfiniment créateur de la vie morale. L'homme, appelé sans cesse à s'appuyer sur la totalité de son passé pour peser d'autant plus puissamment sur l'avenir, est la grande réussite de la vie. Mais créateur par excellence est celui dont l'action, intense elle-même, est capable d'intensifier aussi l'action des autres hommes, et d'allumer, généreuse, des foyers de générosité.[69]

To give another example from the 1910s, taken from the text of the lecture on George Washington held in the United States on 22 February 1917: 'Il y avait en elles je ne sais quelle des réserves de une force invisible, je ne sais quelle puissance indéfinie de rayonnement. Elles étaient chargées d'une espèce d'électricité qui se propageait comme par induction et qui magnétisait et aimantait tout un peuple' ('There was in them [the deeds and words of extraordinary personalities like those of Joan of Arc and Washington himself] I do not know what reserves of an invisible force, I do not know what indefinite capacity for reasoning. They were charged with a kind of electricity that spread by induction, magnetizing and attracting an entire people').[70] But it is in the *Deux sources de la morale et de la religion* (1932), the work in which Bergson extends his reflection to the sphere of the life of man in society, that the idea of the diffusion as if by contagion of a superior ethical-religious message finds its most complete and detailed formulation. The bearer of this message is above all the figure of the mystic and, in particular, of the Christian mystic. Already in the first chapter, the reason why the saints have so many imitators and the great propagators of good manage to influence entire crowds into following them is identified in the appeal exercised by their own existence, an existence in which the mystics permit the flow of a beneficial flux that 'à travers eux' ('through their person') tends to win other men and that takes the form of an outburst of love: 'amour qui pourra aussi bien se transmettre par l'intermédiaire d'une personne qui se sera attachée à eux ou à leur souvenir resté vivant, et qui aura conformé sa vie à ce modèle' ('love which can equally be transmitted through another person tied to them or to their surviving memory, and that has modelled his life on theirs').[71] However, it is in

---

69 Henri Bergson, 'La conscience et la vie', in *L'energie spirituelle*, pp. 815–36 (pp. 833–34): 'The point of view of the moralist is superior. Only in man, and especially in the best of us, does the vital movement unfold without obstacles, launching the infinitely creative current of moral life through that work of art that is the human body, which the vital movement itself has created in passing. Man, constantly called to base himself on the totality of his past in order to have greater weight in the future, is life's great success. But the creator par excellence is the one whose action, intense in itself, is also capable of intensifying the action of other men, and generously igniting clusters of generosity'.

70 Henri Bergson, 'Conférence du 22 février 1917: Anniversaire de Washington devant l'American Club' ('L'éloge de G. Washington'), in *Correspondances* (Paris: Presses Universitaires de France, 2002), pp. 715–20 (p. 715).

71 Henri Bergson, *Les deux sources de la morale et de la religion*, in *Œuvres*, pp. 979–1247 (pp. 1003, 1059–60).

the third chapter — in which there are also, among other things, references to the magnetization and the suggestion caused by hypnosis — that attention is focused precisely on Christian mysticism, on the current of life and love that arises from it, as well as on its means of propagation.[72] And the fourth chapter, in which Bergson again dwells on the diffusion of Christian mysticism, ends with some pages dealing with phenomena — such as 'manifestations télépathiques' ('telepathic manifestations') or those on account of which 'quelque chose passe' ('something passes') from the outside to the inside of both the body and the consciousness — which are concerned with that 'psychic research' which had been the subject of a broader discussion in the above-mentioned 1913 conference.[73]

Influence, diffusion, propagation, transmission…: even when dealing with the important theme of moral exemplarity and mysticism, Bergson therefore uses massively, as we have seen him do in several other places in his corpus, what we can call the lexicon of contagion (and, among other things, he often resorts, on this as on other occasions, to the same analogies — from magnetism to hypnosis — to which those who interpret imitation or social manipulation in terms of 'psychic contagion' resort). It seems, then, that even Bergson, like so many others have done, has taken up a mental scheme belonging to the medical-scientific field to use it in his studies; and the objective presence of the idea of contagion in his writings — which scholars have not failed to notice — seems to confirm this.[74] However, there is another quintessentially lexical fact that must not be overlooked. Unlike those who have spoken of 'psychic contagion' (but also those who have spoken of 'contagious magic', of 'contagiousness of the sacred', and so on), that is, unlike those who have clearly stated their debt to the contagion of infectious diseases, Bergson almost never uses the term *contagion* itself, neither with regard to moral and religious imitation, nor the other times in which he draws abundantly from the lexicon that gravitates around the contagion of infectious diseases. And perhaps this is not accidental. Perhaps his case is different. What we see in Bergson, in fact, does not seem, all in all, to be so much — and simply — an indirect, derivative, and metaphorical use of the idea of contagion (as happens, in fact, in all the other authors), as instead the systematic adoption of a theoretical model of the interpretation of both material and spiritual reality (a model consisting of a sort of dynamic of interaction and transfer) which has almost everything in common with the act of contagion in its proper sense, but which — first of all and

---

72 Bergson, *Les deux sources*, pp. 1158, 1164–65, 1168–79.

73 Bergson, *Les deux sources*, pp. 1238, 1243–45. It is also worth bearing in mind that in the second chapter Bergson, in considering studies of ethnology and anthropology, deals extensively with the belief among primitive peoples in a force that spreads in nature and that allows the exercise of influences of various kinds: pp. 1115–29.

74 For example, there are references to the idea of contagion in Bergson in the following recent works: Andrew Hewitt, *Social Choreography: Ideology as Performance in Dance and Everyday Movement* (Durham: Duke University Press, 2005), pp. 100–01; Joshua Gunn, 'Canned Laughter', *Philosophy and Rhetoric*, 47 (2014), no. 4, pp. 434–54 (pp. 436–37); Wesley H. Burdine, 'Feeling Out of Time: Phenomenal Bodies and Temporality in *fin de siècle*' (Ph.D. dissertation, University of Minnesota, 2016), Chapters 1 and 4. See also Luciana Parisi, 'Biotech: Life by Contagion', *Theory, Culture & Society*, 24 (2007), no. 6, pp. 29–52 (pp. 31, 33–36, 47).

independently from this act, whose so-to-speak official denomination (namely, that of *contagion*) actually rarely appears — constitutes an autonomous conceptual structure, characteristic and recurring, of his own thought.[75] And this is a conceptual structure that underpins his philosophical discourse — as we have tried to show, through some examples — whether dealing with consciousness and psychological states, perception and representation, when focusing on the evolution of life, or dealing with so-called paranormal phenomena, and when the time comes to tackle the ethical and religious issue…

If therefore — as it seems — this is the case, that is, if this conceptual structure really exists and is active in Bergson's thought, then the originality of the position of the author of the *Évolution créatrice* is evident: the idea of contagion is not in fact present in his thought as an external element that is called into question to explain certain phenomena, but is a constitutive aspect of it. In other words: a theoretical option that in practice coincides with the idea of contagion is an organic and essential component of Bergson's philosophy. But precisely for this reason we can then say that, in considering Bergson, we are confronted by a very peculiar case — but no less significant, on the contrary — of the presence of the motif of contagion between the late nineteenth and early twentieth centuries.

75 On contagion in a metaphorical sense, see in particular Donald Beecher, 'An Afterword on Contagion', in *Imagining Contagion*, pp. 243–60.

Bibliography

Lucretius, *De rerum natura*, ed. by Cyril Bailey (Oxford: Oxford University Press, 1978).

***

Adair-Toteff, Christopher, '"Methodological Pestilence": Max Weber's Devastating Critique of Stammler', *Max Weber Studies*, 14 (2014), no. 2, pp. 245–68.

Astell, Ann W., 'Saintly Mimesis, Contagion, and Empathy in the Thought of René Girard, Edith Stein, and Simone Weil', *Shofar*, 22 (2004), no. 2, pp. 116–31.

Bashford, Alison, and Hooker, Claire (eds.), *Contagion: Historical and Cultural Studies* (London and New York: Routledge, 2001).

Beecher, Donald, 'An Afterword on Contagion', in *Imagining Contagion in Early Modern Europe*, ed. by Claire L. Carlin (New York: Palgrave Macmillan, 2005), pp. 243–60.

Benda, Julien, *Une philosophie pathétique* (Paris: Cahiers de la quinzaine, 1913).

Bergson, Henri, *Extraits de Lucrèce*, dixième édition (Paris: Delagrave, undated).

———, *Essai sur les données immediates de la conscience*, in *Œuvres* (Paris: Presses Universitaires de France, 1959; seconde édition 1963), pp. 1–157.

———, *Matière et mémoire*, in *Œuvres* (Paris: Presses Universitaires de France, 1959; seconde édition 1963), pp. 159–379.

———, *Le rire. Essai sur la signification du comique*, in *Œuvres* (Paris: Presses Universitaires de France, 1959; seconde édition 1963), pp. 381–485.

———, *L'évolution créatrice*, in *Œuvres* (Paris: Presses Universitaires de France, 1959; seconde édition 1963), pp. 487–809.

———, 'Le rêve', in *L'énergie spirituelle. Essais et conférences*, in *Œuvres* (Paris: Presses Universitaires de France, 1959; seconde édition 1963), pp. 811–977.

———, *Les deux sources de la morale et de la religion*, in *Œuvres* (Paris: Presses Universitaires de France, 1959; seconde édition 1963), pp. 979–1247.

———, *La pensée et le mouvant. Essais et conférences*, in *Œuvres* (Paris: Presses Universitaires de France, 1959; seconde édition 1963), pp. 1249–1482.

———, 'Sur le pragmatisme de William James. Vérité et réalité', in *Œuvres* (Paris: Presses Universitaires de France, 1959; seconde édition 1963) pp. 1440–50.

———, *Mélanges* (Paris: Presses Universitaires de France, 1972).

———, *Correspondances* (Paris: Presses Universitaires de France, 2002).

———, *Sur le pragmatisme de William James* (Paris: Presses Universitaires de France, 2011).

Brodie, Richard, *Virus of the Mind: The New Science of the Meme* (Seattle: Integral Press, 1996).

Burdine, Wesley H., 'Feeling Out of Time: Phenomenal Bodies and Temporality in *fin de siècle*' (Ph.D. dissertation, University of Minnesota, 2016).

Caeymaex, Florence, 'Les discours de guerre (1914–1918). Propagande et philosophie', in *Annales bergsoniennes VII* (Paris: Presses Universitaires de France, 2014), pp. 143–66.

Camus, Albert, *La peste* (Paris: Gallimard, 2021).

Cariou, Marie, *L'atomisme. Gassendi, Leibniz, Bergson et Lucrèce* (Paris: Aubier Montaigne, 1978).

Carlin, Claire L. (ed.), *Imagining Contagion in Early Modern Europe* (New York: Palgrave Macmillan, 2005).

Céline, Louis-Ferdinand, *Semmelweis* (Paris: Gallimard, 1999).

Cioran, Emil M., *Histoire et utopie*, in *Œuvres* (Paris: Gallimard, 1995), pp. 979–1061.

Conrad, Lawrence I., and Wujastyk, Dominik (eds.), *Contagion: Perspectives from Pre-Modern Societies* (Aldershot: Ashgate, 2000).

Dawkins, Richard, *The Selfish Gene* (Oxford: Oxford University Press, 1976; second edition 1989).

Deleuze, Gilles, and Guattari, Félix, *Mille plateaux. Capitalisme et schizophrénie 2* (Paris: Les Éditions de Minuit, 1980).

Dennett, Daniel C., *Consciousness Explained* (Boston: Little, Brown & Co., 1991).

Durkheim, Émile, *Les formes élémentaires de la vie religieuse. Le système totémique en Australie* (Paris: Presses Universitaires de France, 1990).

Foucault, Michel, *Naissance de la clinique. Une archéologie du regard médical* (Paris: Presses Universitaires de France, 2007).

———, *Histoire de la folie à l'âge classique* (Paris: Gallimard, 2017).

———, *Surveiller et punir. Naissance de la prison* (Paris: Gallimard, 2020).

Frazer, James, *The Golden Bough: A Study in Magic and Religion* (London: Palgrave Macmillan, 1990).

Freud, Sigmund, *Massenpsychologie und Ich-Analyse / Die Zukunft einer Illusion* (Frankfurt a. M.: Fischer, 1993).

García Márquez, Gabriel, *El amor en los tiempos del cólera* (Barcelona: Bruguera, 1985).

Giono, Jean, *Le hussard sur le toit* (Paris: Gallimard, 1995).

Girard, René, *La violence et le sacré* (Paris: Grasset, 1972).

———, 'The Plague in Literature and Myth', *Texas Studies in Literature and Language*, 15 (1974), pp. 833–50.

Givone, Sergio, 'Quando contagioso è il linguaggio', in *Metafisica della peste. Colpa e destino* (Torino: Einaudi, 2012).

Grandone, Salvatore, *Lucrezio e Bergson. La ricezione del 'De rerum natura' in Francia nel XIX secolo* (Rome: Aracne, 2018).

Gunn, Joshua, 'Canned Laughter', *Philosophy and Rhetoric*, 47 (2014), no. 4, pp. 434–54.

Hatfield, Elaine, and others, *Emotional Contagion. Studies in Emotion and Social Interaction* (Cambridge: Cambridge University Press, 1994).

Healy, Patrick, 'The Birthing of Things: Bergson as a Reader of Lucretius', *Footprint*, 8 (2014), pp. 29–39.

Hewitt, Andrew, *Social Choreography: Ideology as Performance in Dance and Everyday Movement* (Durham: Duke University Press, 2005).

James, William, 'Great Men, Great Thoughts, and the Environment', *The Atlantic Monthly*, 46 (1880), no. 276, pp. 441–59.

———, 'The Importance of Individuals', *Open Court*, 4 (1890), pp. 2437–40.

———, *The Varieties of Religious Experience. A Study in Human Nature* (Cambridge: Cambridge University Press, 2011).

Jarcho, Saul, *The Concept of Contagion in Medicine, Literature, and Religion* (Malabar: Krieger, 2000).

Klemperer, Victor, *LTI. Notizbuch eines Philologen* (Berlin: Aufbau-Verlag, 1947).

Le Bon, Gustave, *Psychologie des foules* (Paris: Presses Universitaires de France, 2020).

London, Jack, *The Scarlet Plague* (New York: Macmillan, 1915).

Lucci, Antonio, 'Ansteckung. Plädoyer für eine Ethik der Kontingenz', in *Die Corona-Gesellschaft. Analysen zur Lage und Perspektiven für die Zukunft*, ed. by Michael Volkmer and Karin Werner (Bielefeld: transcript Verlag, 2020), pp. 357–67.

Lynch, Aaron, *Thought Contagion: How Belief Spreads through Society* (New York: Basic Books, 1996).

Madelrieux, Stéphane (ed.), *Bergson et James. Cent ans après* (Paris: Presses Universitaires de France, 2011).

Malaparte, Curzio, *La pelle* (Milano: Adelphi, 2010).

Mann, Thomas, *Der Tod in Venedig* (Frankfurt a. M.: Fischer, 1992).

———, *Der Zauberberg* (Frankfurt a. M.: Fischer, 2003).

Massimilla, Edoardo, 'La "pestilenza metodologica" e la "maledizione del rospo": Max Weber lettore di Gustav Meyrink', *Archivio di storia della cultura*, 31 (2018), pp. 263–72.

Nutton, Vivian, 'The Seeds of Disease: An Explanation of Contagion and Infection from the Greeks to the Renaissance', *Medical History*, 27 (1983), pp. 1–34.

Pagnol, Marcel, *Les Pestiférés* (Paris: Éditions de Fallois, 2020).

Parisi, Luciana, 'Biotech: Life by Contagion', *Theory, Culture & Society*, 24 (2007), no. 6, pp. 29–52.

Pernot, Camille, 'Spiritualisme et spiritisme chez Bergson', *Revue de l'enseignement philosophique*, 15 (1964), no. 3, pp. 1–23.

Petyx, Vincenza, *Bergson e le streghe di Macbeth. Dagli 'écrits de guerre' a 'Les deux sources de la morale et de la religion'* (Alessandria: Edizioni dell'Orso, 2006).

Ranger, Terence, and Slack, Paul (eds.), *Epidemics and Ideas: Essays on the Historical Perception of Pestilence* (Cambridge: Cambridge University Press, 1992).

Rigoni, Mario A., 'Contaminazione totale', in Emil M. Cioran, *Storia e utopia* (Milan: Adelphi, 1982), pp. 147–59.

Russo, Maria Teresa, *Esperienza ed esemplarità morale. Rileggere 'Le due fonti della morale e della religione' di Henri Bergson* (Pisa: ETS, 2017).

Saramago, José, *Ensaio sobre a Cegueira* (Lisbon: Caminho, 1995).

Sighele, Scipio, *La folla delinquente* (Milan: La Vita Felice, 2015).

Snowden, Frank M., *Epidemics and Society: From the Black Death to the Present* (New Haven: Yale University Press, 2019).

Soulez, Philippe, *Bergson politique* (Paris: Presses Universitaires de France, 1989).

Tarde, Gabriel, *Les lois de l'imitation. Étude sociologique* (Paris: Alcan, 1890).

Trochu, Thibaud, 'Bergson et Freud: la "recherche psychique" et l'"exploration de l'inconscient"', in *Bergson et Freud*, ed. by Brigitte Sitbon (Paris: Presses Universitaires de France, 2014), pp. 197–215.

Weber, Max, 'Beitrag zur Werturteildiskussion im Ausschuß des Vereins für Sozialpolitik', in *Max Weber-Gesamtausgabe*, I/12: *Verstehende Soziologie und Werturteilsfreiheit. Schriften und Reden 1908–1917*, ed. by J. Weiß und S. Frommer (Tübingen: Mohr, 2018), pp. 329–82.

Weininger, Otto, *Über die letzten Dinge* (Munich: Matthes & Seitz Verlag, 1997).

Worms, Frédéric, 'Bergson et James, lectures croisées', *Philosophie*, 64 (1999), pp. 54–68.

Concepts and Theories

CARLO BRENTARI

8. Zoonosis

▼ **ABSTRACT** This contribution has two main objectives. The first is to isolate and define a particular trait of the COVID-19 pandemic, namely its zoonotic character, in order to evaluate its importance in relation to other characteristics of this global health crisis. The second is to consider how the widespread awareness of the zoonotic character of the pandemic can change the view that the human species has of itself — its 'perceived identity', so to speak. Finally, we will try to understand whether the relationships, both practical and axiological, that the human species has with non-human animals can be influenced by this identity transformation.

1. Introduction

Like every age of crisis, the contemporary pandemic includes, alongside changes in the historical and material conditions of the human beings involved, certain factors of redefinition of their self-perception. Moreover, since COVID-19 is a global crisis, this redefinition can lead, or at least contribute, to a profound re-signification of the perceived identity of the human species as a whole. Among the different perspectives assumed by philosophers in the history of Western thought, the approach developed by the German philosophical anthropology in the twentieth century is one of the best equipped to grasp changes of this kind. This stream of continental philosophy includes three main thinkers (Max Scheler, Helmuth Plessner, and Arnold Gehlen),[1] as well as two other philosophers (Ernst Cassirer and Susanne Langer) who, at least partially, can be assimilated to it.[2] The interdisciplinary ability of German philosophical anthropology to investigate, on the one hand, the human species as a

1 See Max Scheler, *The Human Place in the Cosmos* (Evanston: Northwestern University Press, 2009); Helmuth Plessner, *Levels of Organic Life and the Human* (New York: Fordham University Press, 2019); Arnold Gehlen, *Man. His Nature and Place in the World* (New York: Columbia University Press, 1988).

2 See Ernst Cassirer, *Gesammelte Werke* (Hamburg: Felix Meiner Verlag, 2001–), XXIII: *An Essay on Man. An Introduction to a Philosophy of Human Culture* (2006); Susanne Langer, *Mind: An Essay on Human Feeling*, 3 vols (Baltimore–London: The John Hopkins University Press, 1983), II.

Epidemics and Pandemics, ed. by Michele Nicoletti and Alessandro Palazzo (Turnhout: Brepols, 2024), pp. 217–234
BREPOLS PUBLISHERS 10.1484/M.STPH-EB.5.136412

natural form of life, spread across the entire surface of the Earth, and, on the other, the variety of its symbolic, cultural, and identity forms of existence can be found in many contemporary authors. One of them is Yuval Noah Harari, as we shall see, who considers the human species as a life form that is wholly natural in its origins and evolution and, at the same time, peculiar in terms of the life forms it has developed through the cultural elaboration of the possibilities offered by the environment.[3]

Moving from this theoretical background, this contribution aims to achieve two key goals. The first is to define and 'isolate' a particular trait of the COVID-19 crisis — i.e., the zoonotic character of the pandemic that triggered it. The second is to study the implications of the zoonotic nature of the pandemic in the two directions we have recognized as pertinent to philosophical anthropology. On the one hand, we will discuss its transformative potential towards human identity, with particular regard to the possibilities of changing the image humans have of themselves and of modifying their axiological reference points; on the other, we will try to unearth some concrete environmental and bioethical implications of this transformation process of the anthropological identity. The multifaceted relationship between human beings on the one side, and non-human animals on the other, will be our guiding thread in this recognition of the contemporary self-perception and experience of the world.

2. Definition and First Approach to the Topic

Zoonoses are 'human infectious diseases caused by pathogens shared with wild or domestic animals'.[4] According to a monographic issue that *The Lancet* dedicated to the topic in 2012, more than 60% of infectious diseases affecting humans derive from pathogens we share with domestic or wild animals.[5] In addition to COVID-19, these diseases include rabies, Ebola haemorrhagic fever, HIV (at its first appearance), toxoplasmosis, severe acute respiratory syndrome (SARS), type A influenzas, Rift Valley fever, and many others. The pathogens that cause them are often enzootic (i.e., permanently present) in animal populations. After their transversal passage in the human species — an event called cross-species transmission, or spillover — they can become endemic in the human species or disappear after short periods. This depends on many factors, which range from the level of transmissibility inside the human species to the duration of the asymptomatic incubation period (in the case of COVID-19, both factors favour the circulation of the pathogen on a global scale). A relevant element of zoonoses is the presence of vectors, i.e., organisms that transmit the pathogen from the animal population in which it is enzootic to humans. Based on this criterion, zoonoses can be divided into vector-borne and non-vector-borne diseases. To the former belong malaria, dengue, Lyme disease, and many other

3 Yuval N. Harari, *Sapiens. A Brief History of Humankind* (London: Vintage, 2019).

4 William B. Karesh and others, 'Zoonoses 1. Ecology of Zoonoses: Natural and Unnatural Histories', *The Lancet*, 380 (2012), pp. 1936–45 (p. 1936).

5 Karesh and others, 'Zoonoses 1. Ecology', p. 1936; see also Kate E. Jones and others, 'Global Trends in Emerging Infectious Diseases', *Nature* 451 (2008), pp. 990–94.

pathologies; to the second AIDS, Ebola, COVID-19, and others. Both types of zoonoses can result in endemic diseases — for the diseases of the first group, when their vectors are very common and/or difficult to eradicate; for those belonging to the second group, when the pathogens that cause them develop a high human-to-human transmission capacity. Zoonoses can arise from pathogens belonging to all *taxa* that can enter *Homo sapiens*' microbiome: viruses, bacteria, fungi, protozoa, etc. Those that evolve into pandemics, however, are mainly due to viruses.[6]

From this first description, it is clear that zoonoses must be understood as inter-specific processes involving at least two life forms (the pathogen and the host); in many cases, however, the biological species involved are three: the pathogen, the vector, and the host. Therefore, since it seeks to grasp the complexity of living systems, the ecological perspective proposes itself as a valid stance for studying zoonoses; not surprisingly, the term 'eco-epidemiological' is rapidly spreading in the specialized literature on zoonoses.[7] On the epistemic level, an initial consequence is that an adequate consideration of the phenomenon has to rest on the awareness that, inside an ecosystem, the effects of every intervention are often non-linear and difficult to predict (see below, in section 4.3.1, the discussion of a particular kind of zooprophylaxis involving human intervention on the interspecies balance). Furthermore, the eco-systemic consideration of zoonotic diseases is particularly relevant since it requires the assessment of the impact of a particular type of host, i.e., humans, on the rest of the ecosystem. Many cases of zoonosis are, in fact, linked to the form taken by the human activities of gathering, breeding, or transforming natural resources. As we shall see, the mosaic-like deforestation of tropical forest areas, in order to make room for crops, creates the ideal situation for contact between wild animals (such as bats) and domestic animals, which then transmit the pathogens to humans.[8] To give another example, the use of antibiotics in intensive farming has a selective effect on the pathogens, which, therefore, reach the human beings in variants that are already resistant to drugs.[9]

Alongside the medical and eco-systemic perspectives (and closely intertwined with them), a third standpoint is involved in understanding zoonoses: the perspective of the humanities (where we include history, cultural anthropology, geopolitics, and geo-sociology). The humanities are particularly fruitful when it comes to understanding the conditions of the transformation of a local zoonosis into a pandemic. A particularly clear and effective example of the contribution these disciplines can make to the study of zoonoses is David Quammen's account of the origins of the AIDS

6 Stephen S. Morse and others, 'Zoonoses 3. Prediction and Prevention of the Next Pandemic Zoonosis', *The Lancet*, 380 (2012), pp. 1956–65 (pp. 1957–58).

7 Huai-Yu Tian and others, 'How Environmental Conditions Impact Mosquito Ecology and Japanese Encephalitis: An Eco-epidemiological Approach', *Environment International*, 79 (2015), pp. 17–24; Elvira Matassa, *Zoonosi e sanità pubblica. Un approccio interdisciplinare per un problema globale* (Milano: Springer Italia, 2017), pp. 11–13.

8 David Quammen, *Spillover. Animal Infections and the Next Human Pandemic* (London: Vintage Books, 2013), p. 157.

9 Karesh and others, 'Zoonoses 1. Ecology', p. 1940.

pandemic. Relying on research by Michal Worobey and others,[10] Quammen identifies — in a biopsy report from 1908 — the first evidence of the presence of HIV-1 in the population of Kinshasa. Research on primates shows that the primary source of HIV-1 was probably a chimpanzee; the spillover did not need vectors (HIV-1 is not a vector-borne disease) and it probably occurred by direct contact between the blood of a chimpanzee killed for food and a wounded human being (possibly a hunter). Where the humanities step in is not here, but in understanding what happened later, between 1908 and the global diffusion of AIDS in the 80s. With an anthropologist's viewpoint, Quammen highlights the role of the transformation of the practice of prostitution from forms similar to concubinage (which were traditional in Congolese society) to the commercialization of sex on a large scale in the second half of the twentieth century. This transformation, in turn, relies on the urbanization model resulting from the previous colonial history in Congo and Cameroon. Other factors in Quammen's account can be approached through the humanities: the mass health policies carried out by the colonial authorities between 1921 and 1959, which aimed to fight trypanosomiasis and venereal diseases but led to the common practice of the re-use of syringes;[11] in the 1960s, as a consequence of the decolonization process, the presence in Congo of Haitian teachers, who later returned to Haiti carrying the virus with them; and finally, the Haitian migration towards the United States. Although some passages remain incomplete and the discussion is still open about the relative weight of the various factors, it is clear that many of the factors that made the HIV-1 a zoonotic pandemic belong to fields such as the history of medicine, the sociology and anthropology of sexuality, colonial and post-colonial studies, migration studies, etc.

3. Philosophical-Anthropological Implications

This paper arises from the conviction that also philosophy, and in particular, philosophical anthropology, can make a valuable contribution to the understanding of some key aspects of zoonoses, and especially of the COVID-19 pandemic. These aspects are mainly linked to transformations in the identity of such subjects (the human beings) that can experience the pandemic also on a symbolic level. This pandemic, in other terms, is a crisis that has to be not only medically overcome, but understood as a possible self-perception shift. In the following two sections I will try to highlight two COVID-related fracture lines in the identity of contemporary human beings.

---

10 Michael Worobey and others, 'Direct Evidence of Extensive Diversity of HIV-1 in Kinshasa by 1960', *Nature*, 455 (2008), pp. 661–64.

11 Here the author refers to Jacques Pepin and Annie-Claude Labbé, 'Noble Goals, Unforeseen Consequences: Control of Tropical Diseases in Colonial Central Africa and the Iatrogenic Transmission of Blood-borne Diseases', *Tropical Medicine and International Health*, 13. 6, (2008), pp. 744–753.

3.1. Species Identity

The first question to tackle is what kind of identity we are dealing with. We are not referring to a hypothetical ontological basis, or essence of identity, which would be the substratum for other personality traits (according to the metaphysical model of the soul). The perspective adopted here is rather a pragmatic one. We will consider as the core of the personal identity the trait (or traits) of the self that the individual *perceives* as characterizing what (s)he is. This kind of re-perceived identity is what human beings try to grasp and define when faced with the question 'who are you?' — a question that, albeit fundamental on the existential level, does not necessarily imply a metaphysical theory on the general essence or basis of identity. In her/his spontaneous response to this question, each human being will usually privilege one of the many possible layers of identity: be that familiar, professional, national, or religious. Even in the dimension of perceived identity, indeed, there can be hierarchies, based on the individuals' familiar and cultural context and on the biographical events experienced by them. Even inside a model of identity in which the traits of the self are free from ontologically fixed hierarchical relationships, there are some traits that exert hegemony and others that are rather subordinate. In other words, in the answer to the question 'who are you', one identity layer plays the role of a substratum for the others (it is one thing to answer, 'I am a Protestant German'; another is 'I am a German Protestant').

On the basis of this model, in which personal identity is seen as a biographical construction that freely employs the materials of the self- and world-experience, our focus falls on the fact that, among the many possible layers of identity, there is also our identity as a biological species. Most people are aware they belong to the *Homo sapiens* species; some also know that *Homo sapiens* is not the unique species within the genus *Homo* but coexisted, to limit ourselves to two examples, with *Homo neanderthaliensis* up to 30,000 and with *Homo floresiensis* up to 13,000 years ago. This layer, however, rarely rises to the status of supporting core of the lived identity — that hegemonic substratum that, in answering the question 'who are you?', bears the other qualifications. In most cases, species identity remains in the background of personal identity and does not exert any influence on individual choices, which are largely entrusted to other layers and value networks (familiar background, cultural traditions, religious affiliations, etc.). Religion, in particular, continues to be an influential source of meaning, to which many people refer, at different levels of self-awareness, in seeking the answer to questions of identity. In the traditional paths of identity construction, in other words, the awareness of belonging to the *Homo sapiens* species remains abstract and inactive; it does not become a source of values and purposeful behaviours. The kind of challenges human beings have to face today, however, demands not only a sober and scientific consideration of the place of *Homo sapiens* in the ecosystem but also the placement of the species identity into the core of contemporary personal identity.

3.1.1. On the Notion of the Immune Self

In order to define the approach we have chosen, it is appropriate to make two clarifications. The first one is the distinction between the proposal of the integration of the species identity into personal identity and the notion of the immune self, much discussed in the last fifty years in philosophy of biology and philosophical anthropology.[12] The notion of the immune self is based on the analogy between personhood, or selfhood, and the immune system; this analogy aims to propose a view of personal identity as a holistic and self-organized system for the selective inclusion of alterity. In reality, depending on the different authors, the notion includes both aspects: microbiome, and the symbolic and value elements of the personality. The self, in other words, is seen as a dynamic filter of external forces and elements, both at the microbiological level, and at the level of personal identity.

It is interesting to note that the elaboration of this position also requires a reinterpretation of the functions of the immune system itself — which appears now as a sense organ, capable to discriminate and 'decide' what has to be included in the self.[13] The main task of the immune system, in other words, is no more the 'insular' defence against external pathogens, but the institution and preservation of a healthy microbiome, of a dynamic internal ecology. Given that microorganisms very often come from other biological species, it follows that the microbiological part of the self is zoonotic by nature. In their synthetic reconstruction of this shift of paradigm, at least as far as continental philosophy of biology is concerned, Bartlomiej Swiatczak and Alfred Tauber move from Claude Bernard's 'insular construct' of the organism's immune system; according to the authors, Bernard's 'depiction of the immune self as disconnecting the organism from its surroundings harmonized with a particular Western cultural experience of seeing "ourselves as entities, separate from the rest of the world — as containers with insides and outsides"'.[14] On the basis of the common opposition towards the overestimation of the organism's separation, Swiatczak and Tauber identify a series of authors whose arguments seriously affect the model of 'insularity and autonomy'.[15] Some of them (Michel Foucault, Susan Sontag, Donna Haraway, Giorgio Agamben, Roberto Esposito, and Peter Sloterdijk) pursue the intent of a postmodern deconstruction of subjectivity; others, less known, try to re-centre on relationality the contemporary philosophy of biology (Richard Lewontin, Gérard Eberl, Angelina M. Bilate, and Juan J. LaFaille;[16] to the aforementioned

12 See Alfred I. Tauber, *The Immune Self. Theory or Metaphor?* (Cambridge: Cambridge University Press, 1994).

13 Enzo Soresi, *Il cervello anarchico* (Milano: UTET, 2013), p. 48.

14 Bartlomiej Swiatczak and Alfred I. Tauber, 'Philosophy of Immunology', *The Stanford Encyclopedia of Philosophy*, ed. by Edward N. Zalta, available at https://plato.stanford.edu/archives/sum2020/entries/immunology/ (last accessed 11/09/2021). For the internal quote see George Lakoff and Mark Johnson, *Metaphors We Live By* (Chicago-London: University of Chicago Press, 1980), p. 58.

15 The hendiadys recurs several times in Swiatczak and Tauber, 'Philosophy of Immunology'.

16 For a concise review of the most relevant publications of the mentioned authors, from the point of view of the immune self theory, see the 'Bibliography' section in Swiatczak and Tauber, 'Philosophy of Immunology'.

authors Lynn Margulis should be added, due to her relevance in evolutionary studies on symbiosis and the intraorganic biome)[17].

If the reinterpretation of the function of the immune system (from insularity to the management of the organism's internal ecology) is scientifically valid,[18] the recourse to the concept of the immune self to think about personal identity must, however, be taken with caution. On the one hand, we must be aware that, at least in the twentieth century if not earlier, many other relational conceptions of identity had already been proposed; think only of Didier Anzieu's *The skin-ego* (1985), in which the self was compared to another dynamic system managing the interchange with the outside: the skin.[19] On the other hand, it should not be forgotten that a theory of personhood linked to the model of the immune system remains based on a metaphor, or, at best, on an analogical transposition;[20] it is, therefore, exposed to many epistemological risks. With regard to the ontological specificity of its fields of application, the main risk of this notion remains that of a leap in level: a category that is valid at a physiological and intraorganic level cannot be transposed directly to identity dynamics of a political, social, or cultural kind.[21] Ultimately, a greater awareness of the immune components of identity can prepare, integrate, or strengthen the self-perception in terms of species identity, but it cannot be its core.

3.1.2. *Against Reductionism*

The second clarification of the approach we are putting forward here is about the way we can refer to the species *Homo sapiens* in the making of personal identity. What needs to be clarified is whether the foundational reference to the species identity in the construction of personal identity does, or does not, hide reductionist intentions. Following the reflection of Nicolai Hartmann, we can understand by reductionism the tendency to see in the processes of a determined level of reality 'nothing but' derivative, or epiphenomenal forms of lower level processes.[22] In the case of the

---

17 Lynn Margulis, *Symbiosis in Cell Evolution: Microbial Communities in the Archean and Proterozoic Eons* (New York: W.H. Freeman, 1993).

18 This is shown by the promising developments in the medical field of fecal transplantation; see, in this regard, Yosuke Kurashima and Hiroshi Kiyono, 'Mucosal Ecological Network of Epithelium and Immune Cells for Gut Homeostasis and Tissue Healing', *Annual Review of Immunology*, 35 (2017), pp. 119–47.

19 Didier Anzieu, *The Skin-ego* (London: Karnak Book, 2016).

20 This epistemological problem was clearly outlined already at the beginning of the debate on the notion of the immune self; see Alfred I. Tauber, *The Immune Self. Theory or Metaphor?* (Cambridge: Cambridge University Press, 1994).

21 The initiator of the debate, Alfred Tauber, shows that he is well aware of this problem in Alfred I. Tauber, 'Immunity in Context: Science and Society in Dialogue', *Theoria: An International Journal for Theory, History and Foundations of Science*, 31. 2 (2016), pp. 207–24. From the epistemological point of view, Nicolai Hartmann's idea of the ontological autonomy of the different layers of being remains central here, especially in the transitions from the organic to the psychic layer and from the latter to that of social and cultural formations; see C. Brentari, 'The Role of the Missing Reason: the Search for a Stratum-Specific Form of Determination in Nicolai Hartmann's Theory of Life', in *New Research on the Philosophy of Nicolai Hartmann*, ed. by Keith Peterson and Roberto Poli (Berlin-Boston: De Gruyter, 2016), pp. 65–80.

22 Nicolai Hartmann, *New Ways of Ontology* (Chicago: Henry Regnery Company 1953), p. 89.

reference to species identity, many possibilities of reductionism open up: first the idea (typical of the Darwinism of the late nineteenth and early twentieth centuries, but certainly not of contemporary evolutionism) that every species-specific trait has to be directly functional to the survival and reproduction of the members of the species. This is not the right place to outline the process of thought by which evolutionism overcame the naive functionalism of its first phase. It is enough to remember that concepts such as Susanne Langer's 'tolerant evolution'[23] or Stephen Jay Gould's 'exaptation'[24] allow us to think about the spaces of autonomous development that evolution grants to biological species. In this perspective, language, imagination, culture, art, rituals, and the search for sense of philosophers and scientists, etc., appear as the particular path that the species *Homo sapiens* has taken to interact with its environment — a natural expression of cognitive biodiversity which, in addition to allowing survival in even very hostile sectors of the planetary environment, opens up wide spaces for further knowledge and self-expression. In short, the possible traits of the species identity may include a wide range of cognitive, cultural, and ethical elements — in stark opposition to the narrative of the survival of the species at the expense of other species and the environment. The contact with a nature as intact as possible, for example, is felt by an increasing number of individuals as a species-specific need — not a condition for 'survival', nor a nostalgic ideal, nor even a mere opportunity for recreation or 'elevation', but a crucial part of our being human.

3.2. COVID 19 and Species Identity

If it is clear that the proposed integration of species identity into personal identity does not aim at placing — as a founding value — the mere survival of the species, it is also evident that this re-orientation of identity will not be free from conflicts of other kinds. The aforementioned re-centring of the layers of personal identity around a new pole of hegemony, in fact, does not happen without individual and collective resistances. While the acute phase of the pandemic was underway, for instance, religious rites involving a lowering of the level of distancing (such as the bathing in the Ganges or the mutual shaking of hands in the Catholic rite) suddenly appeared in a different light. Under the pressure of prevailing collective interests, priorities were revised, and the health of the population overcame the symbolic and eschatological value of the rite — relativizing, in this way, the commonly assumed superiority of the values to which religious rites refer. The axiological alternative between the categories of 'health' and 'salvation' was shown in clear terms, for many for the first time.[25]

Obviously, not only religious rites become problematic in times of pandemics — think only of the social practice of political voting. For our analysis of identity

23 Langer, *Mind* II, p. 400.

24 Stephen Jay Gould, *Challenges to Neo-Darwinism and Their Meaning for a Revised View of Human Consciousness*, (Cambridge University: Clare Hall, 1984), pp. 66–67.

25 See section 5 of chapter 13 of this volume on how reactions to the pandemic have discredited some religious leaders.

conflicts, however, they are a very interesting case. The traditional claim for absoluteness of the religious dimension (and the consequent perception of rituals as mandatory) clashes with the cogency of anti-COVID regulations. When rites reminiscent of the belief in eternal life, or reincarnation, are suspended to safeguard the health of individuals, the meaning of the rite is relativized; its performative valence, so to speak, wins over its symbolic meaning. This kind of relativization pertains to the core values the rite refers to, which are often hegemonic in the construction of traditional personal identities. Not only that, given the global dimension of the pandemic, people have witnessed the same conflicts between religious-communal life and medical safety in every part of the world. This adds a new dimension to the individual processes of critical thought: if I approve the subordination to the sanitary norms of the rites of others' religions or confessions, I don't feel justified if I oppose the subordination of my rituals to the same prescription. In a long-term perspective, and in a more concrete form than the abstract awareness of religious and cultural plurality, the contemporary experience of the global subordination of the collective practices to the higher cause of the health of the population can stimulate a change in the collective self-perception of practitioners; when faced with the question 'what are humans', people could start to answer 'a species with rites and religions' (it is too early to say, and it is beyond the scope of this contribution, what this turning point might imply with regard to the truth value ascribed to religious beliefs).

Being an infection of zoonotic origin, COVID-19 can significantly strengthen the awareness of the (risky) closeness of human to non-human life forms. This awareness, in turn, is one of the possible ways of re-centring human self-perception around species identity. And, if species identity moves to the core of the self, a deep redefinition of the axiological priorities could follow, with a chain effect that may be explosive both inside personal identity, and on the social and cultural level. Self-perception in terms of species identity can imply the acceptance of a whole series of implications and corollaries: the contingency of the presence of humans on the planet Earth, the absence of teleology in hominization, the absence of special projects or destinies that would separate human beings from other life forms and human history from ecology, and the fact that death and extinction are the norm, and duration of life forms rather an exception.

If the anthropological turning point of self-perception in terms of species identity has not yet been achieved, the current pandemic has contributed to one of its preparatory steps, a more concrete awareness of our unity as a species.[26] All over the

26 The German philosopher Jürgen Habermas recently felt the need to begin his analysis of the 'pandemic state of exception' from the firm statement that the Sars-CoV-2-related crisis concerns 'the members of the *homo sapiens* species [*der Species* homo sapiens] [*sic.*] all over the planet Earth' and is a 'war of species vs. species [*eine Kriegsführung von Species gegen Species*]' (Jürgen Habermas, 'Corona und der Schutz des Lebens. Zur Grundrechtsdebatte in der pandemischen Ausnahmesituation', *Blätter für deutsche und internationale Politik*, 66. 9 [2021], pp. 65–78 [p. 65]). Without over-interpreting Habermas' text, whose focus is not on species identity but on the debate on human rights and the role of the state, it is, however, significant to point out the lexical shift from the term *Gattung* (genus), which Habermas used in previous works (for example, about the implications of biomedical and genetic treatments on the self-understanding

world, people have experienced the same fight against the virus (and, later, against the same variants of the virus). Due to the unprecedented level of global digital interconnection, peoples from different backgrounds have established between their own experience and that of others, not abstract relationships, but precise, immediately transposable correspondences. They have witnessed the advance of the pandemic as one can do with a natural phenomenon on a smaller scale, such as a flood that engulfs neighbouring villages one after another, until it reaches their own. Although with different national and cultural styles and inside different governance systems, people have discussed the same containment measures. On the figurative level, the images of people wearing masks in every part of the world have managed to make concrete the idea of a common challenge that, by its very nature, must be addressed as a species — and without the distractions linked to the supposition of any higher destinations of humanity.

The traits of the pandemics that make of it a key event for the establishment of the species identity are the same that make inappropriate the analogy with war and the World Wars. If it is true that aggression and propensity to war are species-specific traits as well, it is also true that, contrary to the pandemic experience, they tend to build identity upon oppositional units. Using Erik Erickson's terminology, later taken up by Konrad Lorenz, war and intergroup aggression are both a condition and an effect of the human tendency to cultural pseudo-speciation. As we know, pseudo-speciation is a radical form of ethnocentrism that can be found in the self-perception of many pre-modern cultures; it consists in considering the members of one's own human group (a tribe, a nation) as the human species par excellence (in some cases, as among the Inuit, the very name of the population simply means 'humans'). Consequently, the members of other groups are potentially de-humanized. War, in other words, both exploits and enhances the tendency to ideological division and dehumanization of the enemy.

The enormous ethological importance of pseudo-speciation, however, should not lead to neglecting the prefix 'pseudo-' that makes up the term in question. Pseudo-speciation is a cultural analogue of biological speciation, not an unchangeable trait of the human species (that would compel human beings to predetermined behaviours). It affects self-perception, not 'nature', and can therefore be opposed by reinforcing alternative ways of constructing personal and collective identity. In a context of deeply changed global conditions, the tendency towards ethnocentric closure, which proved to be (relatively) effective in the past history of humanity, can be overcome by unifying collective experiences. COVID-19 may well be one of the latter. Some of the factors supporting this thesis have been mentioned above: the immediate transposability of individual experiences on the global scale, the consequent perception of a common task, and the increasing awareness that the challenge has to be faced by humans on the basis of the similarity of their life form.

of human beings), to the term *Species*. See, in this regard, Jürgen Habermas, *Auf dem Weg zu einer liberalen Eugenik? Der Streit um das ethische Selbstverständnis der Gattung*, in Id., *Die Zukunft der menschlichen Natur. Auf dem Weg zu einer liberalen Eugenik? Erweiterte Ausgabe* (Frankfurt a.M.: Suhrkamp, 2002), pp. 34–163.

4. Environmental-Ethical Implications

As discussed above, the ecological perspective is one of the most valid approaches to understanding zoonoses on a scientific level. Moreover, this standpoint offers numerous possibilities for reflecting on the moral implications of the human action towards the other components of the natural world. The assumption of a systemic perspective applied to zoonoses has, in other words, a great relevance for ethical-environmental thought and, in general, for the discipline of the human/animal studies. In this section we will indicate two lines of reflection that ecological analysis of zoonoses can offer.

4.1. The Risks of Mosaic-like Penetration in Wildlife Areas

First, the ecological perspective helps us to rethink the relationship between human animals and the resources of their environment. Many of the aforementioned studies on the spreading of zoonoses stress the role played by the transformations in land-use in the industrial and post-industrial age. As reported by Karesh and others, 'many zoonoses can be linked to large-scale changes in land use that affect biodiversity and relations between animal hosts, people, and pathogens. Land modification, irrespective of reason, changes vegetation patterns, vectors and host species dynamics (e.g., abundance, distribution, and demographics), microclimates, and human contact with domestic and wild animals'.[27] The most favourable situation for the rising of zoonoses is where a growing population makes massive, but unplanned recourse to the resources of a habitat that is still largely intact and rich in biodiversity. The fragmentation of wild nature areas and the formation of mixed zones, in which small and large plots of cultivated land alternate with forest areas of different sizes, creates the ideal situation for humans and domesticated animals to come into contact with the vectors of pathogens (whose primary hosts are frequently wild animals).

To mention a concrete case study, this mosaic-like situation has led to the recrudescence of a particular type of malaria in Malaysia and Borneo. The disease is due to the unicellular parasite *Plasmodium knowlesi*, which belongs to the same subgenus as the more widespread *Plasmodium falciparum*. The parasite infects primarily the long-tailed macaque (*Macaca fascicularis*), the pig-tailed macaque (*Macaca nemestrina*), and the Sumatran surili (*Presbytis melalophos*). Infection occurs through mosquitoes belonging to two species, *Anopheles hackeri* in the Malaysian peninsular and *Anopheles latens* in Sarawak. As reported by Quammen, who refers to Janet Cox-Singh and Balbir Singh's research, the massive transmission of *Plasmodium knowlesi* from the primary hosts to humans is due to the fact that, during the harvest period, the farmers of these areas spend the nights guarding the fields they have opened in the forest, trying to prevent the macaques from plundering them.[28] The increase in the

27 Karesh and others, 'Zoonoses 1. Ecology', p. 1936.

28 Janet Cox-Singh and Balbir Singh, 'Knowlesi Malaria: Newly Emergent and of Public Health Importance?', *Trends in Parasitology*, 24. 9 (2008), pp. 406–10; Quammen, *Spillover*, p. 157.

possibility of zoonoses, therefore, appears as one of the arguments that can be used to oppose unplanned mosaic-like deforestation.

4.2. The Zoonotic Risk in the Historical-Anthropological Evaluation of Agriculture

Second, the ecological and systemic consideration of zoonoses can stimulate a critical reflection on the form of life and the resource management adopted by *Homo sapiens* since the agricultural revolution (about 12,000–9,000 years ago). From James C. Scott's *Against the Grain*[29] to Noah Harari's *Sapiens*, many historians of the prehistoric age are seriously calling into question the traditional description of the passage from the hunter-gatherer phase of mankind, characterized by seasonal displacements over large territories, to the agricultural and urban phase of human history. 'The narrative of this process' — writes Scott programmatically — 'has typically been told as one of progress, of civilization and public order, and of increasing health and leisure. Given what we now know, much of this narrative is wrong or seriously misleading'.[30] Scott and Harari put forward numerous elements in favour of this thesis. The transition to agriculture would have impoverished both the diet and the variety of experiences of the members of the species;[31] agriculture would have led to an increase in the number of populations, but at the same time would have worsened their average state of health and made them more susceptible to diseases;[32] dependence on a single food source (the type of cereal grown) would have exposed human groups to a terrible risk, that of losing stocks and crops due to wars or extreme natural events.[33] Among these elements, the increased danger of zoonosis also plays a prominent role. If it is true that hunting and gathering also involved the possibility of contact with primary hosts and vectors, a lifestyle in close contact with domestic animals and in conditions of poor hygiene seems to have been much more favourable to the onset of diseases of zoonotic origin. Even with today's awareness of the ecological sources of zoonoses, infections due to pathogens' spillover from wild primary hosts to domestic animals, and then to humans, have certainly not ceased. In some cases, the situation is aggravated by the practice of intensive farming, which increases the spread of pathogens among animals and forces farmers to use antibiotic and antiviral drugs —

29 James C. Scott, *Against the Grain. A Deep History of the Earliest States* (New Haven-London: Yale University Press, 2017).

30 Scott, *Against the Grain*, p. 2.

31 Scott, *Against the Grain*, p. 86: 'Is it the case, for example, that like their domesticates, sedentary, grain-planting, domus-sheltered people have experienced a comparable decline in emotional reactivity and are less intently alert to their immediate surroundings?'; Harari, *Sapiens*, p. 58: 'The forager economy provided most people with more interesting lives than agriculture or industry do'.

32 Scott, *Against the Grain*, p. 21: 'A second great and unanticipated burden of agriculture was the direct epidemiological effect of concentration — not just of people but of livestock, crops, and the large suite of parasites that followed them to the domus or developed there'; see Harari, *Sapiens*, p. 60, p. 99.

33 Harari, *Sapiens*, p. 59: 'By not being dependent on any single kind of food, they [*foragers*] were less liable to suffer when one particular food source failed'; see Scott, *Against the grain*, p. 63.

which, as is now known, have among their effects the selection of resistant strains of pathogens.[34]

4.3. New Ways of Thinking about the Relationship between Human and Non-Human Species

This is not the place to propose a solution to the global reduction of the remaining 'wild nature' areas and the increasing invasiveness of human activities on the planet. These phenomena are linked on the one side to the models of economic growth, and, on the other, to the choices made by human beings about parenting; and both issues are too vast to even be sketched. What can be done, following a path opened by Hans Jonas in *The Imperative of Responsibility*,[35] is to show the inadequacy of the way many people still tend to think about the relationship between 'nature' and urbanized areas. As Jonas points out, in the Greek and Roman classic age, the city (including the agricultural area that surrounded it) was seen as an island of 'civilization' — that is: a portion of territory subjected to a high level of human transformation — in the middle of a vast 'sea' of untouched nature. If, on the one hand, this hermeneutic model celebrated the transformative capacity of human beings, on the other it was accompanied by the perception of the city as a fragile entity, constantly threatened by the return of nature (whose great power, after all, couldn't even be scratched by humans).[36] After the industrial revolution, the increase in the transformative power of human technique (a power which reaches as far as the climatic conditions of the Earth), has made this hermeneutic model extremely dangerous. Narratives focused on the conquest of nature — similar to those that nourished the European imagination in the age of the geographic explorations and are still well attested in common sense — often underestimate the extension of the anthropized areas, keeping alive the illusion that, in a not better defined 'elsewhere', there would be wide areas of virgin nature. Moreover, the classical model usually overestimates the self-regenerative capacities of nature, its ability to recover after human interventions, thus hindering the sober and scientific consideration of the damages the latter bring with them.

Today, the model of the pre-modern world is unsuitable for grasping the real relationship between non-human nature and man-transformed areas. On the one hand, global climate change puts in doubt the residual legitimacy of the concept of 'intact' nature. Even if one wants to limit the scope of this concept to areas with a limited impact of human transformative action, still, however, the model Jonas attributes to classicism must be reversed — 'islands', today, are the wilderness areas, that have to be preserved through the concession of a special juridical status. The failure of the nature-culture dichotomy favours models centred on hybridization processes, mosaic-like configurations, species migrations, and interspecies contaminations

34 Karesh and others, 'Zoonoses 1. Ecology', p. 1938, p. 1941.

35 Hans Jonas, *The Imperative of Responsibility. In Search for an Ethics for the Technological Age* (Chicago-London: University of Chicago Press, 1984).

36 Jonas, *The Imperative of Responsibility*, pp. 2–4.

— in short, on various forms of interaction between more-anthropized and less-anthropized ecosystems. The Earth appears as a changing network of territories of different species; due to climate change and human activities, their boundaries are subjected to a constant process of mixing and refusion, which, in many cases, prevents the achievement of long-term equilibria similar to those antecedent to the Anthropocene.

4.3.1. In Praise of Complexity

At this point, many of the threads that run through our reflection on zoonoses intersect. The re-centring of personal self-perception around species identity, in fact, should be accompanied by the awareness of the constant imbalance of contemporary interspecific relationships. Species identity, in other words, must not be considered as a definitive datum — as if there were some unrecognized anthropological features that could give *Homo sapiens* a secure ecological place, thus helping to find the way towards environmental sustainability. On the contrary, the adoption of the species identity perspective makes interspecific coexistence appear in the right light — that is, as a highly complex field. Every action of the human species is a risky intervention in a delicate network of contingent processes, interwoven with causal relationships that should be patiently unravelled before making decisions.

For instance, as remarked by A. Marm Kilpatrick and Sarah Randolph, in the fight against vector-borne diseases, the eradication of the primary hosts (one or more wild species) could appear as a viable solution. Also leaving ethical motivations aside, however, the adoption of the complexity paradigm helps us understand that the outcomes of these wildlife management operations are very uncertain. The decrease in the number of the primary hosts could lead to an increased density of the vectors feeding on each of them, with a possible growth in infections (if the few remaining primary hosts were infected). Likewise, the search for 'dilution effects' through the introduction of new primary host species could have unpredictable outcomes, according to the idea of the ecological cascade effect. As the authors point out, 'feeding on additional alternative hosts sometimes results in increased vector densities, which could result in higher transmission even if a smaller proportion feed on people'.[37] In short, adopting and using an eco-epidemiologic approach, based on the paradigm of interspecific complexity, often means accepting that the outcomes of human interventions may not be linear.[38]

---

37 A. Marm Kilpatrick and Sarah E. Randolph, 'Zoonosis 2. Drivers, Dynamics, and Control of Emerging Vector-Borne Zoonotic Diseases', *The Lancet*, 380 (2012), pp. 1946–55 (p. 1953).

38 The eco-epidemiological approach adopted in this contribution is characterized by a moderate level of holism and by the tendency to see in the human species the only actor capable of planning and adopting long-term strategies of global environmental restoration. Other models, that refer programmatically to James Lovelock and move from the view of the whole planet Earth as a symbiotic and self-regulating system, support more pronounced forms of holism. For a relevant application of this second type of holistic models to COVID-19, see Roberto Cazzolla Gatti and others, 'Diversity lost: COVID-19 as

5. Concluding Remarks

In our analysis, the global experience of COVID-19 zoonosis has shown a great transformative potential towards the identity of human beings and their relationships with other animal species and with the environment. If a leading thread can be identified for the reflections we have put forward, it is the idea of the inversion of the 'axiological sign' of the status of human beings. Traditionally, the fact that human beings belong to a biological species was seen as a starting point to be overcome by history, or as an annoyingly limiting factor to be technically circumvented. The proposal of this contribution is the sober acceptance of the fact that humans are primarily members of the *Homo sapiens* species and that their history arises from a particular way of interacting with the environment: culture, our species-specific biodiversity.

This axiological inversion does not necessarily involve changes in the lines of action to be adopted. The search for treatments and vaccines to oppose zoonoses can continue with the same commitment whether we consider the biological condition and the consequent exposition to cross species pathogens as a limiting condition ('unfortunately, humans are *also* animals'), or whether we place species identity at the core of personal identity. In the face of broader tasks, however, which involve rethinking our way of inhabiting the Earth, the adoption of a species perspective as a hegemonic trait of the person could have decidedly positive effects. To use Arnold Gehlen's anthropological lexicon, humans' identity is mediated by the tasks of the moment; identity should neither be discovered nor defended, but built up in relation to collective needs. In the present moment of the history of *Homo sapiens*, the phase of pseudo-speciation seems to lie behind us; our needs, therefore, appear more clearly as the needs of one species inside an irreplaceable ecological environment. If it is so, then the construction of identity should follow this path, relativizing other layers of identity — the same for which humans, for millennia, have separated into groups and been willing to kill and die. At the present moment, while the pandemic is still running its course, the COVID-19 zoonosis is likely to constitute a species-unifying experience to a much greater extent even than the ecological crisis due to climate change. With regard to the latter, collective reactions range from denial to the search for local solutions, often in the guise of the nationalistic closure towards the outside. This is linked to different factors: the variability of the effects of climate warming (which, on a local scale, can even lead to temporary positive effects for some populations); the different severity with which different countries are affected by it; and the fear of migrations due to climate emergencies, etc. Yet, no perspective would be more adequate towards climate change than the one which stresses our species-specific ability to modify — and, implicitly, to preserve or re-equilibrate — its global environment.

---

a Phenomenon of the Total Environment', *Science of the Total Environment*, 756 (2021); DOI: https://doi.org/10.1016/j.scitotenv.2020.144014 (last accessed 11/09/2021).

Bibliography

Anzieu, Didier, *The Skin-ego* (London: Karnak Book, 2016).

Brentari, Carlo, 'The Role of the Missing Reason: the Search for a Stratum-Specific Form of Determination in Nicolai Hartmann's Theory of Life', in *New Research on the Philosophy of Nicolai Hartmann*, ed. by Keith Peterson and Roberto Poli (Berlin-Boston: De Gruyter, 2016), pp. 65–80.

Cassirer, Ernst, *Gesammelte Werke* (Hamburg: Felix Meiner Verlag, 2001–).

———, *An Essay on Man. An Introduction to a Philosophy of Human Culture* (2006).

Cazzolla Gatti, Roberto, and others, 'Diversity lost: COVID-19 as a Phenomenon of the Total Environment', *Science of the Total Environment*, 756 (2021), https://doi.org/ (last accessed 11/09/2021)10.1016/j.scitotenv.2020.144014

Cox-Singh, Janet, and Balbir Singh, 'Knowlesi Malaria: Newly Emergent and of Public Health Importance?', *Trends in Parasitology*, 24. 9 (2008), pp. 406–10.

Gehlen, Arnold, *Man. His Nature and Place in the World* (New York: Columbia University Press, 1988).

Gould, Stephen Jay, *Challenges to Neo-Darwinism and Their Meaning for a Revised View of Human Consciousness*, (Cambridge University: Clare Hall, 1984).

Habermas, Jürgen, 'Corona und der Schutz des Lebens. Zur Grundrechtsdebatte in der pandemischen Ausnahmesituation', *Blätter für deutsche und internationale Politik*, 66. 9 (2021), pp. 65–78.

———, *Auf dem Weg zu einer liberalen Eugenik? Der Streit um das ethische Selbstverständnis der Gattung*, in Id., *Die Zukunft der menschlichen Natur. Auf dem Weg zu einer liberalen Eugenik? Erweiterte Ausgabe* (Frankfurt a.M.: Suhrkamp, 2002), pp. 34–163.

Harari, Yuval N., *Sapiens. A Brief History of Humankind* (London: Vintage, 2019).

Hartmann, Nicolai, *New Ways of Ontology* (Chicago: Henry Regnery Company 1953).

Jonas, Hans, *The Imperative of Responsibility. In Search for an Ethics for the Technological Age* (Chicago-London: University of Chicago Press, 1984).

Jones, Kate E., and , 'Global Trends in Emerging Infectious Diseases', *Nature* 451 (2008), pp. 990–94.

Karesh, William B., and , 'Zoonoses 1. Ecology of Zoonoses: Natural and Unnatural Histories', *The Lancet*, 380 (2012), pp. 1936–45.

Kilpatrick, A. Marm, and Sarah E. Randolph, 'Zoonosis 2. Drivers, Dynamics, and Control of Emerging Vector-Borne Zoonotic Diseases', *The Lancet*, 380 (2012), pp. 1946–55.

Kurashima, Yosuke, and Hiroshi Kiyono, 'Mucosal Ecological Network of Epithelium and Immune Cells for Gut Homeostasis and Tissue Healing', *Annual Review of Immunology*, 35 (2017), pp. 119–47.

Lakoff, George, and Mark Johnson, *Metaphors We Live By* (Chicago-London: University of Chicago Press, 1980).

Langer, Susanne, *Mind: An Essay on Human Feeling*, 3 vols (Baltimore–London: The John Hopkins University Press, 1983).

Margulis, Lynn, *Symbiosis in Cell Evolution: Microbial Communities in the Archean and Proterozoic Eons* (New York: W.H. Freeman, 1993).

Matassa, Elvira, *Zoonosi e sanità pubblica. Un approccio interdisciplinare per un problema globale* (Milano: Springer Italia, 2017).

Morse, Stephen S., and , 'Zoonoses 3. Prediction and Prevention of the Next Pandemic Zoonosis', *The Lancet*, 380 (2012), pp. 1956–65.

Pepin, Jacques, and Annie-Claude Labbé, 'Noble Goals, Unforeseen Consequences: Control of Tropical Diseases in Colonial Central Africa and the Iatrogenic Transmission of Blood-borne Diseases', *Tropical Medicine and International Health*, 13. 6, (2008), pp. 744–753.

Plessner, Helmuth, *Levels of Organic Life and the Human* (New York: Fordham University Press, 2019).

Quammen, David, *Spillover. Animal Infections and the Next Human Pandemic* (London: Vintage Books, 2013).

Scheler, Max, *The Human Place in the Cosmos* (Evanston: Northwestern University Press, 2009).

Scott, James C., *Against the Grain. A Deep History of the Earliest States* (New Haven-London: Yale University Press, 2017).

Soresi, Enzo, *Il cervello anarchico* (Milano: UTET, 2013).

Swiatczak, Bartlomiej, and Alfred I. Tauber, 'Philosophy of Immunology', *The Stanford Encyclopedia of Philosophy*, ed. by Edward N. Zalta, https://plato.stanford.edu/archives/sum2020/entries/immunology/

Tauber, Alfred I., *The Immune Self. Theory or Metaphor?* (Cambridge: Cambridge University Press, 1994).

———, 'Immunity in Context: Science and Society in Dialogue', *Theoria: An International Journal for Theory, History and Foundations of Science*, 31. 2 (2016), pp. 207–24.

Tian, Huai-Yu, and , 'How Environmental Conditions Impact Mosquito Ecology and Japanese Encephalitis: An Eco-epidemiological Approach', *Environment International*, 79 (2015), pp. 17–24.

Worobey, Michael, and , 'Direct Evidence of Extensive Diversity of HIV-1 in Kinshasa by 1960', *Nature*, 455 (2008), pp. 661–64.

MICHELE NICOLETTI

9. Fear and Dispossession

▼ **ABSTRACT** The pandemic has represented the return of 'large-scale death' on the public scene of the world. This essay analyzes the nexus between fear, society, and politics in general terms and, more specifically, in the time of pandemics. The fear of self-dispossession is identified as a feature common to contemporary societies. The COVID-19 crisis has emphasized this fear and has limited the opportunities for enjoying personal liberties and rights. Within this context, the essay maintains that an important role can be played by a vigorous re-proposal of the principle of 'self-belonging', understood as, on the one hand, the aspiration that one's dignity be respected, and, on the other, that the irreducibility and inviolability of the Self be recognized. This principle can serve as the foundation for not only an existential perspective of the liberty and relationality of the individual, but also a vision of society based upon respect for basic universal rights and a democratic practice which extends from the local to the global level. The principle of self-belonging is seen as an alternative to the authoritarian and paternalistic approaches to the pandemic crisis.

Events related to the Covid-19 pandemic have enormously challenged, and continue to challenge, the preparedness and resilience of present-day societies. Arguably for the first time since World World II, the challenge of a deadly threat has again come to the fore on a global scale. While death can be regarded as an object of a mechanism of psychological repression in modern societies, it has claimed its place back, in particular in the form of 'large-scale death'. For many months, the media has been filled with news regarding the merciless 'countability' of death. To be sure, compared with the Spanish flu of the early twentieth century, figures related to the Covid-19 pandemic have not reached apocalyptic levels thus far. The Spanish flu resulted in a number of deaths reaching the tens of millions (around 50 million, according to some), with a world population totalling 1.8 billion at that point in history. The number of Covid-19 casualties at the time of writing is approximately 6 million with a current population level at 7.7 billion, though the calculation of casualties is fairly

Epidemics and Pandemics, ed. by Michele Nicoletti and Alessandro Palazzo (Turnhout: Brepols, 2024), pp. 235–252
BREPOLS PUBLISHERS 10.1484/M.STPH-EB.5.136413

complex in the Covid context.[1] Still, this is not only a matter of numbers. This is about the phenomenon of 'large-scale death' as such, which has returned to the world's great astonishment.

In the following pages I will attempt to analyze the impact of 'large-scale death' on society and contemporary politics through three steps by looking at: (1) how the pandemic has fuelled a return of fear onto the political stage; (2) how the pandemic and the measures adopted to fight against it have touched on the rights of persons; (3) which kind of principle can be deployed to articulate an idea of democratic politics capable of dealing with the pandemic and with further challenges beyond the health crisis.

1. Death, Fear, and Politics

The Covid-19 pandemic has represented a return of large-scale death at the global level. Before the crisis, people had died 'one by one' as single individuals and, on average, without much clamour. As an individualized and privatized event, death was somehow repressed.[2] During the pandemic, instead, people have died as part of collective entities, and single deaths have been announced publicly as an admonishment and reminder for all. But such announcements have not reminded citizens that everyone 'has' to die; rather, they have reminded them that everyone 'may' die. Death as an anticipated possibility has come back onto the public stage, which has been challenged by such a diffuse, widespread death. Political actors have been confronted with the need to take a public position with respect to death. Some have endeavoured to deny death, others to challenge it, and most to contain it. All three positions have prominent predecessors among past 'negationists', 'agonists', and 'rescuers'.

Contagion has returned as well. Contagion entails that death can be transmitted from one person to another without intention or violence and possibly, conversely, through a simple hug. The possibility of sickness and death crept into human relationships: the other may be a threat, and we can be a threat to the other. Not proximity but distance and distancing have been imposed as a necessary measure. And isolation has thrown many into a condition of anxiety. It is as if the collective unconscious had been carved by the words of Hannah Arendt, who described isolation practices as presuppositions for the obliteration of the public sphere, and thereby for totalitarianism: 'Isolation and loneliness are not the same. I can be isolated — that is in a situation in which I cannot act, because there is nobody who will act with me — without being lonely; and I can be lonely — that is in a situation in which I as a person feel myself deserted by all human companionship — without being isolated. Isolation is that impasse into which men are driven when the political sphere of

1 David Adam, 'The Pandemic's true death toll: millions more than official counts', *Nature*, 601 (2022), pp. 312–15.

2 Geoffrey Gorer, *Death, Grief and Mourning* (London: Cresset, 1965); Philippe Ariès, *Western Attitudes Toward Death: From the Middle Ages to the Present* (Baltimore: Johns Hopkins Univ. Press, 1975); William M. Spellman, *A Brief History of Death* (London: Reaction Books, 2014).

their lives, where they act together in the pursuit of common concern, is destroyed'.[3] There has been a further comeback, the idea that non-human forms of life, such as viruses, can be a real threat to human life. Mankind had tamed and subjugated other beasts and confined them to nature parks. Now there are forms of life that are not subject to human control. Right when the 'Anthropocene' was emerging as a powerful discourse focusing on the absolute centrality of human agency, human hubris has been humbled.[4]

1.1. The return of Fear

The return of death on the public scene has increased the general pessimism about the human condition which stalks the globe from the beginning of the twenty-first century.

People are feeling threatened and therefore afraid. And fear leads them to support the politics of security, of protection — politics, in other words, of closure rather than of openness.

This is not a recent phenomenon related to the Right Wing Populist Parties.[5] Some of the most important figures of Western political thought — Machiavelli, Hobbes, Schmitt, and others — have written at length on the deep — indeed inextricable — connection between politics and the fear of death and on the extent to which the modern State — from its ideologies to its structure — was constructed around this idea. Their ideas remind us that politics is — above all — an association against death and that when our politics cannot effectively protect our material lives there is an inevitable increase in the sense of insecurity and mistrust.

And precisely because there is this deep connection between fear and politics, fear can be instrumentalized. As Friedrich Neumann has shown, there exists both a true anxiety and a neurotic anxiety,[6] the latter generated by imaginary dangers, which are depicted as being devastating. This neurotic anxiety — such as developed during the twentieth century with regard to an imagined 'Jewish conspiracy' — is a 'manufactured' anxiety designed to cause the Ego to regress to a state of such confusion that it feels driven to follow the herd, to identify emotionally with a charismatic leader, and to give up any attempts at the autonomous exercise of reason. The unprecedented condition of the contemporary individual — who suffers from loneliness and the loss of identity and is thus in constant search of connections and of ways in which to reclaim — or recreate — their identity — makes it all the easier to manufacture anxiety.[7]

---

3 Hannah Arendt, *The Origins of Totalitarianism* (New York: Meridian Books, 1958), p. 474.

4 See the remarks on how the pandemic has changed human identity in chapter 8 of this volume.

5 Ruth Wodak, *The Politics of Fear: What Right-Wing Populist Discourses Mean* (New York: Sage, 2015).

6 Franz Neumann, *The Democratic and the Authoritarian State* (New York: Free Press, 1957).

7 On the pandemic's capacity to exacerbate conspiracy thinking, see especially section 4 of chapter 10 of this volume.

Before the pandemic, the typical objects of neurotic anxiety were immigrants and foreigners, who were perceived as threats to the health and safety of our communities. Once again, as when racist ideologies were first emerging in the nineteenth century, some people have spread the idea that the 'decadence' of rich countries is linked to the presence, or arrival, of 'foreigners' who are contaminating our lives, polluting them, poisoning them, that they are carriers of sickness and disease. And once again, a politics of 'hygiene' was being invoked.[8]

The arrival of the pandemic has brought back the real anxiety, generated by the real, mortal threat of the virus. But the neurotic anxiety has not disappeared. On the contrary, the real necessity of physical hygiene has increased the social emphasis on hygiene and society has become a perfect laboratory for new procedures and practices of hygienification. Our anxiety has received a new, 'natural' foundation. And to make matters worse, after the pandemic, the war. The fears have multiplied.

1.2. *The Dispossession of the Self*

Now, after the pandemic, our fears are many, and various. Every continent, social group, and individual has their own particular fears and to imagine otherwise is not just difficult, but a wrong-headed and dangerous simplification. That said, to postulate a common — or at least dominant — thread can, I feel, help us in our discussion.

The contemporary fear of the *dispossession of the self* is — I believe — one such commonality. To conquer the Self has been one of the prime objectives of both Western and Eastern culture throughout the centuries. Although many different methods have been attempted to attain this goal, all share the idea that the realization of one's own true existence and the attainment of happiness are only possible through self-discovery, self-knowledge and self-fulfilment within this life — in other words, in a set of actions that affirm, or negate, or transcend the Self — depending on the particular ethical and philosophical view adhered to. Underpinning all these views is the idea of the conquest of the Self — in other words, possession of the Self. Perhaps it is also because of this constant emphasis on self-knowledge and self-possession as the way to realization in the world that the Ego today seems so uncertain and disorientated, in the face of what it sees as the greatest of all dangers: the dispossession of the Self.

Fear of dispossession assumes different forms: one can be dispossessed of one's body, as happens to so many battered women; the migrants who are raped or violated; all the victims of human trafficking — some of whom have their very organs harvested; to all who are ill and whose lives are prolonged against their will, when they have lost their ability to express their own desires — or whom others allow to die because they are tired of caring for them, or want to get their hands on an inheritance.

8 Michel Foucault, *Il faut défendre la societé*. Cours au Collège de France 1975–1976 (Paris: Gallimard, 1997); Roberto Esposito, *Immunitas: The Protection and Negation of Life*, trans. by Z. Hanafi (London: Polity Press, 2011).

One can be dispossessed of one's wealth, of one's work, of one's future — as is happening to an unthinkable number of young people today. One can be dispossessed of one's identity, one's environment, one's food, language, and traditions, by cynical actors who dominate today's unregulated markets, commodify everything, and homogenize or erase qualities and differences which have no market value. One can be dispossessed of one's dignity, interiority, privacy — invaded by external observers, controllers, watchdogs, or merchants of souls. And one can be frightened of being dispossessed of one's savings — by the banks or by the mysterious machinations of international finance. One can fear being dispossessed of one's land or hard-earned situation in life — dispossessed by the newcomers: the young, or migrants who threaten our right of 'original occupancy' in time and in living space. Then there are the 'parasites', who have never done a day's work, and who envy 'our' prosperity/well-being, and, of course, those inefficient, corrupt governments… We are frightened of being dispossessed of our very right and ability to decide our own destiny and the destiny of our communities — by technology, by bureaucracy, by the State, by Europe, by the international order — by, in fact, any and all of the myriad entities that control our lives from distant places.

It is not an accident that one of the most recurrent themes is that of 'surveillance': from Foucault's surveillance society through to Zuboff's surveillance capitalism, this expression points to a widespread feeling of being observed, controlled, watched.[9] The tracking practices adopted by some governments to detect the trails of contagion have intensified this feeling. And hostility towards vaccination practices has become entrenched due to fear that external agents could be injected into one's body. With respect to the situations of illness as well as vaccination, the human body has been perceived as a place under threat of invasion by external agents.

This has led to a widespread fear and a general retreat into isolationism — people are seeking to protect themselves from external forces and somehow to shield whatever they feel remains of their selfhood — maybe the personal, or family, or tribal, or national self — in the conviction that the world — that history — wants to sweep us all away and that we, every one of us, are in the hands of others.

So, the overriding fear of our times can perhaps be described as a fear of a general dispossession — the fear of being controlled by others. And this fear leaves us gazing out, through sullen, suspicious eyes, at the world around us. Suspicion is the most common reaction to a sense of dispossession: suspicion which spills into interpersonal relationships, of course, but also, above all, poisons the social structure and its institutions, science included.

9 Shoshana Zuboff, *The Age of Surveillance Capitalism. The Fight for the Future at the New Frontier of Power* (London: Profile Books, 2019).

1.3. A Well-worn Theme — Alienation

Nothing new here — in fact, 'dispossession', 'being in the hands of others' are phrases that lead us to a term which we know all too well: alienation. To become disaffected. To belong to others. To be in the hands of the others.

We are dealing with a phenomenon that can be traced throughout most of human history, in both interpersonal and social dynamics: not new and, indeed, somehow integral to the very story of the human spirit, as Hegel's powerful analyses set out to demonstrate.[10] But, according to Hegel, alienation is not only negative — the crushing and deprivation of the human spirit — it is also a time of necessary set-back before which the liberation of the individual, or of a society, cannot take place. An eternal phenomenon, in a certain sense, although in modern — and particularly in capitalist — societies it is unusually pronounced: not just a pathology of the system, but the way in which the system itself functions — by uprooting and dispossessing and thus creating the conditions for new conquests, at the cost — however — of untold alienation and the relegation of countless people to irrelevance. This analysis is not only Marx's: numerous other observers — both conservative and liberal — have reached the same conclusion.

Placing their faith in the responses to the 'wild' capitalism of the nineteenth century — above all the creation of democratic and socialist movements: the institutions of democracy, state intervention and welfare systems, mechanisms for market regulation — many people underestimated the forces of alienation in contemporary society. Only now — on the verge of being overwhelmed by global market forces — are they waking up — only to be almost paralyzed by the terrifying extent to which self-dispossession — whether real or feared — already surrounds us. Most guilty of this underestimation are the progressives. The very people who — more than any others — analyzed — and devised effective strategies to overcome — the phenomenon of alienation. Strategies born out of enormous struggle and suffering, whose successes were due to an extraordinary human commitment to solidarity. The manufacturers of fear — the shock troops of the dispossessors — were thus allowed to run rampant, while progressives, unable to devise new, genuinely emancipatory policies for those who were being serially dispossessed, were caught in the middle, between the merchants of alienation and their stubborn opponents. They made no real effort to understand what was actually happening and didn't know how to reimagine their previous victory, how to create a more sophisticated balance between democracy and the market, a more human order for economic and social relations in this era of globalization and finance capitalism. Globalization can, of course, open up huge opportunities. But only if there are rigorous mechanisms in place that are strong enough to withstand the immense pressures exerted by global actors.

The human governance of affairs needs time. A more advanced equilibrium cannot be achieved in an instant. The evolution of the emerging forces shatters old

---

10 Georg Wilhelm Friedrich Hegel, *The Phenomenology of Spirit* (1807), trans. by Peter Fuss and John Dobbins (Notre Dame, IN: University Press, 2019).

conceits — our long-inhabited carapaces — and before a new order can be built, humanity is left exposed to the rapacious greed of the predators among us. It means little to say that 'in the long term' the benefits of the system will be shared by all when the present is so full of distress and social dislocation. One of the progressives' strengths in the past was their ability to combine visions of the future with short term strategies — this ensured that whole generations did not have to be sacrificed in the building of a system which would only be in place when they were too old — or too dead — to enjoy it. The blending of prophetic vision with historical gradualism was key to the progressives' past victories. Without a sense of history, in other words, it is hard to be progressive — being open to the future is necessary — being open to the hope that human activity — over time — is not entirely meaningless, purposeless, useless, or downright harmful, but can instead make our lives better. Today, this sense of history seems to have vanished: we lack not only a sense of gradualism, but also — it seems — any clear ideas of what might constitute a prophetic vision, what sort of world we want to build.

The pandemic has crippled any radically progressive vision of history. This experience of health crisis has clearly proved that the ordeal of the pandemic is destined to characterize our future and cannot simply be projected into a remote past, when historical plagues occurred. There will never be a future entirely free of this evil. The mantra reiterated by epidemiologists has been the following: 'we must learn to live with pandemics'. Humanity's future will be inhabited by illness. Medical science may save a number of lives and contain damages but may not liberate us from every evil entirely.

Thus, a paradox has occurred: at the very time in which medical science has turned into the new religion of humankind, it has secularized itself and shown its earthly and mundane face. Arguably, the evolution of humanity in the twenty-first century is being marked precisely by the predominance of progress in the field of *medical science*. In terms of its 'epochal' importance, medical science has replaced earlier areas of fundamental human activity, which, in Carl Schmitt's description, included *theology* (for the sixteenth century), *metaphysics* (seventeenth century), *ethics* (eighteenth century), *economy* (nineteenth century), and *technology* (twentieth century).[11] This invites reflection on the enormous success of biopolitical thinking in contemporary debates.

Yet medical science, at the very moment of asserting itself as a supreme faith, seems to secularize itself and dodge the role of new religion. There are, of course, priests of medical science, as well as their opponents, i.e., the anti-vax movement at the edge between religion and superstition. Still, overall, medical science is forced to declare itself as being mere imperfect knowledge, far removed from 'gnosis'. The success of medical science in producing the Covid vaccine, the most formidable tool for combating the pandemic, has simultaneously illustrated how that tool is limited. Far from being a sort of collective purification capable of providing salvation, vaccination is a sheer practical instrument. While powerful, this instrument, like any

11 Carl Schmitt, 'The Age of Neutralizations and Depoliticizations' (1927), *Telos*, 96 (1993), pp. 130–42.

other, is limited in space and time. Faith in science and technology, including medical science and technology, has definitely remained the most widespread form of belief globally in the wake of the pandemic, yet it would be overstated to argue that this new 'faith' generates a new 'trust' as well.[12] The world remains disenchanted.

Traditional religious beliefs, which have lost ground to the faith in science and technology, do not appear to have regained any stamina during the pandemic. Quite the contrary: they have promptly given up their public spaces and even silenced their hope for eternal life. When it comes to eternal life, what could have been a better opportunity for debate than the return of large-scale death? As a way of consolation, if nothing else. Still, nobody has addressed the issue of eternal life. Poor Self has been dispossessed of its eternity as well.

2. Rights under Challenge

The experience of the pandemic has elicited not only fear of the dispossession of the Self. People have experienced a process of gradual dispossession of fundamental human rights, which constitute the pillars of our social existence. The return of large-scale death onto the public stage has not only shaken our daily lives in their diverse aspects; it has also questioned life itself in its radical nature, that is, the existence of individual lives along with the meaning itself of collective social existence. Since the early stage of the pandemic, the challenge of the pandemic has been accompanied by the challenge represented by the measures taken by national and international public authorities to address the pandemic. Such measures have impacted individual and collective life in a significant and radical manner.

Not surprisingly, this experience has posed, and continues to pose, an 'unprecedented' challenge to human rights, as stated in the report *The Coronavirus Pandemic and Fundamental Rights: A Year in Review* by the European Union Agency for Fundamental Rights. From this report, two elements especially come to the fore: the radical novelty of the challenge, which has unveiled contemporary societies' overall lack of preparation vis-à-vis major pandemics; and the complexity of such a challenge, which has seen human rights being restrained not only by the pandemic but also, if in different ways, by the measures adopted to contain the pandemic.

The first right to be challenged has been the right to life and to a dignified death. The pandemic has reminded us that the right to life must be fulfilled not only by ensuring freedom from violent and nefarious interferences, but also through due care and assistance. *Care* means not only medical service for healing a condition of illness; more generally it means attentiveness, consideration, and the taking of responsibility, without which human life cannot be reproduced. Compared with other forms of vegetal and animal life, the reproduction and preservation of human life essentially relies on the *care of others*, as biologically visible in the lengthy processes of gestation

12 Luca Savarino and Paolo Vineis, *La salute del mondo: ambiente, società e pandemie* (Milano: Feltrinelli, 2021), p. 42.

and weaning in the human species. To be truly exercised and enjoyed, the right to life requires 'positive' action by other human beings in addition to 'negative' medical action meant to neutralize pathologies. This applies not only in the early stages of life, but at every moment, until the end. To be celebrated with humanity, the end of life requires, once again, attentive care and the accompanying of those who are departing life.

While the right to life may have a biological basis, the right to a dignified death is an entirely human creation. Dignified death, as epitomized in burial rites and the attempt to protect the dead human body from animals, has been regarded as a historical indicator of the birth of human civilization. During the pandemic, both the right to life and the right to a dignified death have been impacted. To be sure, every human body has been respected and buried, but the most dramatic phases of the crisis have seen a lack of care as is usually due, and a lack of human company in the moment of extreme difficulty and farewell. This has been a pain for humanity and a further instance of dispossession.

In terms of human rights, not only the pandemic, but also the response to it has come with novel challenges to the enjoyment of the rights. Individual and social freedoms have been restricted at all levels, from personal freedoms through to economic, religious, cultural, and political freedoms. Simply by going through the rights listed in constitutions and international conventions, it becomes apparent that virtually all such rights have been impacted by anti-Covid measures: the right to universal access to medical care; the right to freedom and security; the respect for private and family life and the protection of sensitive data; the right to religion, information, freedom of expression, association, and assembly; not to mention the freedom of movement and residence. Social rights have been affected enormously: from the right to education, with school and university activities suspended for lengthy periods or continued only remotely, to the right to work, which has been hit both in the area of free enterprise and that of salaried employment; the right to healthcare and social security, which must be protected to counter not only Covid but any kind of illness and distress. Within this broad spectrum of denied or restricted rights, the heaviest burden has been placed on vulnerable groups, such as women, children, the elderly (especially those living in nursing homes), persons with disabilities, detainees, as well as migrants, asylum-seekers, the Romani population, and the homeless. Further rights have been affected too, such as the right of access to justice.

2.1. Lessons from the Pandemic

The first lesson from the pandemic concerns the unity and indivisibility of human rights. Although this unity was already visible in the Universal Declaration of Human Rights and has been reiterated by the United Nations since, there is still no consensus regarding the inherent relationship between so-called civil and political rights on the one hand, and social and economic rights on the other. It is well-known that these types of rights differ in terms of the material resources required to make them effective. The right to health is more costly than the freedom of assembly. These rights also differ since some rights are fulfilled by mere non-interference by the state, whereas others demand active intervention by a variety of actors. For the latter rights, right-bearers themselves along with social groups must be able to play a key role within a logic of subsidiarity conducive to universal protection and real equality of opportunities. Yet the victim of a violation or restriction of rights, or the person who is otherwise denied the possibility of enjoying the rights, is unique. In this person the unity and indivisibility of the rights is immediately visible and tangible. Being deprived of a home or being unable to go to school and to get a job or decent healthcare does not touch on a single side of human personality but on its entirety, and certainly it affects the social and political dimension of the self as a whole. It is hoped that this lesson will be understood internationally and domestically alike. Following the extremely severe financial crisis of 2008, which especially hit the most vulnerable strata of the population in some European countries, it took nearly ten years for the European Union to bring into focus the relevance of social rights at the Gothenburg Summit of 2017. And only the recent need to respond to the Covid crisis has resulted in a substantial change of attitude to the issue of European solidarity. But it is essential that the large financial resources now available be used not only to sustain economic recovery, but also to support the most vulnerable groups in European societies.

The second lesson from the crisis pertains to the deepening of inequalities. International organizations, from the United Nations to European institutions, are unanimous in identifying this as a key concern. In every area of society and in every country of the world, the impact of the pandemic has worsened existing hardships and widened the inequality gap in virtually every sector. As a result the response to the pandemic has raised an enormous and urgent question of justice, that is, the necessity of granting universal access to medical care and organizing medical services accordingly, beginning from efficient general medical services. To be sure, once vaccination was publicly recognized as the primary tool for fighting the pandemic, vaccines have been distributed based on a universalistic principle, at least in Italy and other European countries, also thanks to strong European commitment in this respect. There remains the open question of considerable international imbalances, as well as the question of how to manage vaccinations in the event of a prolonged pandemic. Furthermore, there are unresolved questions regarding the use of public funding in private medical research and production and the patentability of vaccines. Uncertainties also remain as to an effective universal access to vaccines, which is currently questioned at least in relation to some groups, notably foreigners without social security, as well as regarding adequate medical assistance for pathologies other than Covid.

The increase of inequalities has affected not only the area of healthcare services. Think of the huge gender gap in several countries. The pandemic has radically and adversely affected women's rights, which had already been under attack prior to the Covid emergency: think of women engaged in healthcare and social services, who have been among the most exposed and hit by the pandemic; the higher percentages of women who lost their jobs and income compared with men; and the rise in domestic violence and delayed access to justice and medical care, not to mention the scarce representation of women in the decision-making bodies in charge of dealing with the pandemic. This tragic exacerbation of inequalities has surfaced for every vulnerable group: from children and adolescents who are systematically regarded as marginal elements of society in both ordinary and extraordinary times, through to the elderly and migrants, persons with disabilities and those deprived of freedom, and those without a home.[13]

The third lesson from the Covid emergency concerns recourse to emergency legislation. Some have misrepresented extraordinary measures and the proclamation of a state of emergency as a 'health dictatorship'.[14] This position neglects the fact that, from a human rights perspective, governments acting within constitutional and international legal frameworks are under a democratically-grounded *obligation* to protect first and foremost the right to life and health of *all* citizens. Therefore, healthcare policies in times of a pandemic must be oriented to limiting casualty figures as much as possible. This does not mean that the right to life should be viewed as an absolute right that obliterates any other fundamental freedom. Rather it means that, in a political system grounded on freedom and equality, the legislator can never ignore the need to protect all citizens' equal opportunity to stay alive.[15]

To be sure, emergency legislation has regrettably entailed hasty procedures, regulatory messes, and abuses, especially in some countries, including in Europe, where the event of the pandemic has been instrumentalized to weaken the rule of law, and the rights of opposition parties and civil society. The role itself of parliaments has been significantly diminished. A paternalistic and top-down culture of government has emphasized public authorities' capability of protecting the nation rather than the particular resources made available by ordinary citizens, local communities, and civil society, which have been essential for countering the pandemic. Nevertheless, it would be a mistake to confuse 'emergency' with 'exception' and to suggest an 'exceptionalistic' reading of the emergency. Accurate analyses of the measures actually adopted by governments show that an exceptionalistic reading is not tenable.[16] To the contrary, there have been cases of worrying inaction by governments, and some commentators have complained about *executive underreach*.[17]

International institutions have rightly called on governments to limit recourse to emergency measures and to rather resort to legislation that is proportionate, temporary, non-discriminating and strictly necessary. It is key that institutional actors and civil society monitor public responses to the crisis and promptly denounce any

---

13 As chapter 13 of this volume shows, these issues hit especially hard in the Middle East and North Africa.

14 Giorgio Agamben, *Where Are We Now? The Epidemic as Politics*, trans. by Valeria Dani (Washington DC: Rowman & Littlefield, 2021).

15 Jurgen Habermas, 'Corona und der Schutz des Lebens. Zur Grundrechtsdebatte in der pandemischen Ausnahmesituation', *Blätter für deutsche und internationale Politik*, 9 (2021), pp. 65–78.

16 Tom Ginsburg and Mila Versteeg, 'The Bound Executive: Emergency Powers During the Pandemic', *International Journal of Constitutional Law*, 19, 5 (2021), pp. 1498–1535.

17 David E. Pozen and Kim L. Scheppele, 'Executive Underreach', *American Journal of International Law*, 114, 4, *Pandemics and Otherwise* (2020), p. 608.

abuse. Parallel to this, it is fundamental to empower the most vulnerable groups to achieve conditions of effective equality within society. Now, the question arising is precisely how the human can be empowered to that effect.

3. The Principle of Self-belonging

If there's a new departure point — I suggest — it's to reaffirm the principle of *self-belonging*, common to all human beings: the fact that everyone belongs to themselves and to no other human being, and nothing, else. This is a more radical principle than that of self-determination, which is usually understood within the sphere of action. Here, the intention is to affirm that the being of each person is inalienable, it is not in the hands of others, nor can it be put in the hands of others — just like personal freedom, which vanishes in the instant that it is ceded to another. Nobody can command another completely. Human beings do not derive their meaning from other human beings: the essence of their being lies within. It is within that the dignity — and thus the inviolability — of the human being originates.

To affirm the principle of self-belonging — to possess oneself — is, of course, to do the exact opposite of dispossessing oneself. It is not, clearly, just a question of affirming principles — in a theoretical world of ideas and values: this alone would not be an adequate response to the fear that surrounds us. It is a question of reaffirming the subjectivity.

Therefore, it is a question of taking action, of really safeguarding the legal and social rights of the human being — in all areas of life — thereby strengthening the tools needed to protect people — starting with the most fragile — from physical abuse, but also from future pandemic threats — and to ensure that their personal spheres are protected from criminal invasion, including that perpetrated by speculators, and to counter the total commodification of labour which aims to separate the provision of a service from relationship, and to obliterate countless products of human activity — everything from food products to intellectual creation, from bank savings to personal and family projects.

This is not a question, clearly, of denying the necessity of a moment of objectification and communication of the self, of its activity and the products that result from this activity; the intention is rather to limit the alienating and destructive effects of this objectification in order to increase the realizable potential of the Self. In other words, it is not the insertion of the Self into the external world that is destructive, and a source of anxiety — it is the loss of control of one's Self that accompanies this process. Not the fact of being with others, of being for others, suffering for others — but the experience of being in the hands of others, and not being able to possess — or repossess one's Self — as happens in forms of modern and — sometimes — advanced slavery.

In this sense, the principle that every human being belongs to him or herself is not an individualistic one. Quite the opposite, and the experience of the Covid-19 crisis has clearly demonstrated it. The human being is born and develops in a literal state of (initially also biological) connection — 'co-being' — cradled within a web of nurturing human relationships. Nobody can be born, nobody can develop, outside an existing relational context. Even the movement of becoming 'this' person and thus the awareness and mastery of Self — irreducible to the sum of the relations which has produced it — a unique being who is, as it were, 'extraterritorial' — is only possible within a web of relationships.

One *becomes* an individual, a person, one attains self-belonging through positive social relations which recognize — through a dialectical process — the otherness of the other, the irreducibility of each. And maybe this is why — and I believe it is important to recognize this — the fear of dispossession becomes more acute in times stalked by loneliness and neglect, when to the fear of loss of Self is added the fear of losing one's affective ties.

We all want to be recognized in our otherness, in our difference from everyone else; we all want equality of respect for our bodies, for our personalities, our liberty; we all want to have the opportunity to create relationships and ties of solidarity. On this basis — of recognition and equal respect — a politics of equality can be built. Not a politics which seeks to equalize and must thus deny difference, but rather one which is based in the struggle against all forms of discrimination. This is the aspiration for justice that is intrinsic to humanity: the yearning for the just recognition of our being and activity (retributive justice) and the need to be respected by all other human beings (distributive justice). The principle of self-belonging can thus be understood as a convergence point between various anthropological traditions, both religiously inspired and secular. We see it — in, of course, many different forms, and subject to very different interpretations, from Self-ownership to *Selbstgehörigkeit* — in both the Christian tradition of personalism (from Aquinas to Guardini) and the liberal and libertarian traditions (from Locke to Kant to Nozick).

Nor does the principle of self-belonging isolate the human subject from 'nature', understood as the biological substrate of which they are constituted and as the 'environment' which nourishes them. On the contrary: in (re)taking possession of themselves the subject also takes possession of the nature of which they are formed and recognizes themselves as part of that nature.

The deepest roots of alienation today lie in this alienation of the human subject from human nature, which then inevitably culminates in the artificial reduplication of life. But the proper response to this process is not to try to melt the Self into an uncontaminated, undifferentiated, unattainable primeval nature — to dissolve the human into something assumed to be 'natural' which precedes them and exists independently of them. No — what is required of us is to construct a Self which 'humanizes' nature, while respecting all that is nonhuman within the natural realm. In other words, not nature's devastation, or utter negation, but an understanding that it is the origin of both humanity and all that is other than human. And therefore its domestication, its evolution, but also respect for its wildness. Here 'co-being' — rather than referring just to a common humanity, widens and deepens and takes in the sphere of all living beings.

3.1. Self-belonging and Rights

The principle of self-belonging thus allows for the affirmation of both the centrality of — indivisible — civil and social rights and the crucial importance of rights linked to humanity's connection with nature and the environment. For years we have considered social rights to be secondary — adjunctive — forgetting that their content — access to vital goods such as food, clothing, shelter, health, education — has always — both philosophically and within the historical context — been a precondition for all claims to, and the enjoyment of, fundamental civil and political rights.[18]

The fact that access to these vital rights is a necessary precondition for the exercise of other rights is very evident: unless we are alive, we cannot express ourselves freely. Morally, therefore, situations in which poverty or disease threaten people's very existence establish absolute obligations: Hans Jonas expresses this powerfully, using the example of a tiny baby who, by its very existence and its total inability to survive alone, creates a situation in which everyone around it is absolutely obliged to provide for its survival.[19] The case of the 'injured person on the roadside' is the same — here, too, we have an absolute obligation to stop and help: this injunction is so strong in our civilization that indifference is considered culpable and failure to help is a crime. So, access to the opportunity to feed ourselves, to receive adequate medical care, and to build affective and family relationships are all clearly preconditions for the exercise of all vital functions and therefore for our very existence.

But if the principle of self-belonging is a dynamic one, if our self-appropriation is a process in time, this process develops through an enriching of knowledge and of experience, through knowing and doing. In this sense, the principle of self-belonging inevitably involves a strong claim to the right to health, education, and work, since without these it's delusional to imagine genuine paths to emancipation.

Perhaps nowadays we pay insufficient attention to the critical importance of education and work on the anthropological — and not only the social and political — plane. In previous centuries, the centrality of the rights to education and work was obvious — they were seen as fundamental not only to a just society but also — and above all — to the process of self-realization. Universal access to these two basic rights should — I believe — return to the top of today's agendas.

The affirmation of civil — and social — rights cannot — of course — be left to individuals and social movements: institutions and the State also have a crucial role to play. Here we see that the principle of self-belonging, as a universal right, cannot merely be declared as an individualistic and passive concept — it requires the active regulation of economic and social life, particularly — for the reasons given above — in order to guarantee the rights to health, education and work.

18 Norberto Bobbio, *The Age of Rights* (Cambridge: Polity Press, 1995).

19 Hans Jonas, *Das Prinzip Verantwortung. Versuch einer Ethik für technologische Zivilisation* (Frankfurt a. M.: Suhrkamp, 1979).

3.2. *Self-belonging and Democracy*

In political terms, the principle of self-belonging corresponds to the fundamental principle of democracy understood as that of the self-belonging and self-government of a community of individuals who aspire to the recognition of their basic liberty, and respect for their equal dignity.

Just as individuals fear the dispossession of self and the condition of being in the hands of others, today's communities and peoples are at risk of being deprived of their capacity to govern themselves. We are therefore called upon to reassert — at the social level, too — the principle of self-belonging, relaunching the ideal of democracy on this basis — at all levels, from the local to the international — in order that every — admittedly necessary — process of objectification and opening up to the Other does not bring with it a permanent loss of control over our lives, and the lives of our communities. I do not here deny the need for wide societies, and for opportunities to go beyond the traditional boundaries of our original communities — i.e., usually, our native countries. Nor — still less — do I deny the need for mediation between the Self and organs of government, represented, at the political level, by associations, parties, and institutions. The crucial thing is to ensure that the individual can influence the government of his or her community, at any and all levels. To have — in other words — the possibility — at all times — to be a political 'subject', not just an 'object' — an actor with the ineradicable power — however small — to shape the decisions that affect his or her life. In this way the nature of the 'Self' of each person is preserved in the power relations between individuals. The infinite dignity of each person is revealed not only when he or she is an object to be protected, but also when he or she is a co-deciding subject in matters which affect their lives, whether at the local level or internationally. The future of democracy depends on the preservation of a genuinely open space for co-decision, to ensure that democracy — the highest form of 'self-belonging' — does not itself become a place of alienation — thus risking democratic disaffection and an illusory escape into other forms of discourse and authoritarian or populist political structures.

The current socio-political landscape calls urgently for the reaffirmation of democracy as a system based on moral freedom, equality (between all citizens, and between the governed and their governments), and reasoned debate. This means not only representative elections (i.e., democracy by appointment) but also forms of collective decision-making (participatory democracy)[20] through processes of information, discussion, and deliberation (deliberative democracy). Just as human subjectivity is constantly changing — its moral, cultural, and social dynamics are just that — never static — so, too, political subjectivity is always nourished, despite the proliferation of phenomena of political alienation and political disaffection, fatal to democracy itself.

Today's retreat into nationalism in the face of Europeanist and internationalist ideals has partly been caused by the growing sense of a loss of control and even the impossibility of influencing the governance of a public sphere which has become so

20 Pierre Rosanvallon, *Le bon gouvernment* (Paris: Seuil, 2015).

vast and apparently distant and remote. If, however, we consider the fact that the nature of contemporary phenomena — from the global economy to terrorism, from environmental issues to migration and pandemics — is transnational, it is evident that the democratic challenge cannot be met by a regression to lower levels. Instead, we must try to foster the democratization and constitutionalization of power at the international level, strengthening, not weakening, the forms — however limited and sometimes contradictory they may be — of international democracy that have so far been established.

Although human rights protection at the international level is at times chaotic and ineffective, the efforts to affirm them have — whatever their immediately success, or apparent failures — served to strengthen them, precisely because they have affirmed that fundamental rights are not entirely in the hands of the national legislatures and governments. The irony, of course, is that these — national — bodies are — at the moment — the only ones that can ensure that — international — rights are actually respected. This clearly demonstrates the importance of the concept of the cosmopolitical right, which can act as a complement to existent rights within and between states according to the lesson of Kant.

As Sloterdijk has stated: 'The victory of one's own, of the holy egoisms of cities, nations and faiths, could always be purchased with the defeat of the external other. With the deterioration of Earth's fragile atmospheric and biospheric systems, externalization has reached its absolute limit. [...] The operational imperative of the future calls for a new consciousness, new habits of the heart, of cooperation and solidarity with others and nature in order to survive and thrive. I call this "co-immunism"'.[21]

And it is — perhaps — on this belonging to common humanity — the basis of each individual's humanity, and that which obliges us all to treat each other with humanity — that we must again insist in this era of resurgent nationalisms and alarming politics of discrimination. In so doing, we must be careful not to turn humanity into an ideology that is imposed on the citizenry, or a weapon to brandish in the political struggle. We must not succumb to the illusion that the whole of humanity can — or should — become a single political subject. The secret is to be able to look at the Other, and recognize ourselves. In this era of fear and hate, we must rediscover not only the principle of self-belonging but also the fact that each human being shares their humanity with everyone else.

This is the strongest anthropological legacy left to us by the great religious and secular traditions which have always cherished the democratic vision when racial discrimination threatens it. Living together is not easy: effort is required to 'co-be', and this effort is often expressed in fear of the Other. On the other hand, it is important to recognize that this 'co-being' can heal our fear of loneliness and isolation and thus

21 Peter Sloterdijk, 'Co-Immunism in the Age of Pandemics In The Age Of Pandemics and Climate Change', *Noema*, June 12 (2020), available at https://www.noemamag.com/co-immunism-an-ethos-for-our-age-of-climate-change/ (last accessed 17/06/2022).

give individuals new energy and hope for life. And this is precisely the expansive, optimistic energy with which we can defeat hatred, oppression and suffering.

This happens wherever the sense of 'co-being' is grounded in the inextinguishable liberty of each individual, in the recognition that everyone is unique and in the according of equal respect to all. This combination of recognition and respect needs to have policies and systems in place which can guarantee its existence — it requires something more in terms of social justice. This 'more social justice' — when aspired to and realized by each human being — is that which, in the fear of the dispossession of self, can restore to society and to its institutions their true 'sense', and thus reconcile them with the deepest aspirations of everyone.

Bibliography

Adam, David, 'The Pandemic's true death toll: millions more than official counts', *Nature*, 601 (2022), pp. 312–15.

Agamben, Giorgio, *Where Are We Now? The Epidemic as Politics*, trans. by Valeria Dani (Washington DC: Rowman & Littlefield, 2021).

Arendt, Hannah, *The Origins of Totalitarianism* (New York: Meridian Books, 1958).

Ariès, Philippe, *Western Attitudes Toward Death: From the Middle Ages to the Present* (Baltimore: Johns Hopkins Univ. Press, 1975).

Bobbio, Norberto, *The Age of Rights* (Cambridge: Polity Press, 1995).

Esposito, Roberto, *Immunitas: The Protection and Negation of Life*, trans. by Z. Hanafi (London: Polity Press, 2011).

Foucault, Michel, *Il faut défendre la societé*. Cours au Collège de France 1975–1976 (Paris: Gallimard, 1997).

Ginsburg, Tom, and Mila Versteeg, 'The Bound Executive: Emergency Powers During the Pandemic', *International Journal of Constitutional Law*, 19, 5 (2021), pp. 1498–1535.

Gorer, Geoffrey, *Death, Grief and Mourning* (London: Cresset, 1965).

Habermas, Jürgen, 'Corona und der Schutz des Lebens. Zur Grundrechtsdebatte in der pandemischen Ausnahmesituation', *Blätter für deutsche und internationale Politik*, 9 (2021), pp. 65–78.

Hegel, Georg Wilhelm Friedrich, *The Phenomenology of Spirit* (1807), trans. by Peter Fuss and John Dobbins (Notre Dame, IN: University Press, 2019).

Jonas, Hans, *Das Prinzip Verantwortung. Versuch einer Ethik für technologische Zivilisation* (Frankfurt a. M.: Suhrkamp, 1979).

Neumann, Franz, *The Democratic and the Authoritarian State* (New York: Free Press, 1957).

Pozen, David E., and Kim L. Scheppele, 'Executive Underreach', *American Journal of International Law*, 114, 4, *Pandemics and Otherwise* (2020), pp. 608–617

Rosanvallon, Pierre, *Le bon gouvernment* (Paris: Seuil, 2015).

Savarino, Luca, and Paolo Vineis, *La salute del mondo: ambiente, società e pandemie* (Milano: Feltrinelli, 2021).

Schmitt, Carl, 'The Age of Neutralizations and Depoliticizations' (1927), *Telos*, 96 (1993), pp. 130–42.

Sloterdijk, Peter, 'Co-Immunism in the Age of Pandemics In The Age Of Pandemics and Climate Change', *Noema*, June 12 (2020), https://www.noemamag.com/co-immunism-an-ethos-for-our-age-of-climate-change/

Spellman, William M., *A Brief History of Death* (London: Reaction Books, 2014).

Wodak, Ruth, *The Politics of Fear: What Right-Wing Populist Discourses Mean* (New York: Sage, 2015).

Zuboff, Shoshana, *The Age of Surveillance Capitalism. The Fight for the Future at the New Frontier of Power* (London: Profile Books, 2019).

NIDESH LAWTOO

10. The Mimetic Faculty Reloaded: Contagion, Immunization, Conspiracies in the Age of Viral Reproduction*

▾ **ABSTRACT** This chapter argues that the human, all too human vulnerability to mimesis (imitation) is a central and so far underdiagnosed element internal to the COVID-19 pandemic crisis. Supplementing medical accounts of viral contagion and providing an alternative to theories of mimetic desire that treated epidemics metaphorically in the past century, I develop a genealogy of the concept of mimesis — from antiquity to modernity to the present — that is attentive to both its pathological and therapeutic or patho-*logical* properties for the present century. Part of an ERC project title *Homo Mimeticus*, the chapter provides new conceptual foundations for a theory of mimesis that is vital to countering contagious crises that cast a shadow on the present and on the future as well.

The coronavirus, like all viruses, is mimetic in the biological sense that it reproduces itself through other living beings. But what is the link between the ancient concept of *mimēsis*, viral contagion, and immunity? And if there is a link, how can an apparently unoriginal concept often translated as 'imitation', or 'representation', help us reflect critically, philosophically, and thus diagnostically, on contagious cultural pathologies such as crowd behaviour and conspiracy theories that do not simply misrepresent the truth about the virus online, but also cast an affective shadow that undermines immunization and amplifies the spread of viral contagion offline? I would like to suggest that the old and protean concept of 'mimesis' can provide, if not a magical immunization, at least a longstanding philosophical perspective to reflect critically on

* This project has received funding from the European Research Council (ERC) under the European Union's Horizon 2020 research and innovation programme (grant agreement n°716181: *Homo Mimeticus: Theory and Criticism*). This is a revised version of an article that appeared in *Paragrana* 30 (2021) and as a chapter in *Homo Mimeticus: A New Theory of Imitation* (Leuven University Press, 2022). I am grateful to both *Paragrana* and Leuven UP for allowing me to reproduce it with some modifications here.

Epidemics and Pandemics, ed. by Michele Nicoletti and Alessandro Palazzo (Turnhout: Brepols, 2024), pp. 253–278
BREPOLS PUBLISHERS 10.1484/M.STPH-EB.5.136414

cultural pathologies that, in times of the pandemic crisis but not only, are in urgent need of transdisciplinary diagnostics attentive to the human, all too human tendency to imitate others — what I also call, for lack of a more original term, *homo mimeticus*.[1]

After the speed with which virologists produced medical vaccines, or *pharmaka*, to contain and hopefully eventually immunize the world population against the COVID-19 pandemic, a plurality of broader social, political, anthropological problems — among others — amplified the pandemic crisis on a plurality of fronts. These include, for instance, the problem of equal vaccine distribution in an increasingly uncertain world plagued by social inequality, racist/sexist discrimination, (new) fascist leaders, and last but not least, conspiracy theories. These among other problems made clear that an epidemic may generate a contagious *undifferentiation* in the general sense that all humans are equally vulnerable to infection in theory; and yet, a number of *differentiating* factors render some humans more vulnerable than others in practice. As the SARS-CoV-2 virus keeps mutating via genetic differentiations that increase the speed of contamination at the viral level (omicron being the latest variant as I revised this piece in January 2022), the COVID-19 pandemic generates a plurality of cultural differences that are equally slowing down immunization in complex (from *complexus*, interwoven) ways, urging cultural theorists and philosophers to stress what should have been clear from the beginning: namely, that a pandemic is a '"total" social phenomenon'[2] that concerns not only virologists, immunologists, medical experts, and healthcare workers fighting the virus on the front lines; it also infects and affects all aspects of social life, from the economy to politics, education to communication to polices of immunization and vaccine distribution that are fully constitutive of a pandemic crisis. As the French sociologist Edgar Morin puts it, relying on a mimetic terminology, the COVID-19 pandemic sets up a 'magnifying glass to social inequalities'.[3]

If we then also consider that a significant segment of the population is composed of pandemic deniers, anti-lockdown protesters, and vaccine skeptics (or antivax) who have fallen prey to conspiracy theories that have gone viral online before retroacting on the population offline in ways that amplify viral infection, a *re*-turn of attention to mimesis is in order. The ancient problematic of false representations of reality can in fact no longer be limited to epistemic and ontological concerns with truth and lies — though these perspectives remain crucial in an age we were perhaps too quick to dub in terms of 'post-truth'. The powers of the false also have political, ethical, pedagogical, affective, and medical consequences that are constitutive of what I call the 'patho(-)logies of mimesis' understood as both mimetic cultural pathologies that spread by mobilizing the register of affect (*pathos*) and critical discourses (*logoi*)

1 *Homo Mimeticus* is an ERC-funded transdisciplinary project that advocates a mimetic turn, or re-turn of mimesis in continental philosophy, critical theory, political theory, literary/film studies, among other perspectives. For outputs, see http://www.homomimeticus.eu/publications/

2 Marcel Mauss, *The Gift: Forms and Functions of Exchange in Archaic Societies* (London: Cohen & West, 1966), p. 78.

3 Edgar Morin (with the collaboration of Sabah Abouessalam), *Changeons de voie: les leçons du coronavirus* (Paris: Denoël, 2020), p. 39.

that give a rational account of this pathos (or patho-*logy*).[4] Since cultural forms of affective contagion are not simply added to viral contagion, but amplify the latter's reach and power of infection, they cannot be considered as external to it, in an old-fashioned 'two-cultures' opposition that is clearly inadequate to account for complex, transdisciplinary problems. On the contrary, a pandemic crisis calls for a plurality of patho-*logical* supplements to account for the joint problematic of contagion and immunization, both at the viral and affective levels, in a spirit of transdisciplinary collaboration. My hypothesis is that in order to account for the complex relation between viral pathologies and cultural pathologies, as well as their respective practices of contagion and immunization, it is useful, perhaps even urgent, to remember that it is not only the nonhuman virus that is contagious; humans' imitative tendencies are imbued with contagious properties that spread contagiously, from self to others as well — for good and ill.

There are a number of symptoms that call for a mimetic turn, or *re*-turn of attention to mimesis central to an interdisciplinary field we call, "mimetic studies."[5] A proliferation of emerging phenomena in social and cultural life, from digital simulations to conspiracy theories, have in fact confirmed Walter Benjamin's insights into the 'significance of the mimetic faculty' to account for magical phenomena of mimicry based on 'sensuous similarities' that via an 'aestheticization of politics, as practiced by fascism', continues to cast a long shadow on the twentieth century.[6] And yet, if Benjamin argued at the dawn of the modernist period that the invention of language may have brought about 'the increasing decay of the mimetic faculty',[7] I will argue that the digital age brought about an exponential growth of what I shall call the hypermimetic faculty and the magical associations it entails. My wager is that the viral contagion internal to an age haunted by pandemic, environmental and other crises sets up a magnifying mirror to *homo mimeticus*. In particular, it reveals an all too mimetic tendency to fall under the pathological spell of emotional contagion in physical crowds on one side and conspiracies theories in virtual publics on the other side. Both sides call for heterogeneous forms of cultural immunization in critical practice.

4 Nidesh Lawtoo, *The Phantom of the Ego: Modernism and the Mimetic Unconscious* (East Lansing: Michigan State University Press, 2013), pp. 6–8.

5 Nidesh Lawtoo, *Homo Mimeticus: A New Theory of Imitation* (Leuven: Leuven University Press, 2022), pp. 9-39.

6 Walter Benjamin, 'On the Mimetic Faculty,' in *Reflections: Essays, Aphorisms, Autobiographical Writings*, ed. by Peter Demetz, trans. by Edmund Jephcott (New York: Schocken Books, 2007), pp. 333–34; Id., 'The Work of Art in the Age of Its Technological Reproducibility' (2nd version), in *The Work of Art in the Age of its Technological Reproducibility and Other Media*, ed. by Michael W. Jennings an others, trans. by Edmund Jephcott and others (Cambridge, MA: Harvard University Press, 2008), pp. 19–55 (p. 42); Nidesh Lawtoo, *(New) Fascism: Contagion, Community, Myth* (East Lansing: Michigan State University Press, 2019).

7 Benjamin, 'On the Mimetic Faculty', p. 334.

1. The Patho(-)Logies of *Homo Mimeticus*

While the COVID-19 pandemic generated a viral contagion that was effectively placed under the lens of epidemiologists and virologists to effectively develop a plurality of vaccines, it has also made clear that a viral pandemic infects and affects the totality of human activities in complex ways that involve the humanities and social sciences as well. In particular, it made visible on a global scale what philosophers from Plato and Aristotle onward considered to be one of humans' defining characteristics, for which there is no single effective immunization: namely, that *homo sapiens* is an extremely mimetic species, not only in the aesthetic sense that humans represent the world via realistic media like painting, theatre, cinema, TV, and now a proliferation of new media with the potential to represent realities that are epistemically false — though in the digital age, in the wake of AI revolutions, we continue to do that well and with alarming efficacy.[8] Humans are also mimetic in the psychological, sociological, anthropological, and political sense that we imitate, often unconsciously, other people, be they real or fictional, embodied or represented, including their emotions, habits, and beliefs, which go viral online and spread 'contagiously', from self to others, offline as well.[9]

The metaphor of 'going viral' is not accidental. Rethinking mimesis in the age of COVID-19 makes us see that imitation turns out to share some important characteristics with viruses: it is linked to a type of reproduction that is not limited to representation but affects and infects human bodies; it does so in ways that operate via microimitations that are imperceptible to the naked eye; it renders bodies vulnerable to a type of contagion that is amplified by proximity with others; and last but not least, it generates effects that go beyond clear-cut categories of good and evil, health and sickness, and cannot be contained within unilateral, universal, and transhistorical diagnostics. For instance, on the one hand, scientifically informed models of behaviour based on a rational knowledge, or *logos*, can be amplified affectively by public personalities (presidents, celebrities, actors) who have the power to turn to (social) media to promote therapeutic or patho-*logical* forms of prevention like social distancing, mask-wearing, and vaccination; on the other hand, the proliferation of pathological cultural models among the same categories of 'exemplary' personalities can also spread irrational sentiments that have nothing to do with the *logos* of science. On the contrary, they are animated by a resentful *pathos* that promotes pandemic-denial, mask-protests, antivax movements, and conspiracy theories that 'go viral' in both the metaphorical sense that they spread, like a virus, in the virtual world of internet simulations, but also in the sense that they retroact, via spiraling feedback

8 See Nidesh Lawtoo, *Homo Mimeticus 2.0: Posthuman Mimesis in Art, Philosophy and Technics* (Leiden: Brill, 2024).

9 As Christoph Wulf and Gunter Gebauer put it, 'the relevance of mimesis is not restricted to the aesthetic [...] its effects press outward into the social world, taking root, as Plato saw it, in individual behavior like a contagion'. Gunter Gebauer and Christoph Wulf, *Mimesis: Culture-Art-Society*, trans. by Don Reneau (Berkeley: University of California Press, 1995), p. 309. See also the special issue on *The Mimetic Condition*, ed. Nidesh Lawtoo, *CounterText*, 1. 8 (2022).

loops, to affect and infect social practices offline in ways that literally disseminate viral contagion in human bodies.

This structural ambivalence entails therapeutic insights that provide a humanistic supplement to the medical sciences. If the vaccine mimics the virus to provide a therapeutic immunity to the infection, leading Judith Butler to rightly note that "both analogy and mimicry are crucial to strengthen the immune system,"[10] this also means mimesis is equally endowed with double pharmaceutical properties. Since classical antiquity, in fact, the all-too-human propensity to imitate others (be they real or fictional) has been considered as both pathological and therapeutic. Already Plato, in fact, considered mimesis as a *pharmakon*, that is, as both 'medicine and/or poison'.[11] Or, to put it in our diagnostic language, the effects are at least double: on one side, the coronavirus generated a form of mimetic contagion that triggered a multiplicity of *pathologies* that affected *homo sapiens* on a multiplicity of levels — biological, psychological, sociological, anthropological, political, economic, etc.; on the other side, it can also serve as a therapeutic and reflective mirror that provides the necessary distance to mobilize different discourses or *logoi* to account for the dynamic of mimetic affects or *pathoi*, including viro-logoi on vaccines that mimic viruses to therapeutic ends — what I call, 'patho-*logies*'. I do so to emphasize the transdisciplinary discourses or *logoi* internal to recent mimetic studies attentive to the contagious power of *pathos*.

Disseminated by globalization, indifferent to national borders, favoured by political inefficiency, and obsessively followed by (new) media, true and false, a pandemic is what Marcel Mauss calls a 'total social fact' [*fait social total*] insofar as this heterogeneous phenomenon is at 'once legal, economic, religious, aesthetic, morphological and so on'.[12] It thus escapes cultural generalizations that aim to contain the proliferating effects of viral and affective contagion within unitary theoretical diagnostics that may still have worked in a relatively secure nation state in the post-war period, but no longer work to ensure immunity in a present interconnected and increasingly precarious world.[13] In the wake of the differentiated reality of the COVID-19 pandemic and the future pandemics that will continue to haunt an increasingly connected body politic, the reality of viral contagion leads us to correct unifying theories of mimetic contagion that were still dominant in the past century.

In the 1970s the French literary theorist René Girard rightly noticed important similarities between the viral contagion internal to epidemics and the affective contagion that follows it, shadow-like. He did so via hermeneutical analyses of renderings

10 Judith Butler, *What World Is This? A Pandemic Phenomenology* (New York: Columbia University Press, 2022), p. 10.

11 Jacques Derrida, 'Plato's Pharmacy', in *Dissemination*, trans. by Barbara Johnson (Chicago: The University of Chicago Press, 1981), p. 70, p. 139.

12 Mauss, *The Gift*, p. 76.

13 For a rich philosophical account of "immunity" as a biopolitical category of protection and negation of life, see Roberto Esposito, *Immunitas: protezione e negazione della vita* (Torino: Einaudi, 2002) and *Immunità comune. Biopolitica all'epoca della pandemia* (Einaudi, Torino 2022). As Esposito's thought on immunity rests on a biopolitical rethinking of community that presupposes minimally an engagement with Foucault, Bataille and Nietzsche to be properly framed, I refer readers to *Roberto Esposito: Biopolitics and Philosophy*, ed. by Inna Viriasova and Antonio Calcagno (Albany, NY: SUNY Press, 2018).

of 'the plague in literature' that uncovered what he considered a referential 'mimetic crisis' behind literary representations of pandemic crises — from Sophocles to Shakespeare, Dostoevsky to Thomas Mann, among others.[14] As Girard puts it: 'Between the plague and social disorder there is a reciprocal affinity' based on the fact that both are 'contagious' in nature; and he adds: 'The appropriateness of the metaphor comes, obviously, from this contagious character'.[15] If the plague is contagious in the viral or literal sense, violence is indeed contagious in the affective, or metaphorical sense. This remains a timely observation. And yet, it is not the direction Girard considers this metaphorical connection. In a striking mirroring inversion of perspective, Girard inverts the relation between reality and metaphor as he claims that the plague in literature does not literally represent the contagious reality of viral contagion. On the contrary, viral contagion 'becomes a transparent metaphor for a certain reciprocal violence that spreads literally like the plague'.[16] According to Girard's metaphorical overturning, it is the contagious nature of violence, not of the plague, that should be taken literally. The plague is a metaphor for social violence. More precisely, the plague as represented in literature turns out to be a mere 'transparent metaphor' for the mimetic violence that is the centre of Girard's theory of violence and the sacred — which does not mean that this metaphorical account of the plague renders us immune from viruses. Metaphorical plague, real violence: this is the decision on which Girard's hermeneutics of contagion stands — or, rather, falls.

Girard's hermeneutical move might be in line with his mimetic theory but is invalidated by viral realities in a way that is at least double. First, writing from the position of a still relatively immune nation state, Girard argues in the 1970s that we 'live in a world less and less threatened by real epidemics', and he adds: 'This fact looks less surprising now, as we come to realize that the properly medical aspects of the plague never were essential; in themselves they always played a minor role, serving mostly as a disguise for an even more terrible threat that no science has ever been able to conquer'.[17] History unfortunately taught us otherwise. From the plague of HIV to the COVID-19 pandemic we have been living in an increasingly precarious world open to infections that are likely to plague an interconnected and interdependent humanity in the future as well. In his last writings, Girard recognized this danger but retained the category of 'undifferentiation' to account for the dynamic of the pandemic,[18] encouraging mimetic studies of the future to supplement his diagnostic — which takes us to the next invalidation.

---

14 René Girard, 'The Plague in Literature and Myth', *Texas Studies in Literature and Language*, 15. 5 (1974), pp. 833–50 (p. 834).

15 Girard, 'The Plague in Literature', p. 836.

16 Girard, 'The Plague in Literature', p. 836.

17 Girard, 'The Plague in Literature,' p. 845.

18 Correcting his diagnostic, the late Girard, confronted with the H5N1 pandemic acknowledged that it is a 'pandemic that could cause hundreds of deaths in a few days and is a phenomenon typical of the undifferentiation now coursing across the planet'. René Girard, *Battling to the End: Conversations with Benoît Chantre*, trans. by Mary Baker (East Lansing: Michigan State University Press, 2010), p. 24. For an initial supplement to Girard, see Nidesh Lawtoo, 'The Cooperative Community: Surviving Epidemics in *The Shadow-Line*', in *Conrad's Shadow: Catastrophe, Mimesis, Theory*, (East Lansing: Michigan State

Second, Girard claims that both viral and affective contagions cause a state of 'undifferentiation' that affects all subjects, equally generating what he calls a 'crisis of differences'. What he suggests is that individual, social, economic, political, national, and other differences are erased by the double dynamic of mimetic contagion, be it literal or metaphorical, in transhistorical ways Girard considers constitutive of 'the eternal ethos of the plague'.[19] Humans are indeed all vulnerable to both forms of medical/affective contagion that erase differences in the sense that all are equally vulnerable to infection in theory; yet the COVID-19 pandemic taught us that the opposite is true in practice. In fact, both viral and social contagion generate an exacerbation of a plurality of medical, social, cultural, economic, and political differences that need to be reconsidered. Contrary to an 'eternal ethos' internal to metaphorical interpretations of the Plague, the type of medical-psychological-social-systemic, etc., violence it causes are different enough. The toll of viral infections, in fact, manifested itself radically differently across the world, depending on age, ethnic group, class, nationality, etc. It was also radically inflected by the politics of each country and the social/economic inequalities that differentiated the levels of infections significantly, as countries like Brazil and India, African Americans in the US, and undocumented migrants in Europe and other parts of the world made strikingly clear, and the unequal rollout of vaccines across the globe confirmed. Rather than 'undifferentiation', then, the COVID-19 pandemic magnified the differential plurality of social pathologies like systemic racism that plague what Frantz Fanon called, 'the wretched of the Earth', while also revealing class inequality, sexism, exclusionary practices that continue to structure patriarchal/racist ideologies, and the violent divide between North and South that deprives silent majorities of what Achille Mbembe calls 'the universal right to breathe'.[20]

From a contemporary perspective, then, we can thus say that violence, which is not only physical, but manifests itself in a number of structural forms of oppression, is visibly at play; and precisely for this reason it is crucial to account for the interplay between two different, entangled, and quite literal and real pathologies such as viral and social pathologies. If Girard's mimetic theory still accounts for the scapegoating mechanisms internal to social crises that routinely direct violence against minorities, it no longer reflects the complex reality of a pandemic crisis, which calls for patho-*logical* supplements. For new voices in mimetic studies concerned with the real and rather heterogeneous implications of a pandemic crisis, COVID-19 gives

---

University Press, 2016), pp. 91–125. If it is easy to critique Girard's metaphorical blunder in 2021, I note that my first concerns with the 'contemporary pandemics that, every year, threaten to contaminate an increasingly globalized, permeable, and precarious world' led me to state, in 2016, that 'the shadow of epidemics looms large on the horizon' (p. 92).

19 Girard, 'The Plague in Literature,' p. 834.

20 Achille Mbembe, 'The Universal Right to Breathe', trans. by Carolyne Shread, *Critical Inquiry*, 47. 52 (2020), *In the Moment* (blog) https://critinq.wordpress.com/2020/04/13/the-universal-right-to-breathe/ (last accessed 16/01/2021). On gender inequality and the pandemic see, Kecia Ali, Julia-Watts Belser, Grace Y. Kao, Shiverly T. J. Smith, 'Living It Out: Feminism During Covid 19', *Journal of Feminist Studies in Religion, 36. 2 (2020), pp. 107–16.*

us an occasion to rethink mimesis for the twenty-first century and theorize contagion again to prepare for crises to come. Rather than a hermeneutic that uncovers a mimetic sameness hidden behind an epidemic plague treated metaphorically, then, genealogical lenses propose a diagnostic of the multiplicity of differences that emerge from the patho(-)logical interplay of social contagion and viral contagion treated quite literally.

A genealogy of mimesis that looks back to the past in order to cast light on the patho(-)logies of the present does not provide a unitary answer, universal structure, or theoretical system to frame a constantly changing phenomenon. Instead of taking its starting point in a triangulation of mimetic desire still of Oedipal inspiration,[21] it foregrounds an all too human vulnerability to what I call mimetic *pathos* (good and evil) and the critical *distance* that can potentially ensue if we step further back to precursors of the mimetic turn. In *On the Genealogy of Morals*, Friedrich Nietzsche calls this paradoxical double movement between mimetic pathos and critical distance, 'pathos of distance'.[22] A central concept in his genealogy of morality that unmasks a magical faith in other worlds 'behind the world [*Hinterwelt*]',[23] Nietzsche informs my genealogy of contagion and immunity, urging us to remain faithful to this world. On his shoulders, I take three genealogical steps in this immanent direction to outline a diagnostic of mimetic patho(-)logies in the age of COVID-19. I take two steps back to reevaluate the relation between mimesis and contagion for the ancients in Plato's philosophy and for the moderns in crowd psychology. These steps back will allow me to leap ahead toward the challenge of immunization in an age dominated by conspiracy theories that reload the contagious powers of false shadows for a digital age constitutive of the *vita mimetica*.

2. *Vita Mimetica:* Ancient Shadows, New Simulations

First step. Origins are never simply pure and singular but given the dominant translation of 'mimesis' as representation or copy of an original model it might be useful to step back to the one of the most influential thinkers who introduced this concept in western thought. According to Plato's philosophical *logos*, mimesis, *pathos*, and cultural pathologies cannot easily be dissociated. Let us in fact recall that when the concept of *mimēsis* first appears on the philosophical scene in Books 2 and 3 of the *Republic*, Plato does not introduce an ontological concept that reduces the phenomenal world to a visual copy, shadow, or 'phantom [*phantasma*]' of transcendental ideas, turning artistic representations into phantoms of phantoms 'at three removes' from

21 See Nidesh Lawtoo, 'Violence and the Mimetic Unconscious (Part I), The Catharsis Hypothesis: Aristotle, Girard, Freud', *Contagion*, 25 (2018): pp. 159–92.

22 Friedrich Nietzsche, *On the Genealogy of Morals*, trans. Douglas Smith (Oxford: Oxford University Press, 1998), p. 12.

23 Nietzsche, *Genealogy of Morals*, p. 5.

the metaphysical world of intelligible Forms.[24] We will have to wait until Book 10 for this famous critique of mimesis qua ontological mirror based on the logic of visual likeness, adequation, and representation to appear, a metaphysical and epistemic critique Plato also theorized via the example of the painter and continues to cast a shadow on contemporary limitations of mimesis to the sphere of realistic aesthetics. Instead, in the *Republic* mimesis is first introduced as a theatrical, dramatic concept in line with its etymological origins — from *mîmos*, 'actor' as well as 'performance' — linked to mimetic impersonations that concern first and foremost the education (*paideia*) of youth in the Greek city (*polis*) in a period still partially dominated by an oral culture. As Eric Havelock argues in *Preface to Plato*, Plato's critique of mimesis must be understood in the context of what he calls an 'oral state of mind' in which the actor or reciter of poetry (*rhapsode*) who speaks in mimetic (first person) rather than diegetic (third person) speech has 'the power to make his audience identify almost pathologically and certainly sympathetically with the content of what he is saying'.[25] Both at the level of form (*lexis*) and content (*logos*) of mimetic spectacles, dramatic impersonations of the *Iliad*, the *Theogony*, or the tragedies and comedies, says in substance Plato, under the mask of Socrates, have a pathological effect on the public not only because they do not represent the truth about the gods (epistemic reasons), but also because the public participates emotionally in these spectacles by sym-pathos (feeling with) endowed with contagious affective properties (psychological reasons). Crucially, according to Plato's patho-logy, it is this affective force that endows mimesis with a contagious, irrational, and magnetic power. Thus, in a related dialogue titled *Ion*, Plato compares the mimetic force of poetry, understood in the broad sense of literature and myth, to a 'magnet' that transmits the property of magnetism to 'iron rings' generating a long 'chain' that goes from the Muses to the poet to the reciter of poetry to the audience that is contagiously and pathologically magnetized by such a mimetic spectacle.[26]

Reframed within this theatrical context, the famous Allegory of the Cave in Book 7 of *Republic* is brought closer to home in this period of seclusion within our private caves, reduced freedom of movement, and intensified mediatized exposure to (mis)representations that shadow reality. Let us thus recall that in the Platonic myth, the chained prisoners are spellbound by a 'puppet show' projected by carriers of simulacra walking in front of a fire and projecting 'shadows cast from the fire on the wall that fronted them [the prisoners]'.[27] The prisoners mistake the shadows for reality because they lack the critical distance of the philosopher who, with the help of a guide, can take rational steps back from the illusory sphere of sensorial perception, break the chain that ties him to these projections, and start the steep, ascending path of philosophical thought. That is a rational, dialectical, and rather vertical logos

---

24 Plato, *Republic* 597e, in *The Collected Dialogues of Plato*, ed. by Edith Hamilton and Huntington Cairns (New York: Pantheon Books, 1963), pp. 575–844 (p. 822).

25 Eric A. Havelock, *Preface to Plato* (Cambridge, MA: Harvard University Press, 1963), p. 41, p. 45.

26 Plato, *Ion* 533d-e, in *The Collected Dialogues of Plato*, pp. 215–28 (pp. 219–20).

27 Plato, *Republic* 514b–515a, p. 747.

that eventually leads, according to the myth, to the real source of light outside the cave: the sun that stands for the idea of the Good and to the unconcealment of truth via the contemplation of the intelligible and transcendental Forms, or ideas, characteristic of the *vita contemplativa* — as a metaphysical tradition that goes from Plato to Heidegger suggests.[28] And yet, depending on how we interpret those mimetic shadows projected in the cave, the myth is also open to alternative, more immanent and embodied perspectives. In particular it welcomes interpretations attentive to the imperceptible dynamic of affective contagion, or pathos, within a cave haunted by the powers of phantasmal simulations that have spellbinding, hypnotic, and magnetic effects — a psychological perspective attentive to what I call *vita mimetica.*[29]

Considered from the immanent, embodied, and experiential condition of the chained prisoners, we should wonder about the type of force, or power, that metaphorically chains and inclines spectators toward those shady projections on the wall. Plato, as the fine dramatist that he is, specifies that due to an 'echo' in the cave, the voices of the carriers of simulacra behind the prisoners generate the impressions that the shadows themselves speak in the first person, via mimetic lexis: 'if their prison had an echo from the wall opposite them, when one of the passers-by uttered a sound, do you think that they would suppose anything else than the passing shadow to be the speaker?'[30] Who, indeed is the speaker? This is not only a narratological question or a metaphysical question — it is, first and foremost, a patho-logical question. Could it be, in fact, that the prisoners remain chained, magnetized, pathologically spellbound by, or bound to, those projections mistaken for true realities, precisely because the spectacle of moving shadows is animated? Thus reframed, the speaking and moving shadows generate a mimetic sym-pathos or affective identification that is magnetic, contagious, and has an immanent psychological power that is at least double: first, the shadows chain spectators to appearances that are far removed indeed from reality; and second, they cast an intoxicating spell on the prisoners generating a contagious pathology. This is, indeed, what Plato 'himself', always under the mask of Socrates, suggests in *Ion* when he specifies that the effect of the magnetic/mimetic chain that goes from the poet to the audience is to generate a state of Dionysian intoxication in spectators who are dispossessed by this magnetic and contagious power. Thus, he compares theatrical spectators to the 'Corybantes' who are 'sized with Bacchic transport' and are 'bereft of their senses'.[31] Dionysian rituals, for Plato, are dramatically entangled with the intoxicating power of poetry.

---

28 Martin Heidegger, *The Essence of Truth*, trans. by Ted Sadler (New York: Continuum, 2002).

29 Informed by Arendt's account of the *vita activa*, a first step in this direction while not focused directly on mimesis can be found in Adriana Cavarero, *Platone* (Milano: Raffaello Cortina Editore, 2018), pp. 129–47. Joining perspectives, Cavarero and I stretched this mimetic connection in Adriana Cavarero and Nidesh Lawtoo, 'Mimetic Inclinations: A Dialogue with Adriana Cavarero', in *Contemporary Italian Women Philosophers: Stretching the Art of Thinking*, ed. by Silvia Benso and Elvira Roncally (New York: SUNY Press, 2021), pp. 183–99, as well as in *Homo Mimeticus*, 69–91.

30 Plato, *Republic* 515b, pp. 747–48.

31 Plato, *Ion* 534 a-c, p. 220.

Among the moderns, Nietzsche is often remembered as an anti-Platonic thinker with respect to his critique of idealist metaphysics, but his opposition to Plato is not as clear-cut as the dominant commentaries make him appear to be. On the contrary, when it comes to mimesis, Nietzsche writes contra/with Plato in the spirit of a Homeric contest I call 'mimetic agonism'.[32] As Nietzsche will make clear at the twilight of metaphysics in *The Birth of Tragedy*, there is a contagious (Dionysian) mimesis that is not confined within the wall of visual (Apollonian) representation. Rather, it transgresses the boundaries between self and other, generating a mimetic pathos that can have intoxicating effects on spectators, depriving them not only of true representations of reality but also of their rational control over their ego. In sum, as a psychological tradition that goes from Plato to Nietzsche indicates, this mimetic pathos has the (will to) power to take possession of spectators, dispossess them of their rational faculty, or logos, and generate mimetic pathologies that are constitutive of the *vita mimetica*.

If we now further our genealogy of mimesis from a more contemporary perspective, this mimetic tradition still helps us to reflect critically on new (social) media that, perhaps more than ever, cast a magnetic, contagious, and intoxicating spell on the human imagination. As film critics from André Bazin onward routinely noted, the Allegory of the Cave anticipates the mimetic powers of cinema to induce what Edgar Morin calls an 'imitation-hypnotic state' in spectators who are emotionally tied to cinematic images via mechanism of 'projection and identification'.[33] As Morin puts it: 'Our needs, our aspirations, our desires, our obsessions, our fears, project themselves not only into the void as dreams and imaginings, but onto all things and all beings'.[34] While cinema reproduces the Platonic scenario of the cave in the twentieth century, in the digital age the mimetic-hypnotic effects of moving shadows continues to operate on a variety of smaller screens, which, from TV to computers to smartphones, intensify the power of Apollonian images to cast a Dionysian spell with the power to generate an intoxicating psychic dispossession of the ego still constitutive of the twenty-first century.

What was true for the Platonic prisoners remains true for contemporary spectators and digital users: mimetic media do not only represent what Plato calls 'phantoms' far removed from reality — that is, copies that are epistemologically false; they also turn the ego into what Nietzsche already called a 'phantom of the ego'[35] — that is, a subject who is psychologically affected by the contagious powers of mimesis. If phantoms of reality disseminated via new media online are often rightly stressed in contemporary discussions of the powers of lies in the age of 'post-truth', it is equally crucial to stress the affective (Dionysian) receptivity of the phantom of the ego that

32 On Nietzsche's mimetic agonism with Plato and his ambivalent evaluation of mimetic intoxication (celebratory at first, critical later) see Lawtoo, *The Phantom of the Ego*, pp. 52–83.

33 Edgar Morin, *The Cinema, or the Imaginary Man*, trans. by Lorraine Mortimer (Minneapolis: University of Minnesota Press, 2005), p. 96, p. 91.

34 Morin, *The Cinema*, p. 85.

35 Friedrich Nietzsche, *Daybreak* trans. by R. J. Hollingdale (Cambridge: Cambridge University Press, 1982), p. 61.

makes *homo mimeticus* vulnerable to (Apollonian) illusions in the first place. These contagious illusions are particularly virulent in periods of crisis, like a pandemic crisis, and can lead to collective intoxications that manifest themselves in social pathologies (pandemic denial, anti-mask/antivax protests, conspiracy theories, etc.) that double and redouble the reach of the viral pathology.

Thus reframed, we are in a better position to reevaluate the relevance of mimesis in the age of viral reproduction. Plato's Allegory reaches in the present as it foreshadows a world of simulation which postmodern critics were perhaps too quick to disconnect from the problematic of mimesis. Contra Plato, Jean Baudrillard, for instance, diagnosed a hyperreal world of simulacra and simulation that no longer rests on 'imitation' but 'liquidates all referents' insofar as the hyperreal 'substitutes the real with signs of the real'.[36] Influential at the twilight of the last century, this postmodern diagnostic of simulation is of loose Nietzschean inspiration. Yet, it does not account for the human, all too human effects generated by a hyperreal world of simulacra, which, while no longer resting on the logic of mimesis as representations, continues to cast a material (Dionysian) shadow on this world, generating not only phantoms of reality but phantoms of egos in the twenty-first century.[37]

The inversion of perspective from mimetic phantoms to mimetic egos that already informed Nietzsche's critique of Platonism is now redoubled by our critique of postmodernism. In light of the discovery of mirror neurons in the 1990s, the neurosciences provide an empirical confirmation that visual representations, no matter how far removed or disconnected from reality, have indeed the mimetic power to generate contagious reflexes; images seen from a visual distance can trigger neurological discharges that generate mimetic pathos via an immediate form of affective communication that is not necessarily mediated by consciousness but generates 'embodied simulations' nonetheless.[38] In light of humans's confirmed receptivity to mirroring reflexes caused by perception of movements (real or represented, true or false), it is thus urgent to provide a mimetic supplement to a postmodern diagnostic of hyperreality prominent at the twilight of the last century that no longer accounts for the catastrophic realities of the present century. In fact, hyperreal simulations disconnected from the logic of mimetic representation have the power to retroact on homo mimeticus via feedback loops that blur the line between truth and lies, originals and copies, facts and alternative facts, digital simulations and embodied imitations, generating shadows that are far removed from reality, indeed; and yet, they can also induce deeply-felt, false, and intoxicating beliefs. The latter trigger contagious actions that are socially pathological endowed with the immanent power to amplify viral contagions in real life. I call this looping effect whereby hyperreal simulations retroact on mimetic reflexes, hypermimesis; and I do so, to stress that the hyperreal may no

36 Jean Baudrillard, *Simulacres et Simulation* (Paris: Galilée, 1981), p. 11.

37 See Lawtoo, *The Phantom of the Ego*, Chapter 1.

38 Vittorio, Gallese, 'Embodied Simulation: From Neurons to Phenomenal Experience,' *Phenomenology and the Cognitive Sciences*, 4 (2005), pp. 23–48.

longer be subordinated to the logic of representation but continues to be rooted in the all too real laws of imitation.

Now that we have reloaded this ancient myth on the contagious powers of mimesis whose intention was to dispel artistic lies as shadows in the past, let us continue to uncover the mimetic truth on the contagious power of simulations in the present. As a significant section of the world population was holed up in private caves during multiple COVID-19 lockdowns in what was the first world pandemic to be shadowed and redoubled by digital media, practices of social distancing in privileged countries protected *homo sapiens* from the epidemic contagion and the viral pathology it entails. Still, *homo mimeticus* was far from immune from affective contagion and the social pathologies a *vita mimetica* also entails. On the contrary, chained to the continuous flow of daily news on a plurality of digital devices that amplified the pathos (from *penthos*, suffering) generated by the increasing number of victims, a contradictory double movement familiar to genealogists of mimesis began to take shape.

With some critical distance increased by the growing number of theoretical reflections on the systemic and highly differentiated implications of the pandemic crisis, this double movement allows us to return to our driving question whereby we started in more specific diagnostic terms. I reframe it as follows. In the case of the COVID-19 epidemic, we are indeed facing a hybrid viral/virtual phenomenon in which the viral pandemic is shadowed by an obsessive media focus on the spread of the virus and its proliferating mutations that not only generates sym-pathos for the real victims; the pandemic also generates a multiplicity of conspiracies theories that question the logos of science and disseminate magical causal explanations that reloaded the mimetic faculty in the age of the Internet. It did so, for instance, by directing responsibility of complex problems toward simple imaginary scapegoats (from Bill Gates to 5G to Corona beer) that made and continue to make a significant part of the population lose the sense of the reality of the pandemic itself.

Given the systemic complexity of the pandemic, even among philosophically-informed perspectives, some wondered: did rational *homo sapiens* driven by the pathos of *homo mimeticus* lose sight of the proportions between the mass-mediatized phenomenon and the pandemic itself — as the Italian philosopher Giorgio Agamben controversially claimed when, at the outset of the pandemic, he compared COVID-19 to a 'normal flu' and condemned the Italian government's disproportionate response qua 'state of exception' from a philosophical distance that condemned what he called a 'religion of health'?[39] Alternatively, and considered from the other end of the spectrum, is COVID-19 a sign that humanity has reached a tipping point and that we are now facing an epochal transformation that is likely to generate even more catastrophes — as Slovenian philosopher Slavoj Žižek writes with pathos in *Pandemic!* when he claims that the virus *will 'destroy the foundations of our lives'*.[40] Or should we rather forge a complex middle path between pathos and distance, as Nietzschean genealogical lenses indicate?

39 Giorgio Agamben, *A che punto stiamo? L'epidemia come politica* (Macerata: Quodlibet 2020), 13.

40 Slavoj Žižek, *Pandemic! COVID-19 Shakes the World* (New York: Polity Press, 2020).

The patho(-)logies of contagion remind us that the (new) media are certainly not a transparent window onto the world but should be framed within the long history of mimesis which I schematically reconstruct as follows: 1) at the dawn of philosophy, Plato (in)famously introduced the trope of the 'mirror' to account for different ontological degrees of reality predicated on a philosophical *logos* that denounces mimesis as a phantom of a phantom; 2) at the twilight of metaphysics, writing with and contra Plato, Nietzsche overturned the diagnostic by relying on the logic of pathos, or patho-*logy* to unmask the power of phantoms to take possession of the modern ego; 3) jumpstarting mimetic theory from a romantic source of inspiration, Girard diagnosed mimesis as a state of undifferentiation predicated on the Dionysian logic of violent pathos (with Nietzsche), while framing this logic in an ideal triangular form that culminates in a scapegoating mechanism that (with Plato) operates as a *pharmakon*; 4) at the end of the metaphysical spectrum, Baudrillard, with Nietzsche, contra Plato, rejected the doubling logic of the mirror at the twilight of mimetic realism by introducing a hyperreal world of simulation that has nothing to do with imitation. This history of mimesis reaches until the twilight of the twentieth century, and it now needs to be updated for the present century.

Building on, while pushing against, this genealogy, I convoke the trope of the magnifying glass to diagnose pathological mimetic phenomena that remain rooted in material process of viral and affective reproduction that infect *homo mimeticus* in differentiated ways. Once doubled by a heterogeneous media landscape, attention to the duplicity of mimetic patho(-)logies reveals how the media, while not having access to a stabilizing essence of truth, can faithfully reproduce a scientific *logos* to inform the population; alternatively they can also spread pathological lies via the power of mimetic *pathos* to deform, and in the case of conspiracy theories, dissolve the contours of reality. Both true and false forms of patho(-)logical communication can in turn generate hypermimetic processes that do not simply mirror an ideal, stable, and immutable reality. After all, the scientific patho-*logy* on the virus must continue to evolve to keep up with a mutating virus. Nor do they reveal a metaphorical truth hidden at the foundation of the world, for both viral and affective pathologies operate on two different but related and equally real levels of contamination. Rather, conspiracies generate spiraling feedback loops between the pathology of viral contagion and affective contagion whereby the latter is not simply an effect of viral contagion but also a cause of it. This dynamic looping effect can in turn lead to pathological effects (as in the case of pandemic denial) and patho-*logical* effects (as in the case of legitimate fear). Everything hinges on the message communicated to human faculties that are as rational as they are mimetic faculties.

Narratives of linear progress based on the *logos* of science affirmed that the vaccine rollout will eventually put this pandemic to a global stop, though we now have sufficient evidence to realize that the agentic properties of the virus should not be underestimated for it can always return in a mutated form. Moreover, this *logos* should not underestimate the looping effects of false accounts of reality that convince by drawing on the intoxicating *pathos* of mimetic contagion to work counter to immunization and preventive measures in insidious ways critical theorists can analyse from a patho-*logical* distance. At its very minimum, a critical *logos* on mimetic *pathos* can be put to use to dispel one of the greatest myths about *homo sapiens* that should have been unmasked by the horrors of the twentieth century but still informs 'scientific' approaches to the human in the twenty-first century: namely, the ideal of a fully rational, autonomous, and self-sufficient creature characteristic of the subject of the *Aufklärung* alias *homo sapiens*. This ideal fails to account for a *vita mimetica* that was already at play in the classical period and makes a massive come-back in the modern period, casting a shadow on the present as well.

3. Modern Contagion: Microbes, Crowds, Publics

Second step. The connection between mimesis and affective contagion became central to sociological reflections in the last decades of nineteenth century, which saw unprecedented numbers of people assembled in cities. The phenomenon of the 'crowd' (*foule, Masse, folla*) gave rise to transnational theories of crowd behaviour that were neglected in the second half of the twentieth century, yet are currently returning to the forefront of critical attention in the present century in the context of political crises.[41] This mimetic, or rather, hypermimetic phenomenon deserves to be revisited in the context of pandemic crises as well. Founding figures of crowd psychology like Gustave Le Bon and Gabriel Tarde in France, Wilfred Trotter and William McDougall in England and, later, Sigmund Freud in Austria, noted that when people are assembled in a physical crowd or, at one remove, become part of a virtual public, while reading newspapers for instance — and today Twitter, Facebook, TikTok, YouTube, etc. — emotions are transmitted from self to other in an irrational, unconscious, and as they would all say, 'contagious' way.[42] As Le Bon puts it in his widely popular, *The Crowd*: 'In a crowd every sentiment and act is contagious, and contagious to such a degree that an individual readily sacrifices his personal interest to the collective interest'.[43] Already prior to Le Bon, Gabriel Tarde had expanded the diagnostic from the crowd to account for the social bond *tout court* by considering society in terms of flows of imitation. Thus, he asks in *The Laws of Imitation*: 'And this similitude [in opinions and emotions] is it not due to a flow of imitation which can be accounted for by needs and ideas disseminated by previous imitative contagions [*contagions imitatives*]?'[44] Well before Girard, then, both Le Bon and Tarde use the concept of 'contagion' metaphorically to indicate an invisible transmission of

41 For this recent revival of interest, see Christian Borch, *The Politics of Crowds: An Alternative History of Sociology* (Cambridge: Cambridge University Press, 2012); Gunter Gebauer and Sven Rücker, *Vom Sog der Massen und der neuen Macht der Einzelnen* (Deutsche Verlags-Anstalt, 2019); Lawtoo, *(New) Fascism*.

42 For Henri Bergson's thoughts on 'contagion' in this same context, see especially section 4 of chapter 7 in this volume.

43 Gustave Le Bon, *The Crowd: A Study of the Popular Mind* (New York: Dover Publications, Inc., 2002), p. 7.

44 Gabriel Tarde, *Les Lois de l'imitation* (Paris: Seuil, 2001), p. 50. On the contemporary relevance of Tarde's theory of imitation see also, Andrea Mubi Brighenti, 'Tarde, Canetti, and Deleuze on Crowds and Packs', *Journal of Classical Sociology*, 10. 4 (2010), pp. 291–314.

emotions that spread, virus-like, from self to others generating an affective contagion that, we should add, has systemic implications for viral contagion as well.

Despite the numerous and still unexplored analogies between crowd psychology and mimetic theory, it is important to stress that the metaphorical use of contagion in crowd psychology differs significantly from Girard's mimetic theory — and in this difference lies the foundation for an alternative theory of homo mimeticus. If Girard read the plague in literature as a metaphor for a more fundamental dynamic of contagious violence, crowd psychologists invert the perspective and draw inspiration from the medical reality of medical contagion to metaphorically account for the psycho-social dynamic of mimetic, or affective contagion. For crowd psychologists, it is not that viral contagion is metaphorical of affective contagion; on the contrary, affective contagion can be metaphorically compared to an all too real viral contagion.

The advantages of this inversion are plural: first, the metaphorical use of the term 'contagion' does not dispute the danger or reality of viral contagion; rather, it draws on the language of medical contagion to account for the disconcerting capacity of emotions in a crowd to spread invisibly, from self to others, like a microbe or virus. Writing in fin-de-siècle France, both Le Bon and Tarde borrowed the concept of 'contagion' (*la contagion*) directly from Louis Pasteur's then relatively new discovery of microbes to account for diseases like cholera and rabies. Second, confronted with the disconcerting emotional suggestibility of urban crowds, social theorists applied the concept of contagion to the collective psyche to account for the unconscious relation, or hypnotic rapport between self and other, a mirroring relation that leads the ego to mimetically reproduce the affects of others in potentially exponential ways that provide an alternative foundation for mimetic studies. Crowd psychology, in fact, proposes a dyadic/rhizomatic rather than triangular/familial structure at the origins of a type of contagion that resembled much more the dynamic of viral infection. In fact, a subject driven not only by mimetic desire but by a mimetic pathos that includes desire and other affects as well, both good and bad, has the power to contaminate others with the same pathos in ways that can expand exponentially to affect and infect the entire mass or crowd. The medical language of contagion is thus well-chosen to account for a dynamic of transmission that operates not only at the intersubjective level but also at the broader social and collective level. Finally, this metaphorical use is relevant for our diagnostic for it shows that the social *logos* on affective contagion and the medical *logos* on viral contagion are genealogically linked, encouraging contemporary theorists to think about the spiraling interplay between viral and social pathologies.

How does *affective* contagion operate? Via a mirroring, mimetic principle that belongs to a pre-Freudian tradition of the unconscious that was marginalized in the past century, yet genealogical lenses are bringing back to account for contagious phenomena for the present century. Both Le Bon and Tarde, in fact, like Nietzsche before them, relied on the model of hypnosis or hypnotic suggestion to account for the contagious dynamic of emotions. For Le Bon, contagion and suggestion are two sides of the same mimetic phenomenon: 'When defining crowds, we said that one of their general characteristics was an excessive suggestibility, and we have shown to what an extent suggestions are contagious in every human agglomeration; a fact which explains the rapid turning of the sentiments of a crowd in a definite direction'.[45] It is because subjects who are part of a crowd are in a psychic state of light hypnosis, or suggestion, that they are prone to mirroring the emotions of others, going potentially as far as turning the idea of others into an action, which is the very definition of suggestion. Gabriel Tarde confirms this point as he zooms in on the neuronal mimetic principles that account for this contagious process as he writes: 'the action at a distance from brain to brain that I call imitation, is assimilable to hypnotic suggestion [*suggestion hypnotique*]'; and he specifies that this mirroring/contagious mechanism via theories of hypnotic suggestion that assume (rightly we know now) that in humans 'nerves imitate nerves, brains imitate brains'.[46] As I have shown elsewhere, for a pre-Freudian psychological tradition, reflex forms of mirroring imitation, much more than dreams, served as a *via regia* to a relational, social, and immanent unconscious I call the 'mimetic unconscious'.[47] If this mirroring principle was discovered in the 1990s and attributed to 'mirror neurons', genealogical lenses reveal that it is more genealogically accurate to speak of a *re*-discovery of unconscious mimetic mechanisms already advocated in the 1890s.

What we must add is that this psychological tradition of the mimetic unconscious, which is attentive to mirroring reflexes, intersubjective bonds, altered states of consciousness, and contagious emotional dynamics, provides a socio-political supplement to account for the interplay between viral and affective contagion. After all, leaders like Mussolini and Hitler were quick to put Le Bon's lessons on how to cast a hypnotic spell on the crowd to fascist use; and there is little evidence that contemporary authoritarian leaders presiding over periods of pandemic crisis do not use the same affective strategies to come to power, remain in power, and in certain cases, downplay pandemic or other crises, thereby undermining immunization and amplifying its power of infection.

The dynamic interplay between viral contagion and affective contagion in an age haunted by the shadow of what I call '(new) fascism' amplifies the viral pathology via pathological political responses. (New) fascist leaders like Donald Trump in the US, and Jair Bolsonaro in Brazil, for example, revealed the plurality of ways in which a pathological politics based on pandemic-denialism that follows conspiracy theories rather than scientific facts aggravated the viral pathology in these countries, amplifying the number of casualties in criminal ways that, along with climate-change denial,

---

45 Le Bon, *The Crowd*, p. 14. On the role of hypnosis and suggestion in the discovery of the unconscious, see Henri F. Ellenberger, *The Discovery of the Unconscious: The History and Evolution of Dynamic Psychiatry* (New York: Basic Books Inc. Publishers, 1970).

46 Tarde, *Lois de l'imitation*, p. 257 n. 1, p. 264.

47 Lawtoo, *The Phantom of the Ego*, and 'The Mimetic Unconscious: A Mirror for Genealogical Reflections' in *Imitation, Contagion, Suggestion: On Mimesis and Society*, ed. by Christian Borch (New York: Routledge, 2019), pp. 37–53.

should be considered as constitutive of (new) fascism in the twenty-first century.[48] And yet, at the same time, the pathological dimension of a (new) fascist response to the epidemic also had the paradoxical effect to generate liberating and positive patho-*logical* forms of anti-fascist contagion. The *pathos* generated by systemic police racism and systemic racial oppression, for instance, ignited anti-racist protests that, under the banner of 'Black Lives Matter' (BLM), also spread contagiously, but via a life-affirmative, non-violent sympathy in the United States and across the world. Similarly, in the UK, protests about systemic violence directed against women sparked solidarity across nations to oppose sexist patriarchal societies which, as recent studies show, render women's lives, just like minorities and illegal immigrants, much more vulnerable and precarious in periods of pandemic crisis.[49]

To move toward our last step, what we must add is that the same (new) fascist rhetoric that privileges the use of images rather than thoughts, emotion or *pathos* rather than reason or *logos*, is very effective in spreading illusory legends among a suggestible crowd, which reach unprecedented proportions in the digital age. As Le Bon already warned:

> The creation of the legends which so easily obtain circulation in crowds is not solely the consequence of their extreme credulity. It is also the result of the prodigious perversions [*déformations*] that events undergo in the imagination of a throng. The simplest event that comes under the observation of a crowd is soon totally transformed [*défiguré*]. A crowd thinks in images, and the image itself immediately calls up a series of other images, having no logical connection with the first. We can easily conceive this state by thinking of the fantastic succession of ideas to which we are sometimes led by calling up in our minds any fact. Our reason shows us the incoherence there is in these images, but a crowd is almost blind to this truth, and confuses with the real event what the deforming action of its imagination has superimposed thereon. A crowd scarcely distinguishes between the subjective and the objective. It accepts as real the images evoked in its mind, though they most often have only a very distant relation with the observed fact.[50]

Credulity, disregard of contradictions, and blind belief in false images, among other tendencies at play in the *vita mimetica*, have, indeed, the magnetic power to render a crowd dangerously vulnerable to legends. This is, after all, an old story. Yet this diagnostic gains new traction in a modern age (dis)informed by hypermimetic media that are mechanically reproduced on a massive scale and generate what Gabriel Tarde calls a 'public'. What Le Bon says of the 'era of crowds' (*ère des foules*) is in fact amplified in what Tarde calls the 'era of the public' (*ère du public*); that is,

---

48 See Lawtoo, *(New) Fascism: Contagion, Community, Myth*. As countries like India are hit by a devastating second wave as I write (April 2021), the criminal implications of downplaying the pandemic, not implementing security measures, and leaving the country disastrously unprepared, also applies to leaders like Narendra Modi, leading the population to call for his resignation.

49 Ali and others, 'Living it Out'.

50 Le Bon, *The Crowd*, 15.

a 'virtual crowd' (*foule virtuelle*) he considers already in 1901 the 'social group of the future' for it is physically dispersed yet mentally connected by a simultaneous exposure to media that generate a 'suggestion at a distance'.[51] Taking the readership of newspapers as a paradigmatic example of a public, Tarde speaks of a mutual suggestion between readers at a distance responsible for the 'unconscious illusion that our sentiment was commonly shared with a great number of others'.[52] Furthering this diagnostic of contagion on the shoulders of Tarde for the digital age, we might add that this suggestibility is aggravated by conspiracy theories that have no relation to facts whatsoever. And yet, they operate on the mimetic unconscious nonetheless by going viral online and generating contagious behaviour offline. In the process, they pose a serious hypermimetic threat to immunization in pathological ways that still require diagnostic investigations and with which I would like to conclude.

4. Conspiracy Theories: The Patho-*logies* of Immunization

Two steps back to the ancient and modern foundations of mimetic studies allow us to make a last step — or jump — ahead to present conspiracy theories about a pandemic that cast a shadow on future crises as well. Isolated by lockdowns, exposed to a plurality of (new) media that rely on algorithms to amplify already held beliefs, *homo sapiens* can easily let go of a rational *logos* to be driven by an irrational *pathos*, shot through by anxiety, fear, and resentment, but also poverty and lack of education. Overwhelmed by conflicting (dis)information, a growing number of the world population is increasingly threatened by the spread of conspiracy theories that go viral online, can now be mass-produced by A.I. chatbots in urgent need of regulations, and, in a spiraling hypermimetic loop, generate contagious pathological effects offline, contaminating a *homo mimeticus 2.0* chained to a multiplicity of new media programmed to amplify exponentially the mimetic faculty in the digital age.

Conspiracy theories provide a new name for an ancient mimetic phenomenon. As Karl Popper made clear in *The Open Society and Its Enemies*, they can be traced back to a collectivist, magical, or as he calls it, 'tribal' or 'closed society' animated by the mimetic faculty and dominated by poetic figures that already worried Plato at the dawn of western civilization. Of course, Popper considers Plato's theory of justice to be tyrannical and antithetical to what he calls the 'open society'. Thus, he spends considerable energy in violently critiquing 'the spell of Plato' in the first part of his *magnum opus* of political theory predicated on the thesis that 'totalitarianism belongs to a tradition which is just as old or just as young as our civilization itself'.[53] Plato's political solution to posit a philosopher king who imposes the *techne* of the *logos* from the top down to censor the *pathos* of mimetic poets is indeed complicit with mimetic pathologies that will be put to devastating fascist practice in the twentieth century.

---

51 Gabriel Tarde, *L'Opinion et la foule* (Paris: Félix Alcan, 1901), p. 11. p. 13. p. 5 (my transl.)

52 Tarde, *L'Opinion et la foule*, p. 4.

53 Karl Popper, *The Open Society and Its Enemies* (Princeton: Princeton University Press, 2020), p. XLII.

That is, the century from which Popper's critique of the closed society in general and magical or mimetic thinking in particular is launched, since he wrote the book during World War II.

And yet, with respect to Popper's specific diagnostic of the contagious powers of mimesis, this agonistic relation with Plato might not be as clear-cut as it first appears to be. Popper, in fact, acknowledges Plato's 'overwhelming intellectual achievement' in terms that convey admiration for what he calls 'Plato's power of diagnosis'.[54] As in the case of Nietzsche but for different reasons, Popper's opposition to Plato should be qualified in terms of *mimetic agonism*, for he fights the exemplary opponent with some of his diagnostic moves.[55] Taking *the* paradigmatic example from Plato's critique of mimesis in Book 3 of *Republic* with which we started, Popper notes that in Homer's *Iliad* the human vicissitudes during the Trojan War were seen as 'enforced by a supernatural will' driven by the gods' decisions located in an Olympic and magical afterworld, or *Hinterwelt*, to use Nietzsche's phrase. As Popper puts it: 'The belief in the Homeric gods whose conspiracies explain the history of the Trojan War is gone. The gods are abandoned. But their place is filled by powerful men or groups',[56] that, we should add, exploit the mimetic faculty in *this* world. *Homo mimeticus* tends to presuppose a magical individual intention to account for big systemic events. As Popper specifies: 'whatever happens in society — especially happenings such as war, unemployment, poverty, shortages, which people as a rule dislike — is the result of direct design by some powerful individuals and groups'.[57] Tribalism, magic, and irrational mimetic associations between great historical events in this world and great transcendental causes animated by powerful forces in other worlds are characteristic of a closed society, which as Plato foresaw, is under the magnetic spell of powerful myths.

But Popper goes further. He foresees that these mimetic powers can resurface with a vengeance in what he calls an 'abstract society'. That is, a technology-mediated, (new) media-dependent, modern society in which people 'have no, or extremely few, intimate personal contacts, [...] live in anonymity and isolation, and consequently in unhappiness'.[58] Popper's avowedly exaggerated thought experiment in the 1940s became a reality in the 2020s and should now ring a bell: 'We could conceive of a society in which men practically never meet face to face — in which all business is conducted by individuals in isolation who communicate by typed letters or by telegrams, and who go about in closed motor-cars'.[59] Needless to say, this has been the very condition of the world population during the first global lockdown in the

54 Popper, *The Open Society*, p. XLI, p. 163.

55 Thus, Popper says in a precise definition of mimetic agonism: 'it is obvious that we must try to appreciate the strength of an opponent if we wish to fight him successfully'. Popper, *The Open Society*, p. XLII.

56 Popper, *The Open Society*, p. 306.

57 Popper, *The Open Society*, p. 306.

58 Popper, *The Open Society*, p. 166.

59 Popper, *The Open Society*, p. 166.

digital age during the COVID-19 pandemic.[60] Given the complexity of an event such as a pandemic, simple intentional explanations have gone viral online: from considering the virus as a biological weapon to linking the vaccine to microchip implants, from blaming 5G technology to scapegoating Bill Gates to considering the pandemic a hoax, the conspiracies are many in what has been called 'an ocean of misinformation'.[61] And given the suggestible status of *homo mimeticus* whose genealogy we have traced, no wonder that the mimetic faculty predicated on the *pathos* of magical thinking was reloaded in a period of crisis — with a vengeance.

What defines conspiracy theories from antiquity to the present is that they provide a simple, unifying, direct, and often grand causal explanation for complex systemic problems that defy singular explanations. As Umberto Eco notes, commenting on Popper, conspiracy theories 'purport to offer explanations in ways that appeal to people who feel they've been denied important information'.[62] More recently, in an informed and heterogeneous collection, Michael Butter and Pieter Knight group conspiracy theories under the heading of 'nothing happens by accident; nothing is at it seems; and everything is connected', and summarize the main characteristics of conspiracy theories as follows: 'they assume that everything has been planned and nothing happens by coincidence; they divide the world strictly into the evil conspirators and the innocent victims of their plot; and they claim that the conspiracy works in secret and does not reveal itself even after it has reached its goals'.[63] Paradoxically, then, as conspiracy theories proliferate online, the public is encouraged to play the role of 'master of suspicion' (Ricoeur's phrase) supplementing Marx, Nietzsche, and Freud in uncovering latent truths behind manifest scientific contents that are, for an increasing number of believers in conspiracies, deemed too factual to be true. No training in hermeneutics is of course presupposed. Consequently, the 'master of suspicion' quickly turns into the slave of conspiracies that appeal to human, all too human suggestibility to a mimetic pathos whose magical-magnetic-mirroring-unconscious powers our genealogy urges to take seriously.

In theory, unmasking the falsity of conspiracy theories should not be a problem for researchers given the former's lack of empirical foundations; and yet since they generate a magical hypermimetic pathos that operates on the mimetic faculty in practice, effectively countering them via a rational *logos* alone is not sufficient — for the power of *logos* is precisely what the *pathos* of conspiracies defies. If we agree with

60 On new, mediated forms of communication that have gained prominence during the pandemic, see chapter 11 of this volume.

61 Richard A. Stein and others, 'Conspiracy Theories in the Era of Covid-19: A Tale of Two Pandemics', *The International Journal of Clinical Practice*, 75 (2021), pp. 1–5 (p. 1).

62 Umberto Eco, 'A Theory of Conspiracies', *Mint*, (2014), available at https://www.livemint.com/Opinion/5lhODHqqZHUCqwOZcw2liL/Umberto-Eco--A-theory-of-conspiracies.html (last accessed 16/01/2022).

63 Michael Butter and Pieter Knight, 'General Introduction', in *Routledge Handbook of Conspiracy Theories*, ed. by Michael Butter and Pieter Knight (New York: Routledge, 2020), pp. 1–8 (p. 1). This is a rich, transdisciplinary collection that opens up multiple perspectives to conspiracy theories, from historical to psychological, semiotic to political, literary to philosophical, among others. This chapter supplements to it a mimetic perspective.

Popper that conspiracy theories are as old as Homer at the level of the message, we should add that (new) media rely on algorithms that amplify the powers of the mimetic unconscious by feeding users' misinformation that reinforces already held beliefs (or confirmation bias), generating bubbles that create, via social media and Internet channels (Facebook, Twitter, YouTube, TikTok etc.), alternative or parallel worlds that can all-too-easily be mistaken for the 'real' world. This challenge is especially visible with respect to the plurality of conspiracies that deny the danger of the pandemic in a period of general crisis, isolation, and hyperconnectivity to a multiplicity of contradictory information, true and false.

Conspiracies not only generate false theories but also pathological practices. They lead *homo mimeticus* to deny the danger of the pandemic, counter safety measures, and spread vaccine hesitancy during an already complex, bumpy, and unequal vaccine rollout. In addition to medical, political, and economic hurdles, not to speak of the virus's multiple mutations, scientific discourse (or logos) find itself undermined by conspiracy-driven affects (or *pathos*) about vaccines. As Butter and Knight confirm: 'psychologists have shown that belief in conspiracy theories about vaccines or global warming leads to a refusal to vaccinate oneself or one's children, or an unwillingness to reduce one's carbon dioxide footprint'.[64] The proliferation of conspiracies on social media, supplemented by increasingly professional-looking documentaries to spread conspiracies, have hypermimetic effects that reach massive proportions in periods of crisis like a pandemic crisis in which everyone is susceptible to pathos.

This is not a minor problem that can be solved from the angle of a scientific *logos* alone, for rational knowledge and empirical methods are precisely what are undermined by conspiracy theories; nor can conspiracies easily be censored, for although some prohibitions are in place (with respect to Holocaust denial, for instance) the right to free speech in an open hyperconnected society escapes censoring mechanisms that already at the time of Plato's relatively closed society could only be imagined in theory. As my genealogy of mimesis from antiquity to modernity tried to show, in broad brush strokes, conspiracy theories call for balancing diagnostic operations that account for the role of *pathos* in reloading the mimetic faculty in the digital age — and perhaps turn the mimetic faculty to patho-*logical* use by relying on the power of positive models or examples to promote the importance of vaccination and preventive measures more generally via both logical and affective means.[65]

In the end, an awareness of the interplay of reason and emotions, *logos* and *pathos*, in the digital age is not only essential to immunization during a pandemic crisis. It is equally vital to confront crises to come. If we consider that conspiracy theories contribute to spreading climate change denial in the epoch of the Anthropocene while also promoting imaginary migrations to other planets behind our own, then

64 Butter and Knight, 'General Introduction', p. 6. For an historical genealogy of 'anti-vax' conspiracies in relation to the Internet, see also Simona Stano, 'The Internet and the Spread of Conspiracies' in *Routledge Handbook of Conspiracy Theories*, pp. 483–96 (pp. 487–93).

65 In addition to scientist and politicians, actors and celebrities play a key mimetic role in pro-vaccination campaigns as an identification with them is already in place.

we have no choice but to heed Zarathustra's warning: '*stay true to the Earth* and do not believe those who talk of over-earthly hopes!'[66] For all humans, be they *sapiens* or *mimeticus*, or an untidy mixture of both, there is no alternative choice. Hence the urgency to join the powers of *logos* and *pathos* to affirm patho-*logical* solutions for the crises of the present that already cast a long shadow on the future.

66 Friedrich Nietzsche, *Thus Spoke Zarathustra*, trans. by Graham Parkes (Oxford: Oxford University Press, 2005), p. 12.

Bibliography

Agamben, Giorgio, *A che punto stiamo? L'epidemia come politica* (Macerata: Quodlibet 2020).

Ali, Kecia, Belser, Julia-Watts, Kao, Grace Y., Smith, Shiverly T. J., 'Living It Out: Feminism During Covid 19', *Journal of Feminist Studies in Religion*, 36. 2 (2020), pp. 107–16.

Baudrillard, Jean, *Simulacres et simulation* (Paris: Galilée, 1981).

Benjamin, Walter, *Reflections: Essays, Aphorisms, Autobiographical Writings*, ed. by Peter Demetz, trans. by Edmund Jephcott (New York: Schocken Books, 2007).

———, 'The Work of Art in the Age of Its Technological Reproducibility' (2nd version), in *The Work of Art in the Age of its Technological Reproducibility and Other Media*, ed. by Michael W. Jennings an others, trans. by Edmund Jephcott and others (Cambridge, MA: Harvard University Press, 2008), pp. 19–55.

Borch, Christian, *The Politics of Crowds: An Alternative History of Sociology* (Cambridge: Cambridge University Press, 2012).

Butler, Judith. *What World Is This? A Pandemic Phenomenology* (New York: Columbia University Press, 2022).

Butter, Michael, and Pieter Knight, 'General Introduction', in *Routledge Handbook of Conspiracy Theories*, ed. by Michael Butter and Pieter Knight (New York: Routledge, 2020).

Cavarero, Adriana, *Platone* (Milano: Raffaello Cortina Editore, 2018).

———, and Nidesh Lawtoo, 'Mimetic Inclinations: A Dialogue with Adriana Cavarero', in *Contemporary Italian Women Philosophers: Stretching the Art of Thinking*, ed. by Silvia Benso and Elvira Roncalli (New York: SUNY Press, 2021), pp. 183–99.

Derrida, Jacques, *Dissemination*, trans. by Barbara Johnson (Chicago: The University of Chicago Press, 1981).

Eco, Umberto, 'A Theory of Conspiracies', Mint, (2014).

https://www.livemint.com/Opinion/5lhODHqqZHUCqwOZcw2liL/Umberto-Eco--A-theory-of-conspiracies.html

Ellenberger, Henri F., *The Discovery of the Unconscious: The History and Evolution of Dynamic Psychiatry* (New York: Basic Books Inc. Publishers, 1970).

Esposito, Roberto. *Immunitas: protezione e negazione della vita* (Torino: Einaudi, 2002).

———. *Immunità comune. Biopolitica all'epoca della pandemia* (Einaudi: Torino, 2022).

Gallese, Vittorio, 'Embodied Simulation: From Neurons to Phenomenal Experience,' *Phenomenology and the Cognitive Sciences*, 4 (2005), pp. 23–48.

Gebauer, Gunter, and Sven Rücker, *Vom Sog der Massen und der neuen Macht der Einzelnen* (Deutsche Verlags-Anstalt, 2019).

———, and Christoph Wulf, *Mimesis: Culture-Art-Society*, trans. by Don Reneau (Berkeley: University of California Press, 1995).

Girard, René, 'The Plague in Literature and Myth', *Texas Studies in Literature and Language*, 15. 5 (1974), pp. 833–50.

———, *Battling to the End: Conversations with Benoît Chantre*, trans. by Mary Baker (East Lansing: Michigan State University Press, 2010).

Havelock, Eric A., *Preface to Plato* (Cambridge, MA: Harvard University Press, 1963).

Heidegger, Martin, *The Essence of Truth*, trans. by Ted Sadler (New York: Continuum, 2002).

Lawtoo, Nidesh, *The Phantom of the Ego: Modernism and the Mimetic Unconscious* (East Lansing: Michigan State University Press, 2013).

———, 'The Cooperative Community: Surviving Epidemics in The Shadow-Line', in *Conrad's Shadow: Catastrophe, Mimesis, Theory* (East Lansing: Michigan State University Press, 2016), pp. 91–125.

———, 'Violence and the Mimetic Unconscious (Part I), The Catharsis Hypothesis: Aristotle, Girard, Freud', *Contagion*, 25 (2018): pp. 159–92.

———, *(New) Fascism: Contagion, Community, Myth* (East Lansing: Michigan State University Press, 2019).

———, 'The Mimetic Unconscious: A Mirror for Genealogical Reflections' in *Imitation, Contagion, Suggestion: On Mimesis and Society*, ed. by Christian Borch (New York: Routledge, 2019), pp. 37–53.

———. *Homo Mimeticus: A New Theory of Imitation* (Leuven: Leuven University Press, 2022).

——— (ed.), *The Mimetic Condition, CounterText*, 1. 8 (2022).

——— (ed.), *Homo Mimeticus 2.0: Art, Philosophy, Technics* (Leiden: Brill, 2024).

Le Bon, Gustave, *The Crowd: A Study of the Popular Mind* (New York: Dover Publications, Inc., 2002).

Mauss, Marcel, *The Gift: Forms and Functions of Exchange in Archaic Societies* (London: Cohen & West, 1966).

Mbembe, Achille, 'The Universal Right to Breathe', trans. by Carolyne Shread, *Critical Inquiry*, 47. 52 (2020), In the Moment (blog),
https://critinq.wordpress.com/2020/04/13/the-universal-right-to-breathe/

Morin, Edgar, *The Cinema, or the Imaginary Man*, trans. by Lorraine Mortimer (Minneapolis: University of Minnesota Press, 2005).

———, (with the collaboration of Sabah Abouessalam), Changeons de voie: les leçons du coronavirus (Paris: Denoël, 2020).

Mubi Brighenti, Andrea, 'Tarde, Canetti, and Deleuze on Crowds and Packs', *Journal of Classical Sociology*, 10. 4 (2010), pp. 291–314.

Nietzsche, Friedrich, *Daybreak*, trans. by R. J. Hollingdale (Cambridge: Cambridge University Press, 1982).

———, *On the Genealogy of Morals*, trans. Douglas Smith (Oxford: Oxford University Press, 1998).

———, *Thus Spoke Zarathustra*, trans. by Graham Parkes (Oxford: Oxford University Press, 2005).

Plato, *Ion*, in *The Collected Dialogues of Plato*, ed. by Edith Hamilton and Huntington Cairns (New York: Pantheon Books, 1963), pp. 215–28.

Plato, *Republic*, in *The Collected Dialogues of Plato*, ed. by Edith Hamilton and Huntington Cairns (New York: Pantheon Books, 1963), pp. 575–844.

Popper, Karl, *The Open Society and Its Enemies* (Princeton: Princeton University Press, 2020).

Stano, Simona, 'The Internet and the Spread of Conspiracies' in *Routledge Handbook of Conspiracy Theories*, pp. 483–96.

Stein, Richard A., and , 'Conspiracy Theories in the Era of Covid-19: A Tale of Two Pandemics', *The International Journal of Clinical Practice*, 75 (2021), pp. 1–5.

Tarde, Gabriel, *L'Opinion et la foule* (Paris: Félix Alcan, 1901).

———, *Les Lois de l'imitation* (Paris: Seuil, 2001).

Viriasova, Inna, and Antonio Calcagno (eds.), *Roberto Esposito: Biopolitics and Philosophy* (Albany, NY: SUNY Press, 2018).

Žižek, Slavoj, *Pandemic! COVID-19 Shakes the World* (New York: Polity Press, 2020).

ĽUDMILA LACKOVÁ

11. Crisis of the Subject in Mediated Communication*

▼ **ABSTRACT** The years 2020 and 2021 have been marked by a pandemic in terms of the unmeasurable damage to health and the economy. While the endangered health of the population is the primary consequence of the COVID-19 pandemic, there are also several secondary ones caused by the security measures taken by the world countries' representatives. First and foremost is the economic loss; apart from that, there is also health damage caused by the lockdown and people's responsibility to stay at home without physical activity or social interactions resulting in general risk for physical and mental health. Besides the health issues, communication is another area which is undergoing a drastic challenge due to indirect COVID-19 pandemic consequences. The traditional forms of mediated communication, widely spread and developed in recent decades thanks to the technological progress, have become, in many cases, the only possible way of human communication. The secondary role of mediated communication over the non-mediated primary communication is questionable in the times we live in. In this chapter, the crisis of the subject of the communication related to pandemic-induced communicational transformation is examined.

1. Introduction: Pandemics and Communication

Concerning the communication aspect of the period of the COVID-19 pandemic, two main features will probably remain in our memories even years after the pandemic is over:
the difficulty of face-to-face communication with masks (visual and auditive) and the mediation of communication through various new media appliances and video

* This publication was funded by the project JG_2024_020 implemented within the Palacký University Young Researcher Grant.

Epidemics and Pandemics, ed. by Michele Nicoletti and Alessandro Palazzo (Turnhout: Brepols, 2024), pp. 279–296
BREPOLS PUBLISHERS 10.1484/M.STPH-EB.5.136415

chats. The former feature, mask-induced worsened communication quality, is not only an effect of the mask impeding the flow of air when pronouncing phonemes. There is also an additional factor mirroring the phenomenon of visual and auditive interconnectedness in perception of speech. The phenomenon was experimentally approached already in 1976.[1] According to the above-mentioned studies, understanding and interpretation of speech is not strictly auditive: visual perception of lip movement plays a very important role in cognitive categorization of phonemes, thus, understanding the pronounced speech and conveyed information. The impact of wearing sanitary masks on speech perception during the period of COVID-19 pandemic was reflected upon by Kopecký.[2]

Sanitary masks worsen the perception of spoken speech but at the same time, they have acquired immense communicative power thanks to the symbolic value they gained during the pandemic.

> As a symbol of heroic resistance against disease, of the care taking of the sick ones and attention to the health of citizens, masks have ended up as selfies of governors, presidents and representatives of institutions, always ready to associate their image with everything that generates consent.[3]

One of the first state representatives publicly wearing a sanitary mask and consequently influencing other important government representatives, becoming a kind of a 'mask idol', was the Slovak president Zuzana Čaputová. Her attitude towards fighting the pandemic ostentatiously expressed by wearing masks, which were even of compelling colours, at official occasions was reflected in many world media as a good example of individual responsibility at the beginning of the era of pandemic for citizens. Being the first female president of Slovakia and generally perceived as an elegant woman, her mask-wearing also became a question of associating the mask with fashion and style.[4] Thus, masks are not only bearers of the meaning of political opinions, representativeness, or attitudes towards the pandemic, but they also convey vogue preferences.

Another aspect of the mutation in communication during the pandemic is the distant form of communication. The restrictions of movement and social isolation

1 Harry McGurk and John MacDonald, 'Hearing lips and seeing voices', *Nature*, 264(5588) (1976), pp. 746–48; see also Mikko Sams and others, 'Seeing and hearing others and oneself talk', *Cognitive Brain Research*, 23. 2–3 (2005), pp. 429–35.

2 Daniel Kopecký, *McGurkův efekt* (Olomouc: Univerzita Palackého v Olomouci, in print, 2022); see also Klára Hájková, 'Jak nošení roušek ovlivňuje naši komunikaci', in *Lingvistika z obýváku*, ed. by Dan Faltýnek (Olomouc: Univerzita Palackého v Olomouci, 2020), available at https://jazykzczk.netlify.app/_book/pm14.html#idea1 (last accessed 21/01/2022).

3 Antonio Santangelo, 'I narcisi mascherati, gli eroi e noi. La parabola dei selfie con la maschera', in *Volti virali*, ed. by Massimo Leone (Turin: FACETS Digital Press, 2020), pp. 39–68 (p. 42). In original 'Così le mascherine, simbolo della resistenza eroica contro la malattia, della cura dei malati e dell'attenzione per la salute dei cittadini, sono finite nei selfie di governatori, presidenti e rappresentanti delle istituzioni, sempre pronti ad associare la propria immagine a tutto ciò che genera consenso'.

4 Sophie Williams, *Coronavirus: How face masks are becoming fashionable*, available at https://www.bbc.com/news/world-52691164 (last accessed 21/01/2022).

went hand-in-hand with the explosion of platforms such as Zoom, Google Meet, Microsoft Teams, and others. Serving mostly for business and work meetings, as simulations of face-to-face communication, these platforms became a part of everyday life for most of the working population, students, teachers, and other public functionaries. The digital environment turned into our new home. Consequently, it might be questionable whether mediated communication stays in a secondary role with respect to unmediated communication. While the communicative power of masks and problems related to wearing sanitary masks were already widely studied,[5] the specifics of the distant form of communication were not paid much attention from the part of communication studies or semiotics. This chapter aims at defining the basic theoretical principles of mediated communication and describing the qualitative differences between traditional unmediated communication and currently widely practiced mediated communication.

2. Mediated Communication and New Media

To begin, let me start with a definition of unmediated communication, or in other words, the face-to-face communicative interaction between two or more individuals:

By unmediated communication we mean communication carried out in the unity of place and time based on the functional presence of only those elements of the communication scheme which have the character of physiologically natural tools, without the participation of any technology but even without the participation of any semiotic means having the character of writing. This means that we consider as unmediated communication such communication that has the character of spoken communication, the channel mediator of which is air as a gaseous environment enabling the spread of sound waves produced physiologically without any technical reinforcement.[6]

Consequently, mediated communication seems to be, according to Kořenský, definable as communication where the air channel mediator is replaced by some technical channel or writing system. The basic schema of mediated communication comprises the two subjects of communication (addresser and addressee) between whom there is a certain (technical) intermediary (regardless of the distance or proximity in time and space).

---

5 *Volti virali*, ed. by Leone.

6 Jan Kořenský, 'Teorie nových médií a transformace prostředku na subjekt?', in *Registre jazyka a jazykovedy* (II), ed. by Jana Kesselová and others (Prešov: Univerzitná knižnica Prešovskej univerzity v Prešove, 2014), pp. 132–36. In original: 'Nezprostředkovanou komunikací míníme komunikaci uskutečňovanou v jednotě místa a času založenou na funkční přítomnosti pouze takových prvků komunikačního schématu, které mají charakter nástrojů fyziologicky přirozených, bez účasti nejen jakékoli technologie, ale dokonce bez účasti jakýchkoli sémiotických prostředků majících charakter písma. Znamená to, že za nezprostředkovanou komunikaci považujeme takovou komunikaci, která má charakter mluvené komunikace, jejímž kanálovým prostředníkem je vzduch jako plynné prostředí umožňující šíření zvukových vln produkovaných fyziologicky bez jakéhokoli technického posílení'.

Let us now consider the question of the extent to which we can speak about an intermediary with the advent of new media. By new media I refer to the media used in communication based on human-computer (or other technological device) interaction. New media are defined in contradiction to 'old' media such as radio, television, etc. The perception and use of the term 'new media' have significantly changed in the last two decades. In his 2001 book, Lev Manovich wrote: 'the popular definition of new media identifies it with the use of a computer for distribution and exhibition, rather than with production'[7] and he pointed to the fact that new media already started undergoing modification by being limited to computer distribution and exhibition, to 'computer-mediated form of production'.[8] In his later book, Manovich[9] directly associated new media with software, and defines the media after 1990 as software-based tools. More concretely, new media are associated, in the last decade, with social network communication. But we should not confound new media with social media: while social media use new media technology, not all new media are social (they do not create networking). The question to be addressed in this chapter, especially in connection to the coronavirus social crisis, is whether the role of new media is the same as the one of 'old' media, with the only difference being the extent of the technological progress and digitalization. In other words, are the digital tools used in new media still 'only' mediators in communication, or do they interfere in some way with the very process of communication and thus transform it?

Although social networks offer seemingly unrestricted freedom of expression for everyone and possible constant involvement in communication, only few people realize that this freedom is limited. Paradoxically and at the same time the danger of new media (I am talking mainly about digital audiovisual social networks, podcasts, and similar platforms for communication) is the restriction and selection of information. The algorithms based on selection of friends and the selection of sites or users that we follow selects the daily influx of information. The most successful social networks such as Facebook or Twitter use complex algorithms which make a selection for us based on our range of interests — they select the information that matches our most-visited pages. In this way, it is no longer just us or other subjects-actors of the communication (communicants), but the social network 'itself' who selects the information we come in contact with (not to mention advertising that works on a similar principle). Therefore, the social network is not only an intermediary, but it also somewhat contributes to the communication and thus becomes another quasi-subject of communication. This viewpoint is not new: the medium as a subject of communication, or technology anthropomorphization, had already been introduced years ago by many scholars.[10]

7 Lev Manovich, *The Language of New Media* (Cambridge, Mass.: MIT Press, 2001), p. 43.

8 Manovich, p. 43.

9 Lev Manovich, *Software Takes Command* (New York: Bloomsbury Academic, 2013).

10 Denisa Kera, 'Globální sítě a mashupy lidí, věcí a dat: Antropomorfizace technologie a dehumanizace lidí', [Global networks and mash-ups of people, things and data: the anthropomorphization of technology and dehumanization of people]' (Plzeň: Antropowebzin, 2007), pp. 9–17; Jan Kořenský, 'Prostor (a čas)

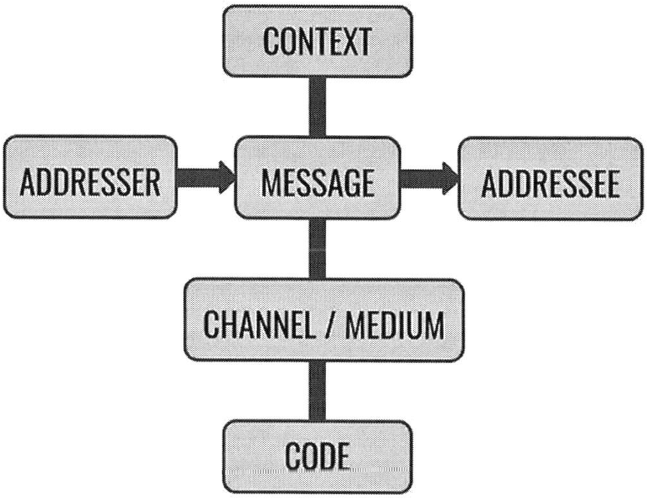

Figure 1. Jakobson's schema of communication

The subject, the addresser of the communication, enters a crisis of identity the moment it merges with the medium. Kera[11] talks about technologization of the subject on one hand and anthropomorphizing of technology on the other hand. While the latter is rather a question to be discussed within the field of robotics or AI, the former is an important issue for communication theory. As will be shown in this chapter, the crisis of the subject in new media communication is more complex than simple technologization of a human subject (which is a logical consequence of the technical progress of our society not only in the area of communication).

I would like to analyse the transformation and crisis of the subject of communication in the new media with the aid of a communication model. The one most frequently used and referred to in the theory of communication is Jakobson's model of communication.[12] It is composed of six main components: addresser, addressee, message, code, context, and channel. For the purposes of this chapter, I will equate the component of channel with a medium.

The classical communication model for mediated communication does not satisfy the requirements for the description of the crisis of the subject in the era of new media. As was already mentioned, by new media I mean the digital social networks in general but also the different platforms for communication that have germinated during the pandemic over the last two years.

---

v komunikaci a jeho proměny v souvislostech s vývojem mediačních prostředků', *Slavistična revija*, 62 (2014), pp. 387–93.

11 Denisa Kera, 'Globální sítě a mashupy lidí', pp. 9–17.

12 Roman Jakobson, *Selected Writings II. Word and Language* (Paris: Mouton, 1962) p. 22.

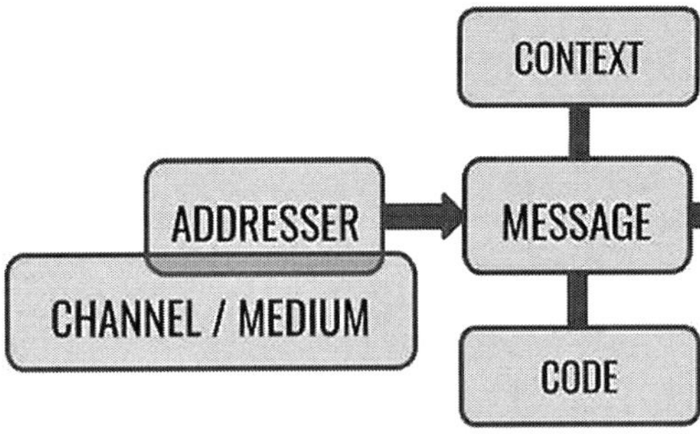

Figure 2. Medium merges with addresser

The above proposal of the communication schema reflects the interference of new media in the structure of communication. A message sender (addresser) who uses a social network, for example, is forced to appear under a social network profile within a social network, and this profile can only be compiled within the limits offered by the social network; the message sender is adapted to the media structure (Figure 2). At the same time, the limits set by the social network or other communication platform might be used by the subject to their proper advantage: the subject can choose what information to present about themselves, what audiovisual material to publish, what kind of identity they can adopt. Therefore, we can talk about the crisis of the new media subject; the subject is no more the same subject, it is necessarily a restricted form of the subject. And the restriction is inevitably meaning-making, in the sense that there is a conscious choice about the content of the restriction.

The crisis of the subject, presented in the form of the merging of subject and medium, is not the only transformation of new media communication. I will briefly comment on two concepts related to the subject which are equally transformed due to the mediation in new media: the visual part of the communication and the emotive function.

Let me first focus on the visual character of new media communication. In many digital social media, the verbal conveying of information is completely or to a great extent replaced by visual such as videos or photographs (Snapchat, Instagram, Tinder). The visual is noticeably directed to visual representation of the face. Faces are the most common visual restrictions of subjects; take profile pictures as an example. This phenomenon was described as the modern 'iconography' of the face by Massimo Leone.[13]

---

13 Massimo Leone, 'The Semiotics of the Face in Digital Dating: A Research Direction', in *Love and Sex in the Digital Age*, ed. by Gianmarco Thierry Giuliana and others, *Digital Age in Semiotics and Communication. Journal by the Southeast European Center for Semiotic Studies*, 2 (2019), pp. 18–40; Massimo Leone, 'Estéticas faciais nas sociedades digitais contemporâneas', in *Contribuições da Semiótica ao ensino de português no mundo*, ed. by Maria Teresa Tedesco and Claudio Correia (Rio de Janeiro: Dialogarts, 2021), pp. 13–22.

When it comes to the emotive function of new media, I would like to demonstrate that it is directly connected to the strong visual component present in this form of communication. There is no doubt that most new media, not only social networks but also digital magazines, journals, etc., have a strong emotional orientation. If we want to recur once again to Jakobson's communication schema and 'play' with his attribution of a specific language function to every constituent of the schema,[14] we can conclude that it is the emotional function — related to the constituent of addresser (see Figure 2) — that is striking an enormous importance in the transformation of communication with the arrival of new media and the parallel crisis of the subject.

Emotive language function had just a marginal role in Jakobson's original model, or better, in Jakobson's understanding of language,[15] but in our adapted new media model, the emotive function is very probably the most important function. We live in the era of communication of emotions, which is probably the most dangerous era of the history of communication. Emotions are the best means of manipulation.[16] It is already a largely discussed fact that the COVID-19 pandemic is a 'media pandemic'. Terms such as 'infodemics' were introduced by large health organizations such as the World Health Organization (WHO 2021)[17] or the Pan American Health Organization (PAHO 2020)[18] in order to mark the spread of disinformation, misinformation, fake news, and conspiracies regarding the coronavirus. This implicitly expresses the fact that the whole spread of emotions of fear, compassion, etc., is easier than ever before and we can only question whether the governments would react to the COVID-19 pandemic in the same manner if the pandemic arrived in historically different times where there was not such an enormous facility to spread emotions all over the world. While during the first wave of the pandemic, the misinformation and conspiracies were mostly linked to the wearing of masks, testing, or the origin of the virus, in the recent months public attention has been oriented towards vaccination.[19]

At this point, let me demonstrate how the emotive part of new media oftentimes corresponds with its visual character. Visual communication is more immediate than verbal communication, so to speak; the visual medium is intuitively 'less mediated'

14 Roman Jakobson, *Selected Writings III. Poetry of Grammar and Grammar of Poetry* (The Hague–Paris–New York: Mouton, 1981), p. 27.

15 Vít Gvoždiak, *Jakobson´s semiotic theory* (orig. *Jakobsonova sémiotická teorie*) (Olomouc: Palacký University, 2014), p. 135.

16 On the manipulation of crowds, see in particular section 3 of chapter 10 in this volume.

17 WHO *Public Health Research Agenda for Managing Infodemics* (Geneva: World Health Organization, 2021).

18 Pan American Health Organization (PAHO), *Understanding the Infodemic and Misinformation in the Fight Against COVID-19* (2020), available at https://iris.paho.org/handle/10665.2/52052 (last accessed 21/01/2022).

19 To learn more about the social media case studies on vaccine narratives across English, Spanish, and Francophone social media, see Rory Smith and others, *Under the Surface: Covid-19 Vaccine Narratives, Misinformation and Data Deficits on Social Media,* available at https://firstdraftnews.org/vaccine-narratives-full-report-november-2020 (last accessed 21/01/2022) or Sahil Loomba and others, 'Measuring the Impact of COVID-19 Vaccine Misinformation on Vaccination Intent in the UK and USA', *Nature Human Behaviour,* 5 (2021), pp. 337–48, available at https://www.nature.com/articles/s41562-021-01056-1 (last accessed 21/01/2022).

than a verbal medium. Maybe this is why visual media are gaining more and more popularity: we deem mediated communication less mediated because of the seeming proximity of the subjects due to their visual exposure. Additionally, visual messages are lacking the linearity related to sequential reading of a written text: when interpreting a visual message, we have the impression of encompassing the whole message at the very first sight whereas a text requires undeniably linear time to get from the first sentence to the last sentence. Due to the illusorily lowered level of mediacy, it is likely that visual media are more suitable for the emotive language function and thus are also more used for the misinformation spread. Case studies focusing on the spread of misinformation have been conducted via visual media platforms such as YouTube.[20] The information about the virus, be it scientifically proven or not, have 'gone viral' on social and new media. The virality of social media is a concept older than the pandemic itself;[21] however, in the context of the COVID-19 it acquires rather sarcastic connotations. Also, the perception of the face — the important bearer of the emotive function in communication — and the different meanings of the human face in the era of pandemic is undergoing a drastic transformation.[22]

In a very simplistic way, the conclusion of the previous sentences is that new media facilitate, favour, and easily convey emotional language function. But if we understand digital media as part of our society,[23] just as we accepted writing systems thousands of years ago, we must accept them as part of our lives, including the new kinds of (or intensity of) emotions they have the power to communicate. Semiotic analysis of the face in digital dating was proposed[24] and some scholars even speak about the 'real' emotions towards digital subjects in computer games for instance.[25]

We have seen that thanks to the emotive function of the new media, the messages conveyed might be modified as emotions may lead to misinterpretation or even fake news. But oftentimes the whole content of the message is reduced to the sole emotion expressed visually: posting photos of subjects (senders) or other visual content very often does not have any informational value other than communicating positive or negative emotions. Posting pictures carries the meaning of 'look at me, today I feel very pretty' or the like. New media favour the role of the subject (addresser) over the role of the message. Or, to put it in simpler words, mostly in the case of social media posts, the message is empty or collapsed into the addresser, for instance when publishing photographs of the very self of the addresser. Likewise, the message itself must correspond to the structure offered by the medium: the visual, audio, but also

20 Caio C. Vieira and others, *Ciência contaminada analisando o contágio de desinformação sobre coronavírus via youtube*, (2020), 10.13140/RG.2.2.27323.03367.

21 *Viralità-Virality*, ed. by Gabriele Marino and Mattia Thibault, *Lexia. Rivista di semiotica*, 25–26 (2016).

22 Leone, *Volti virali.*

23 We can use the term cyberculture, see Martin Charvát, *O nových médiích, modularitě a simulaci* (Prague: Metropolitan University Prague Press and Tongua, 2017).

24 Leone, 'The Semiotics of the Face in Digital Dating', pp. 18–40.

25 *Love and Sex in the Digital Age*, ed. by Gianmarco Thierry Giuliana and others, *Digital Age in Semiotics and Communication. Journal by the Southeast European Center for Semiotic Studies*, 2 (2019).

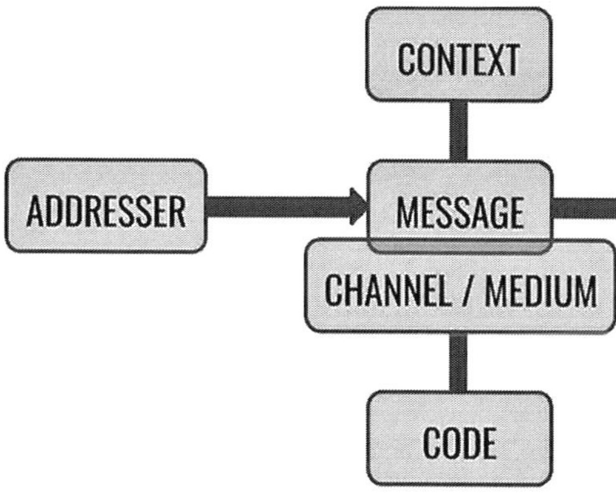

Figure 3. Medium merges with message

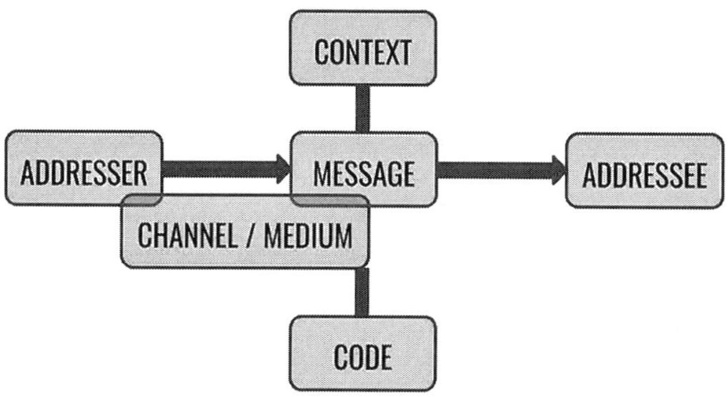

Figure 4. Medium merges with message and subject

the content of the message reflects the possibilities of the medium that transmits it (Figure 3).

If we want to further schematize the aforementioned transformation of the communication mediated by new media with Jakobson's original model of communication, we can conclude that the medium does not fulfill the role of a passive mediator between two subjects, it does not belong to a separate item in the communication schema (Figure 1). On the contrary, the medium coincides with the other components in the communication schema; it overlaps with the subject (addresser) and with the message itself (Figure 4).

The aforementioned findings about Jakobson's model of communication and the inseparability of discrete constituents of the model are but a repetition of what we already know from Gvoždiak. Regardless of the context of new media, Gvoždiak pointed out a paradox of Jakobson's communication model. In the case of the new media, we are dealing with the striking inseparability of the subject from the message and channel, but in accordance with the whole of Jakobon's writings, his model should be understood in terms of the seeming opposition between the code and the message (in contrast with the Saussurean dichotomy of *langue* and *parole*); however, in reality we are dealing with the opposition between the code and the ensemble of communication:

> According to Jakobson's analysis, the complementary part of code is not a message or a parole, but communication or a communication act as a whole, which subsumes all the constitutive components of communication in itself.[26]

Thus, in the words of Gvoždiak, the components of Jakobson's schema are constituting an ensemble of a communicative situation whose decomposability into single components is in fact only artificial. The original model of mediated communication collapses even more with the arrival of new media, and the individual constituents of the model are no longer to hold their privileged status. The discontinuity of the model is broken and merged into a continuum of a subject, media, channel, and message. This also leads to a collapse of the clear distinction between form and substance in Hjelmslevean terms,[27] if we understand the medium as a substantial part of communication.

3. Threats

Before advancing with my argumentation, I would like to mention some general opinions on threats or fears related to the expansion of new media — and their usage — whose number has been exponentially growing since the era of the pandemic. In the previous section I commented on the strong emotional potential of new media — this aspect turns paradoxical when confronted with the critical approach (or worries) of elder generations towards the emotional and social aspect of digitalized new media. Generations not used to new media are to a great extent concerned about the social and emotive lives of the new media generation. Besides the negative emotional impact, another common worry is connected to the risk of decay of our cognitive capacities. In this sense, Umberto Eco was pessimistic about the new media (even if in general terms Eco was known for a rather enthusiastic approach to computers). In an interview for a special issue of the magazine *Alfabeta2*,[28] dedicated to the topic '50

26 Gvoždiak, *Jakobsonova sémiotická teorie*, p. 137. In original: 'z hlediska Jakobsonových výkladů komplementem kódu není zpráva či parole, nýbrž komunikace či komunikační akt jako celek, který v sobě subsumuje všechny konstitutivní složky komunikace'.

27 Louis Hjelmslev, *Prolégomènes à une théorie du langage* (Paris: Minuit, 1971 [1943]).

28 Umberto Eco, 'Apocalittico sarà lei. Intervista a Umberto Eco di Daniela Panosetti', in *50 anni dopo Apocalittici e integrati*, *Alfabeta2*, 2015, available at Apocalittico sarà lei. Intervista a Umberto Eco | Daniela Panosetti (doppiozero.com) (last accessed 21/01/2022).

years after *Apocalittici e integrati*',[29] Eco presents an apocalyptic vision of a society that will cease to have individual memory at its disposal. By inserting our memory into a computer, smartphone, or iPhone, we stop using our biological memory storage — this will eventually result in a society with a huge collective memory stored somewhere on the web, whose individuals will lack individual knowledge; the future development of such a society is uncertain. But as Niola points out, the fear that new media will take our memory is as unfounded as it was in the case of Plato's fear of the invention of a writing system.[30]

Eco is not the only skeptical about new media and their impact on society. There is a general opinion in society that a computer or a mobile phone is something negative if it is used excessively. It is emphasized especially in the context of education: children should not spend too much time in front of computer screens or with smartphones in their hands. Of course, it is important to prevent the loss of our social side at the expense of technology, but it is equally important to realize that the new media, like any other tool mankind has invented, is meant to be useful and is the proof and result of our mental activity. Maybe when the predecessors of today's *Homo sapiens* invented the first primitive tools, they were deemed lazy by their contemporaries who were not used to using tools: instead of fatiguing their hands and cultivating the soil as they properly should, they wanted to make this labour easier with a piece of stone. They might have been afraid that if they started using tools extensively and in excess, over time their offspring would have weaker muscles and they would become deformed, lazy individuals unable to take care of their future. This might be what actually happened somewhat, but it was not damaging for the prosperity of the community; rather the contrary: the invented tools were more and more sophisticated and generally helped the society thrive in the future. New media is nothing but another tool invented by humanity for its own benefit, but this time — rather than assisting with manual tasks — it thinks for us, stores memories, counts, and plans. From an evolutionary point of view, it is a way to ensure the prosperity of the species. Our brain, instead of evolving into a bigger one with more capability to perform demanding computational tasks or with enough storage for the whole of the Babylonian Library, it has transferred this capacity to (external) tools that will do it for us. As Andy Clark notes, 'the brain need not waste its time replicating its capacities. Rather, it must learn to interface with external media. Brains like ours need media, objects and other people to function fully as minds'.[31] Martin Charvát,[32] referring to Lévy, Lyotard, Deleuze, and others, speaks about new-media collective

29 Partial English translation of the volume was published as Umbero Eco, *Apocalypse Postponed* (Bloomington: Indiana University Press, 2000).

30 Marino Niola, 'La delocalizzazione della nostra memoria', *Repubblica*, 41/129, 1 June 2016, p. 29, available at https://ricerca.repubblica.it/repubblica/archivio/repubblica/2016/06/01/la-delocalizzazione-della-nostra-memoria29.html (last accessed 21/01/2022).

31 Andy Clark, *Being There: Putting Brain, Body, and World Together Again* (Cambridge, Mass.: MIT Press, Bradford Books, 1998), p. 220; see also Id. *Supersizing the mind: Embodiment, action, and cognitive extension* (Oxford-New York: Oxford University Press, 2008).

32 Charvát, *O nových médiích, modularitě a simulaci.*

intelligence, which can be understood both as positive (collective intelligence as detached from any kind of totalitarian regime information regulation) or negative (reduction of subjects to a mere transmitter of received information without the capacity of interpret it) output of the digital cyberculture.[33]

The concern about the threat to our cognitive capacities is rather outdated, and the threat to human cognition from the time of Umberto Eco was in the last years replaced by a new one, which is currently widely discussed. The threat of disinformation, or fake news — to use a popular and widely used term — has become the major concern related to new social media.[34]

4. Pandemics

Visual social communication and video communication in the form of vlogs has the already discussed feature of being related to emotive language function, which itself is related to the addresser and his or her self. The problem of the collapse of Jakobson's schema of communication resides in the amorphization of the subject, message, and medium (channel). But how can this collapse be described in semiotic terms? According to Gvoždiak, the components of the communication schema are not to be understood as contradictory to each other but rather as subsuming parts of the whole of the communication. The only binary opposition in this model is the opposition between the code and communication[35] while the code itself is a subsumed component of the communication. We can call this particular binary relation a participative opposition.[36] What remains to be analysed further is the very notion of code. What are the semiotic characteristics of new social media codes? First of all, practically all kinds of new media are multimodal, which makes the characterization of the code quite difficult. But in general terms, and even if multimodal, the most striking feature of the codes of new and especially social media is the visuality. The visual code is widely present in new media, as was already mentioned, and it is related to the emotive language function. What makes visual codes more powerful for expressing emotions compared to other types of codes might be related to their indexical nature. Audiovisual social media communication was reported as indexical

33 Charvát, *O nových médiích, modularitě a simulaci*, pp. 95–119.

34 See Samantha Bradshaw and others, *Industrialized Disinformation. 2020 Global Inventory of Organised Social Media Manipulation* (Oxford, UK: Oxford Internet Institute, 2020) or Dhanaraj Thakur and DeVan L. Hankerson, *Facts and their Discontents: A Research Agenda for Online Disinformation, Race, and Gender*, Center for Democracy & Technology, (2021), 10.31219/osf.io/3e8s5.

35 Gvoždiak, *Jakobsonova sémiotická teorie*, p. 137.

36 Louis Hjelmslev, *Principes de grammaire générale*, (København: Det Kgl. Danske videnskabernes selskab., 1928); Id., 'Structure générale des correlations linguistiques', in Louis Hjelmslev, *Nouveaux essais*, ed. by François Rastier (Paris: Presses Universitaires de France, 1985); Claudio Paolucci, *Strutturalismo e interpretazione* (Milano: Bompiani, 2010), Ľudmila Lacková, 'Participative Opposition Applied', *Sign Systém Studies*, 10.12697/sss.1 (2021).

by Andacht[37] mostly because of the wide presence of visual indexes or symptoms such as psychosomatic features expressed by face or body appearance. Andacht conducted a case study focusing on indexicality of the format of vlog, which was very popular in the first decade of this century. Among the observed symptoms or indexes, we can list facial redness, pallidness, uncontrollable body movements, and other physical expressions of emotional states. These signs are even more powerful or even more indexical in the case of live streaming.

It is evident that indexical signs, among the types of signs of Peirce's famous classification,[38] are the most relevant for emotive language function; because of the direct relation between Representamen and Object, the interpreter has the feeling of immediacy, proximity, and authenticity. Yet in the case of new media, all these usual characteristics of indexes disappear since the communication is mediated; there is no room for immediacy, proximity, nor authenticity. And still the transmission of emotions works perfectly and maybe even better than in the case of unmediated indexes. The very term of mediated indexes is somewhat of an oxymoron, but we can use it for the purpose of this chapter. Thanks to the mediateness of indexes, which also makes them less genuine and more *symbolic*, a whole new space for their abuse opens. The mediateness of the indexical enables the abusive use of these signs; it enables using signs to lie or to fake. Andacht[39] commented on the famous case of a popular 'fake' vlog of a supposed teenage girl with the YouTube nickname lonely-girl155. Interestingly, the popularity of lonely-girl155 did not decrease after it was discovered to be fake, but the fans of the vlog continued watching new episodes. They wanted to know how the story developed. This is a clear example of the primacy of emotions over authenticity or trustworthiness and it perfectly explains why fake news is spreading so rapidly in new and social media: it is not the only consequence of constant reachability but also the emotive nature related to false indexical signs.

With the arrival of the COVID-19 pandemic, mediated new-media-related communication underwent a considerable transformation — this transformation being not qualitative but rather quantitative; we can define it as intensification of the famous Livingstone claim that 'everything is mediated'.[40] The role switching between mediated and unmediated communication happened so fast that we hardly even noticed it and mediated became the primary form of communication. Paradoxically, such a high level of mediation seems to encourage language users to communicate even more. We spend long hours in front of computer or smartphone screens, we contact many people, old friends, former colleagues, and a distant family. The necessity for a high level of mediation makes communication, as it seems, more attractive. There is no communicative alternative, only mediation or the risk of health. Maybe it is the very mediation that facilitates communication: the more media and

37 Fernando Andacht, 'Uma abordagem semiótica e indicial da identidade na era de YouTube' *Intexto*, 79 (2015), pp. 79–98.

38 Charles Sanders Peirce, *Collected Papers of Charles Sanders Peirce*. (Cambridge, Mass.: Harvard University Press, 1931, 1935, 1958).

39 Andacht, 'Uma abordagem semiótica'.

40 Sonia Livingstone, 'On the mediation of everything', *Journal of Communication*, 59. 1 (2008), pp. 1–18.

mediators between the addresser and the addressee, the more involved we are in the act of communication. This is only a seeming paradox, because in fact mediation can make it easier to express desired concepts and to hide those that we want to leave unspoken. Thanks to technology, we have all become masters in communication; technology helps us master the communicative situation and makes us feel more comfortable, because of its possibility of manipulation. There is no more room for ostension; nothing is involuntary or spontaneous anymore. We use filters, we choose the angle from which we want to be seen through the camera lens, and we have constant control over the image of the self we want to expose to others. We will not let anyone exceed the comfort zone; the camera only captures us as long as we permit it. Consequently, the new media crisis of the subject enters even more serious crisis when the mediateness of the communication is the only alternative. Besides the fact that the subject collapses into message and medium and is hardly differentiable from the other components of the communication schema, the subject loses its very subjectivity, the authenticity of its self.

5. Can the Virus Bring Us Where the Semiosis Started?

The fact that the impossibility of unmediated communication does not prevent us from communicating, but rather that some people are more encouraged to communicate, supports the epistemological appeal of non-existence of unmediated signs or impossibility of *intuition*. In his three anti-Cartesian essays of 1868 Peirce argued that the epistemological question of intuitions as the primary source of cognition is incommensurable with his semiotic theory. Peirce's objection to Descartes consists mostly in denying the idea of an absolute beginning of cognition. For Peirce, cognition, as any other semiotic mechanism, builds on an interpretive chain within the unlimited semiosis, which is in direct contradiction to the concept of intuition at the beginning of cognition.

From this criticism emerges the doctrine of the continuity of cognition. The idea of continuity is the opposite of that of an absolute beginning. Synechism is a form of criticism of Descartes. The notion of continuity primarily expresses that no single idea has any meaning by itself. Self-evident intuition is impossible. Peirce defines intuition in terms of the lack of continuity.[41]

Thus, not only communication and language but cognition itself exists exclusively in mediation; its connection to reality is indirect and dependent on signs. We cannot think otherwise than through signs. Everything that is accessible to our consciousness is conveyed in our thoughts in the form of signs that refer to previous thoughts, experiences, and feelings. It is not possible to refer to that primary sign where everything began, where the semiosis process started. We have no access to unmediated contact with reality as it is, we only can access reality as it appears to us based on previous

---

41 Hanna Buczynska-Garewicz, 'Peirce and Descartes', in *Living Doubt: Essays concerning the epistemology of Charles Sanders Peirce*, ed. by Guy Debrock and Menno Hulswit (Dordrecht: Springer, 1994) pp. 151–56.

experience. For instance, it is not possible to perceive the smell of disinfectants and cleaning products we use to protect our homes and ourselves from the virus without consciously or unconsciously, voluntarily or involuntarily, interpreting our olfactory experience. The sweet and pungent odour of chlorine reminds us of childhood trips to the swimming pool with parents where the typical smell of chlorine overwhelmed us as soon as we entered the hall of the swimming pool.

Despite all the semiosis and interpretation chain and the existence of direct contact with reality (not mediated by signs) strictly denied by Peirce, some semioticians believe that the situation is not so bleak. At the end of his career, Umberto Eco decided to 'heretically' contradict Peirce in this direction and argued about the situations with no possibility to refer to previous signs, because either there is no time for interpretation (in that case, it is instincts and intuitive reactions to stimuli by the nervous system) or there are no previous signs/cognitions the subject can refer to (newborns' first experience with the world). Eco addressed these heretical issues with the beginning of semiosis already in 1988[42] *mediately* through the narrative in one of his most successful novels, *Foucault's Pendulum*. In this novel, Jacopo Belbo, the main character, tirelessly attempts to reveal the coded secret of the Templars, following hundreds of signs searching for clues that referred to other clues and those to others until they led him to his own death, at the very point of which he returned, in his memories, to his childhood, to the moment when he, for the first and the only time in life, played the trumpet.[43] When, as a boy, he filled his lungs with air and blew into the instrument, the trumpet proudly pointed toward the blue sky — only in the memory of this moment he realized that he understood everything: the whole essence of the world, there were no more questions or answers, it was just the trumpet and that intimate moment only he knew about and that belonged only to him. This moment was a moment of Belbo's connection with the essence, with pure reality without application of signs, interpretations, and meanings.

I believe that, despite the absurdity of the mediation in which we have found ourselves since the arrival of the pandemic of COVID-19, each of us for at least one moment can become Jacopo Belbo and touch the world in its purest substance (without superfluous forms). For example, when we go out into the streets of an empty city and the lazy morning light of the first spring sunrays softly falls on the facades of the walls of buildings that we have never seen before in their integrity: we have never had the opportunity to see the city in which we live without the presence of other people. The depopulated city reveals its unfamiliar face to us, curiously and from behind the mask we look and enjoy the mild spring sun warming that small exposed part of the face. We feel strange, but we feel like it is something genuine and we feel naked in front of this new world that we are still trying to understand. We do not know how to define the feeling, we only know that it is there and that there is probably an initial point of new interpretation, a point at which a new semiosis begins.

---

42 Umberto Eco, *Kant e l'ornitorinco* (Milano: Bompiani, 1997).

43 Umberto Eco, *Il pendolo di Foucault* (Milano: Bompiani, 1988), p. 509.

Because we are certainly facing a new world with new rules, new limits, new forms of communication, new fears, and new preoccupations.

6. Conclusive Remarks

If someone told us two years ago that we would live in a world attacked by a pandemic, in constant fear and in an omnipresent quarantine, we would hardly imagine the situation. Living in a technological and highly globalized world made us believe that such a scenario can only occur in horror movies. We would probably presuppose that technological and scientific progress would not let an epidemic advance in such an extreme way. Yet paradoxically it is the technological and globalized world that was the ideal precondition for the extreme spread of the pandemic. The crisis we are living in is a crisis with probably very long-term consequences. Communication suffers from the impossibility of unmediated information transition, but the major problem is the consequences this impossibility has on the communicative component of the subject.

Bibliography

Andacht, Fernando, 'Uma abordagem semiótica e indicial da identidade na era de YouTube' *Intexto*, 79 (2015), pp. 79–98.

Bradshaw, Samantha, and , *Industrialized Disinformation. 2020 Global Inventory of Organised Social Media Manipulation* (Oxford, UK: Oxford Internet Institute, 2020).

Buczynska-Garewicz, Hanna, 'Peirce and Descartes', in *Living Doubt: Essays concerning the epistemology of Charles Sanders Peirce*, ed. by Guy Debrock and Menno Hulswit (Dordrecht: Springer, 1994) pp. 151–56.

Clark, Andy, *Being There: Putting Brain, Body, and World Together Again* (Cambridge, Mass.: MIT Press, Bradford Books, 1998).

———, *Supersizing the mind: Embodiment, action, and cognitive extension* (Oxford-New York: Oxford University Press, 2008).

Charvát, Martin, *O nových médiích, modularitě a simulaci* (Prague: Metropolitan University Prague Press and Tongua, 2017).

Eco, Umberto, *Il pendolo di Foucault* (Milano: Bompiani, 1988).

———, *Kant e l'ornitorinco* (Milano: Bompiani, 1997).

———, 'Apocalittico sarà lei. Intervista a Umberto Eco di Daniela Panosetti', in *50 anni dopo Apocalittici e integrati, Alfabeta2*, 2015, https://www.alfabeta2.it/2015/06/27/50-anni-dopo-apocalittici-e-integrati/

Eco, Umbero, *Apocalypse Postponed* (Bloomington: Indiana University Press, 2000).

Giuliana, Gianmarco Thierry, and (eds.), *Love and Sex in the Digital Age. Digital Age in Semiotics and Communication. Journal by the Southeast European Center for Semiotic Studies*, 2 (2019).

Gvoždiak, Vít, *Jakobson's semiotic theory* (orig. *Jakobsonova sémiotická teorie*) (Olomouc: Palacký University, 2014).

Hájková, Klára, 'Jak nošení roušek ovlivňuje naši komunikaci', in *Lingvistika z obýváku*, ed. by Dan Faltýnek (Olomouc: Univerzita Palackého v Olomouci, 2020), https://jazykzczk.netlify.app/_book/pm14.html#idea1

Hjelmslev, Louis, *Principes de grammaire générale* (København: Det Kgl. Danske videnskabernes selskab., 1928).

———, *Prolégomènes à une théorie du langage* (Paris: Minuit, 1971 [1943]).

———, 'Structure générale des correlations linguistiques', in Louis Hjelmslev, *Nouveaux essais*, ed. by François Rastier (Paris: Presses Universitaires de France, 1985).

Jakobson, Roman, *Selected Writings II. Word and Language* (Paris: Mouton, 1962).

———, *Selected Writings III. Poetry of Grammar and Grammar of Poetry* (The Hague–Paris–New York: Mouton, 1981).

Kera, Denisa, 'Globální sítě a mashupy lidí, věcí a dat: Antropomorfizace technologie a dehumanizace lidí' (Plzeň: Antropowebzin, 2007).

Kopecký, Daniel, *McGurkův efekt* (Olomouc: Univerzita Palackého v Olomouci, in print, 2022).

Kořenský, Jan, 'Teorie nových médií a transformace prostředku na subjekt?', in *Registre jazyka a jazykovedy* (II), ed. by Jana Kesselová and others (Prešov: Univerzitná knižnica Prešovskej univerzity v Prešove, 2014), pp. 132–36.

———, 'Prostor (a čas) v komunikaci a jeho proměny v souvislostech s vývojem mediačních prostředků', *Slavistična revija*, 62 (2014), pp. 387–93.

Lacková, Ľudmila, 'Participative Opposition Applied', *Sign Systém Studies*, 10.12697/sss.1 (2021).

Leone, Massimo, 'The Semiotics of the Face in Digital Dating: A Research Direction', in *Love and Sex in the Digital Age*, ed. by Gianmarco Thierry Giuliana and others, *Digital Age in Semiotics and Communication. Journal by the Southeast European Center for Semiotic Studies*, 2 (2019), pp. 18–40.

———, 'Estéticas faciais nas sociedades digitais contemporâneas', in *Contribuições da Semiótica ao ensino de português no mundo*, ed. by Maria Teresa Tedesco and Claudio Correia (Rio de Janeiro: Dialogarts, 2021), pp. 13–22.

Livingstone, Sonia, 'On the mediation of everything', *Journal of Communication*, 59. 1 (2008), pp. 1–18.

Loomba, Sahil, and , 'Measuring the Impact of COVID-19 Vaccine Misinformation on Vaccination Intent in the UK and USA', *Nature Human Behaviour*, 5 (2021), pp. 337–48.

Manovich, Lev, *The Language of New Media* (Cambridge, Mass.: MIT Press, 2001).

———, *Software Takes Command* (New York: Bloomsbury Academic, 2013).

Marino, Gabriele, and Mattia Thibault (eds.), *Viralità-Virality, Lexia. Rivista di semiotica*, 25–26 (2016).

McGurk, Harry, and John MacDonald, 'Hearing lips and seeing voices', *Nature*, 264(5588) (1976), pp. 746–48.

Niola, Marino, 'La delocalizzazione della nostra memoria', *Repubblica*, 41/129, 1 June 2016, p. 29, https://ricerca.repubblica.it/repubblica/archivio/repubblica/2016/06/01/la-delocalizzazione-della-nostra-memoria29.html

Pan American Health Organization (PAHO), *Understanding the Infodemic and Misinformation in the Fight Against COVID-19* (2020), https://iris.paho.org/handle/10665.2/52052

Paolucci, Claudio, *Strutturalismo e interpretazione* (Milano: Bompiani, 2010).

Peirce, Charles Sanders, *Collected Papers of Charles Sanders Peirce*. (Cambridge, Mass.: Harvard University Press, 1931, 1935, 1958).

Sams, Mikko, and , 'Seeing and hearing others and oneself talk', *Cognitive Brain Research*, 23. 2–3 (2005), pp. 429–35.

Santangelo, Antonio, 'I narcisi mascherati, gli eroi e noi. La parabola dei selfie con la maschera', in *Volti virali*, ed. by Massimo Leone (Turin: FACETS Digital Press, 2020), pp. 39–68.

Smith, Rory, and , *Under the Surface: Covid-19 Vaccine Narratives, Misinformation and Data Deficits on Social Media*, https://firstdraftnews.org/vaccine-narratives-full-report-november-2020

Thakur, Dhanaraj, and DeVan L. Hankerson, *Facts and their Discontents: A Research Agenda for Online Disinformation, Race, and Gender*, Center for Democracy & Technology, (2021).

Vieira, Caio C., and , *Ciência contaminada analisando o contágio de desinformação sobre coronavírus via youtube*, (2020), 10.13140/RG.2.2.27323.03367.

WHO *Public Health Research Agenda for Managing Infodemics* (Geneva: World Health Organization, 2021).

Williams, Sophie, *Coronavirus: How face masks are becoming fashionable*, https://www.bbc.com/news/world-52691164

FEDERICO LAUDISA

12. The Epistemology of Models in the Era of Pandemic

▼ **ABSTRACT** The Covid-19 pandemic has dramatically shown the need for reliable modelling capabilities, in order to describe and predict large-scale health processes, both in its biological and social dimensions. In the present paper, I attempt a review on the sort of issues that arise from the pandemic-induced pressure on several prediction and estimate processes made possible by models. After a general introduction on the several roles that models have been playing since the birth of modern science, I will sketch the main traits of the modelling tools that proved effective in the era of the pandemic: in this sketch the inevitably high rate of uncertainty, biases, and predictive limits of these tools will be apparent. I will focus then on these classes of models from the point of view of what they are supposed to mean with respect to the general philosophical problem of the basis of *inductive* inference: from this perspective, I will end with some general reflections on the social implications of the reliance on models for counteracting pandemics.

1. Introduction

A large part of the activity across all areas of scientific investigation is devoted to the design and the implementation of models. These models often played a crucial role in the advancement of science, a circumstance witnessed by their centrality in several scientific domains that are especially active in contemporary times, such as cosmology, biology, climatology, and neurosciences, not to speak of social science areas that have become increasingly sensitive to the use of modelling techniques, such as economics or sociology. Unsurprisingly, models have also attracted philosophers' attention: in addition to the conceptual work devoted to the classification of the many kinds and uses of models in science, models raise questions that are extremely relevant from a philosophical point of view. These questions concern for instance the delicate notion of *representation* (assuming that the models should

Epidemics and Pandemics, ed. by Michele Nicoletti and Alessandro Palazzo (Turnhout: Brepols, 2024), pp. 297–308
BREPOLS PUBLISHERS 10.1484/M.STPH-EB.5.136416

represent something in the natural world, how should we interpret this task?), but also epistemic and ontological issues emerge in connection with the use of models: do we really gain new knowledge through models, and what are we supposed to do with this knowledge? Are models themselves a kind of *entity*?

In recent times, however, the speculative character of some of the above issues had to confront the tragic reality of the pandemic — with its load of serious consequences for the biology, economy, and psychology of mankind — so that some typical traits of models have come to the forefront even more than before. In particular, the role of models not only for understanding the mechanisms of the natural world but also for their *prediction*, and, as a consequence, the role of the models in assisting decision-makers at different stages. In the present paper, I attempt a review on the sort of issues that arise from the pressure that the pandemic puts on several prediction and estimate processes made possible by models. After a general introduction on the several roles that models have been playing since the birth of modern science, I will sketch the main traits of the modelling tools that proved effective in the era of the pandemic: in this sketch the inevitably high rate of uncertainty, biases, and predictive limits of these tools will be apparent. I will focus then on these classes of models from the point of view of what they are supposed to mean with respect to the general philosophical problem of the basis of *inductive* inference: from this perspective, I will end with some general reflections on the social implications of the reliance on models for counteracting the pandemic.

2. Models in Science: A Tentative Taxonomy

Since the very birth of modern science with the so-called Scientific Revolution of the seventeenth century,[1] the enterprise of understanding the natural world and its laws turned out to involve an act of *representation* and, in particular, an act of *idealized description* of this world. The leading figures of modern science developed a clear intuition of what was to become a basic requirement of every scientific investigation: in order to have a general understanding of a phenomenon, it is necessary to construct an abstract and idealized representation of the phenomenon itself. This allows for a useful integration between the logical and the empirical sides of the scientific investigation and, above all, allows for an increasing application of mathematics to natural phenomena. As we now know very well after four centuries of science, the formal power of mathematics can be fully displayed only when applied to simple and idealized descriptions of the phenomena we are after: it is exactly this effort of idealization and abstraction that gives rise to what we nowadays call models.

In the philosophical debates on the role of models in science, philosophers distinguished two general attitudes: in the first — called *Aristotelian* idealization — the idealized object is the outcome of a process in which the object is more and more

1 On the understanding of plague and disease during the Scientific Revolution, see chapter 6 of this volume.

deprived of properties that are evaluated as not relevant to the investigation;[2] in the second — called *Galilean* idealization — the formulation of models as idealized representations involves necessarily a good amount of conscious 'distortion' of something complex with the aim of making it more tractable or understandable.[3] The history and teaching of physics, for instance, delivers completely isolated systems or mechanical processes with no energy dissipation, up to idealizations in social sciences in which markets are populated by agents always fully in command of their rationality and freedom. In addition to these general, meta-theoretical attitudes, there is in fact a wide multiplicity of ways in which a model can be defined, characterized, and employed. A common feature of models lies in their *representational* capacity: models are usually supposed to represent a portion of the natural world, a portion that is usually defined as the model's target system (examples abound, ranging from the semi-classical Bohr model of the atomic structure to the point-particles model of a gas, up to the socio-economic models). From a philosophical point of view, the notion of representation is highly complex and would require a detailed treatment in its own right, which is out of the scope of the present work: for our purposes, it may be useful to recall the several dimensions along which models play their representational role, namely *scale* models, *analogical* models, *toy* models, *phenomenological* models, *exploratory* models, and *data* models, with the implicit recognition that these different categories are far from mutually exclusive.[4]

A scale model is perhaps the most intuitive instance of a model, that is a downsized or enlarged copy of a specified target system. A scale model is taken to be a natural replica or a truthful mirror image of the target but, no matter how detailed the model is supposed to be, even this intuitive notion of a model shares features common to the general notion of a model, namely conventionality and approximation. Even when a model is a faithful representation of the target system (suppose a 1:1000 scale model of a plane or a car), the relation between the properties of the model and the properties of the target is usually far from straightforward. *Analogical* models, on the other hand, are based on the choice of a set of similarities between two (classes of) items: the use of analogical models in science aims at increasing our knowledge of the causal mechanisms underlying phenomena by using the pragmatic strategy of conceiving of these unknown mechanisms in terms of what is already familiar and well understood, that is, by exploiting the analogies between model and target system that have been assumed by hypothesis. By paying attention to the distinction between a model, the source of the model, and the subject, or target, of the model,[5] one may

2 Martin R. Jones, 'Idealization and Abstraction: A Framework', in *Idealization XII: Correcting the Model*, ed. by Martin R. Jones and Nancy Cartwright (Poznań Studies in the Philosophy of the Sciences and the Humanities 86) (Amsterdam–New York: Rodopi, 2005), pp. 173–217.

3 Ernan McMullin, 'Galilean Idealization', *Studies in History and Philosophy of Science Part A*, 16 (1985), pp. 247–73; Angela Potochnik, *Idealization and the Aims of Science* (Chicago: University of Chicago Press, 2017).

4 Roman Frigg, Stephan Hartmann, 'Models in science', *The Stanford Encyclopedia of Philosophy*, 2020, available at https://plato.stanford.edu/archives/spr2020/entries/models-science/ (last accessed 6/02/2022).

5 Mary B. Hesse, *Models and Analogies in Science* (London: Sheed and Ward, 1963).

hope to build an analogical model of the unknown subject or causal mechanism. To take a biological example, Charles Darwin formulated his model of the subject of natural selection by reasoning by analogy from the source of the known nature and behaviour of the process of artificial selection. In this way, analogical models may play an important creative role in theory development (other examples may be the model of chromosomal inheritance, based on an analogy with a string of beans, or the computational models of the mind, based on analogies with the computer).

The class of *toy models* — a typical example is the Lotka–Volterra model in population ecology — includes models that are supposed to represent their target systems in an extremely simplified and strongly distorted fashion, so as to isolate a limited number of causal or explanatory factors.[6] The use of toy models is often taken to be provisional and limited, since they usually perform poorly in terms of prediction and empirical adequacy (a limit that raises the question whether they should be considered as representational at all)[7]. At a different level we find what are defined as *phenomenological models*. According to common wisdom, phenomenological models are taken to represent observable features of their target systems, refraining from assuming underlying — and so far unknown — processes and mechanisms endowed with a deeper explanatory potential. The liquid-drop model of the atomic nucleus, for instance, portrays the nucleus as a liquid drop and describes it as having several properties (surface tension and charge, among others) originating in different theories (hydrodynamics and electrodynamics, respectively). Certain aspects of these theories —although usually not the full theories — are then used to determine both the static and dynamical properties of the nucleus. This example shows that often phenomenological models, while not strictly derivable from a theory, rely in different ways on principles and laws associated with specified theories. With *exploratory models* the scientific literature on models usually means models which are not put forward explicitly in order to investigate a specific target system, but rather as a starting point of further explorations in which the model is modified and refined. As an example, Gelfert[8] mentions early models in theoretical ecology, such as the Lotka–Volterra model of predator–prey interaction, which does not give an accurate account of the behaviour of any actual population, but provides a starting point for the development of more realistic models. Finally, in this far-from-complete list, we find what are called *models of data*, an expression which refers to the procedures by which the so-called raw data are treated, so as to make them suitable for proper scientific investigation. Models of data are often assumed to play a relevant role in the issue of theory confirmation, since it is the *model* of data, and not the mere raw data, on the background of which theories are put to the test.

---

6 Alexander Reutlinger and others, 'Understanding (with) Toy Models', *The British Journal for the Philosophy of Science*, 69 (2018), pp. 1069–99.

7 Joshua Luczak, 'Talk about Toy Models', *Studies in History and Philosophy of Science Part B: Studies in History and Philosophy of Modern Physics*, 57 (2017), pp. 1–7.

8 Axel Gelfert, *How to Do Science with Models: A Philosophical Primer* (Cham: Springer International Publishing, 2016).

3. Epidemiological Models: Uncertainty, Biases and Predictive Limits

In the wide area of scientific research in which the recourse to models is part and parcel of everyday activity, the sub-area of epidemiology shares for instance with climatology the design and use of models that are not only an end in themselves from the point of view of gaining knowledge but are also supposed to assist policy makers in their job. As a matter of fact, there are two basic approaches to epidemiological modelling, that in some sense figure as two extremes among which several variations on the theme can be found: the *SEIR Compartmental Models* and the *Agent-Based Models*. The former derive their label from the assumption according to which a population is divided into 'compartments': the susceptible (S), the infected (I), and the recovered (R), to which we need to add the exposed (E), due to the incubation period of the COVID-19. This class of models relies on the use of the mathematical tool of differential equations, whose basic idea is to represent the change of a certain quantity, such as the number of cells or the concentration of a particular molecule, as a function of other quantities. The equations that represent these relations are then studied in different dynamical regimes, in order to provide predictions about the behaviour of the target system in different initial conditions. In the context of the SEIR epidemiological models, the formulation of a suitable system of differential equations enables model users to see how persons may change compartment over time, namely how the respective size of the compartments changes over time: for instance, a parameter may express the average number of potentially able to transmit contacts of some person belonging to the S compartment, and so on. On the basis of the differential equation machinery, if we feed the model with input values indicating the initial size of the compartments, the model may deliver good estimates of the size of compartments at subsequent times. Suppose we set $S(t)$ to be the number of people who are not immune to the virus at time t, $E(t)$ the number of people who are incubating the virus but not yet contagious at t, $I(t)$ the number of people who can transmit the virus at t, and $R(t)$ the number of people who recover or die at t. The size of these different compartments may vary according to a number of parameters or variables such as in these very general patterns:

- a fraction of $S(t)$ may shift to $E(t)$, as far as parameters like the number of contacts per person per unit time and the probability of transmission per contact are concerned;
- a fraction of $E(t)$ may shift to $I(t)$ as far as parameters like incubation period and asymptomatic case percentage are concerned;
- a fraction of $I(t)$ may shift to $R(t)$ as far as parameters like infectious period or infection fatality rate are concerned;
- a fraction of the recovered $R(t)$ may turn out to belong again to $S(t)$ as far as parameters like the period of time for which immunity lasts and for which is effective.

As is customary with models, there are relevant factors of idealization and abstraction. Not only do these models share the usual limitation of the differential equation approach, that is, often only the average behaviour of systems can be modelled, so that information about *individual* instances is unavailable; they also disregard biological details of the virus itself (the very mechanisms underlying the virus action) and the effects on the ill people. Moreover, they assume homogeneity for the people in the different groups, rather regular patterns of social interaction among individuals, and basically no difference among individuals in terms of susceptibility to the virus.

Agent-based models (ABM, for short) follow an alternative approach. The models in this class try to describe and predict the evolution of dynamic systems by simulating the behaviour of what they assume to be their constituent 'agents' (individual parts). The ABM drop any description in terms of averages and provide each agent with a program including both data and behavioural rules operating on this data. Thus, ABM represent dynamic systems in the sense that they *simulate* them: in particular, the ABM simulations represent the evolution over time of the target systems *through agent interactions* and with a small amount of a priori assumptions, and the systems' behaviour at a macroscopic scale is observed as an *emergent* behaviour. It turns out as no surprise that the ABM, attempting to capture the behaviour of individuals within an environment, are decisively more intuitive than the differential equation models: 'in particular, the richness of detail one can take into account in ABM makes this methodology very appealing for the simulation of biological and social systems, where the behaviour and the heterogeneity of the interacting components are not safely reducible to some stylized or simple mechanism'.[9] Thus ABM for COVID-19 randomly associate a profile with each agent, where the profile depends on information gathered about the population modelled (age, occupation, mobility habits, and so on). Then, with the aid of massive machine computations, the agents' interactions are simulated over and over, in order to estimate the virus spreading among the agents and evaluate the trends that can affect infections, hospitalizations, deaths, and so on. There is no such thing as a free lunch, though. ABM for COVID-19 'simulate individuals, including their interactions, daily activities and how the virus itself might affect them if they get infected. [...] This granularity allows the model to capture some of the inherent heterogeneity and randomness that get abstracted away in the simplest SEIR models — but at a cost: Scientists need to gather more data, make more assumptions, and manage much higher levels of uncertainty in the models'.[10]

There are recurrent problems for the reliability of this large family of models. A first problem is that the very initial act of collecting data is far from being uncontroversial. Even if we put aside both the natural problems connected with the very act of 'measurement' (which are bound to affect the consistency and reliability of

9 Filippo Castiglione, 'Agent based modelling', *Scholarpedia*, 1 (2006), p. 1562.

10 Jordana Cepelewicz, 'The hard lessons of modeling the coronavirus pandemic', *Quanta Magazine* (2021), available at https://www.quantamagazine.org/the-hard-lessons-of-modeling-the-coronavirus-pandemic-20210128/ (last accessed 6/02/2022).

the 'raw' data) several errors and biases can arise from the summary and analysis of such data[11] — especially when analysis is supposed to lead to such sensitive tasks as the formulation of predictions and causal inferences. Moreover, there is the well-known problem of the use of large quantities of 'Big Data', whose status is methodologically complex and controversial. At the dawn of the Big Data era, a new scientific revolution was supposed to take place. In 2008 Chris Anderson boldly claimed that '"Correlation is enough". We can stop looking for models. We can analyse the data without hypotheses about what it might show. We can throw the numbers into the biggest computing clusters the world has ever seen and let statistical algorithms find patterns where science cannot',[12] whereas Danah Boyd and Kate Crawford focused on the epistemological side: 'Big Data creates a radical shift in how we think about research. [...] Big Data reframes key questions about the constitution of knowledge, the processes of research, how we should engage with information, and the nature and the categorization of reality'.[13] According to several scientists and researchers, the new Big Data scientific paradigm proves to be attractive in many respects, in particular: (i) Big Data-based science would need no theories, models, or *a priori* hypoteses; (ii) with the aid of suitable analytical tools, the data would 'talk by themselves', without any reliance on the biases determined by the theoretical stance of researchers; (iii) the results obtained with these tools would be independent from the specific research contexts of traditional science, and, as a consequence, might be uniquely interpreted by anyone who is able to read statistical data. The subsequent debate has shown, however, that the optimism underlying claims such as those quoted above is bound to face serious problems, connected to the specificity of scientific communities. First of all, the modalities of *production* and *acquisition* of Big Data are far from 'neutral' and 'objective', but take place on the basis of specific aims, assumptions, and viewpoints. The regularities that are isolated by statistical algorithms do not acquire a meaning magically — data do *not* talk by themselves — namely, they become meaningful through a process of choice of specific keys that affects their interpretation; moreover, the claim that statistical skills are sufficient to read the data overlooks the influence exercised by individual scientific training over the very act of reading the data: researchers themselves are embedded into research and knowledge networks whose relevance cannot be ignored.[14]

This kind of epistemological concerns issue of Big Data leads to a further issue, namely that of the alternative between *theory-based models* and *data-driven models*.

---

11 Timothy L. Lash and others, 'Good practices for quantitative bias analysis', *International Journal of Epidemiology*, 43 (2014), pp. 1969–85; Joshua R. Goldstein and Serge Atherwood, 'Improved measurement of racial/ethnic disparities in COVID-19 mortality in the United States', *medRxiv* (2020) pp. 1–13, available at https://www.medrxiv.org/content/10.1101/2020.05.21.20109116v2.full-text (last accessed 6/02/2022).

12 Chris Anderson, 'The End of Theory: The Data Deluge Makes the Scientific Method Obsolete', *Wired*, 23.06.2008, available at https://www.wired.com/2008/06/pb-theory/ (last accessed 6/02/2022).

13 Danah Boyd and Kate Crawford, 'Critical questions for big data', *Information, Communication and Society*, 15 (2012), pp. 662–79 (p. 665).

14 Rob Kitchin, 'Big Data, new epistemologies and paradigm shifts', *Big Data & Society*, (2014), pp. 1–12.

The former may have a significant potential for simulating the possible impact of variation or change in disease transmission, and for evaluating hypothetical alternative interventions[15]. In practice, however, no modelling can be entirely theory-based since any such theory relies at least in part on empirical knowledge concerning disease biology. When such knowledge is less than reliable (as was the case during the early stages of the COVID-19 pandemic), strictly theory-based modelling can generate projections that deviate markedly from the observed (or expected) numbers of infections, cases, and deaths. Moreover, the underlying theory can be itself flawed: this can lead to projections that may significantly diverge from reality even when the observed data to which these are compared have been collected and summarized competently, consistently, and accurately.[16] At the other extreme, exclusively data-driven modelling — which involves attempts to fit functions that best represent any apparent trend amongst the available data — is also rarely used in the exclusive ('data-driven') sense; even though recent advances in computational power and the availability of 'Big Data' have made data-driven modelling techniques very popular in 'predictive analytics'.

4. Models and Induction: Philosophical and Social Implications

Each member in this wide family of models employs methods that, in a broad sense, are instances of a method that philosophers know quite well, namely the *inductive* method. Unlike the deductive method, upon which traditionally mathematics and abstract disciplines in general are supposed to be based, induction is typical of most scientific reasonings concerning the *natural* world. The basic motivation for the philosophers' interest lies in the fact that induction, while providing researchers with the possibility of *enlarging* knowledge, is taken to be affected by an unavoidable rate of uncertainty; for any inductive method is exactly characterized by inferences from known data to unknown hypotheses, a class of inference whose uncertainty led celebrated philosophers of science — such as Karl R. Popper — to reject induction altogether as a plausible tool of research. In the era of the pandemic, this skeptical attitude may have cooperated with a much less philosophical but much more socially serious circumstance, namely an increasing sense of distrust toward science itself. A contemporary philosopher of science aptly remarked in this vein:

> Might philosophers, with their ineradicable scepticism, have contributed to this distrust in scientific expertise? It is not unreasonable to think that the relativism and post-truth-ism propagated not only by continental philosophy but also by the strong programme and the related field of science and technology studies have

15 David Adam, 'Special report: the simulations driving the world's response to COVID-19', *Nature*, 580 (2020), pp. 316–18; Nicholas P. Jewell and others, 'Predictive mathematical models of the COVID-19 pandemic: underlying principles and value of projections', *Journal of the American Medical Association*, 323(19) (2020), pp. 1893–94.

16 J. Luo, 'Predictive monitoring of COVID-19, Data-Driven Innovation Lab', (2020), available at https://www.newsbeast.gr/files/1/2020/05/COVID19PredictionPaper.pdf (last accessed 6/02/2022).

harmed the status of science. Their practitioners, after all, tend to see science as 'just one of the many stories we tell each other'. Why not, in our current situation, believe a story with less inconvenient consequences, one that, for instance, allows us to go about without masks?[17]

The major conceptual source of this debate, clearly, is Hume's argument concerning the foundations of induction. According to a widespread reading of this argument, induction cannot be justified deductively, since induction cannot provide us with certainty. But it cannot be justified inductively either, since trying to do that would involve the use of induction, and that proves to be circular. There has been a long and wide debate on the possible ways out, but a recent interesting proposal has been put forward in recent times by the philosopher of science Gerhard Schurz, for example in his 2019 book.[18] According to Schurz, the mistake of Hume and all later commentators has been the attempt to find *an argument* to show that that induction is reliable. Schurz claims that, in order to justify our reliance on induction, we need to show that induction is optimal, namely that we cannot do better than to rely on it. Schurz's approach is two-fold. First, using formal results from the field of prediction with expert advice, he is able to justify analytically (what he calls) meta-induction, that is, induction over inductive methods. The proof consists in showing that, in every possible world, we can never do better than if we rely on meta-induction (that is, choose our inductive methods on inductive grounds). The second part of the demonstration then consists of an application of meta-induction to incontrovertible empirical findings about the past predictive accuracy of our actual inductive practices as compared to various non-inductive methods. On the basis of Schurz's work, Douven himself was then able to show that we should expect to be good at inductive reasoning, supposing our reasoning capacities are the result of an evolutionary process of selection and variation — as evolutionary epistemologists have long argued — and supposing social epistemologists are right that the pursuit of truth is an essentially collective endeavour. Douven's results have been based on computer simulations, modelling an evolutionary process in which epistemically interacting inductive reasoners are selected to reproduce on the basis of their success at getting at the truth accurately (how close do they get to the truth?) and quickly (how long does it take them to get close to the truth, if they get there at all?). The hope is that results like these might restore confidence in induction and, as a consequence, in science. Here is how Douven, again, comments on this perspective:

> It does not follow from these findings that evolution made us successful inductive reasoners. But at least they show how we might may become such reasoners. Will the doubters now start paying more attention to what scientists have to say about how we ought to navigate our way through the current crisis? You may

17 Igor Douven, 'Covid-19, Induction and Social Epistemology', (2021), available at https://www.thebsps.org/short-reads/douven-socialepistemology/ (last accessed 6/02/2022).

18 Gerhard Schurz, *Hume's Problem Solved: The Optimality of Meta-induction* (Cambridge, Mass.: MIT Press, 2019).

> think the point is still too subtle to sway the demonstrators. You may be right. However, research by cognitive psychologists has shown that people are more likely to accept that something is so when it is pointed out to them why it is so or how it came to be.[19]

This kind of reflection is useful also to emphasize the connection between the purely theoretical side in the treatment of uncertainty and the wider implications of such pandemic-related uncertainty from the social point of view. This connection shows that the pandemic dramatically pointed out how limited the traditional underpinning of contemporary science can be, with its frequent reliance on linear models of thought that may prove totally unfit to face deep global challenges. It has been argued even recently that a 'new epistemology of science' might be needed, an epistemology 'that can serve the public good in times of systemic crises'.[20] These authors interestingly suggest three basic principles of this new epistemology. First, the development of new theoretical frameworks and tools that can support the processes of action and decision-making: these should try on the one hand to preserve the quality of the involved research at a level comparable to the research quality assessment that takes place in ordinary times, but on the other hand they can help to produce inferences in support of urgent decisions at fast timescales based on incomplete knowledge. Second, the increase of scientists' contribution to the public discourse, with a corresponding increase — mainly on the scientists' part — of the willingness to shape the science-society interface. Lastly, a decisive impulse for taking into account a wide diversity of voices for equity, diversity, and inclusion in the scientific process. These principles can be an important contribution of history and philosophy of science and science studies to ongoing transformations of the scientific enterprise.[21]

19 Douven, 'Covid-19, Induction and Social Epistemology'.

20 Guido Caniglia and others, 'COVID-19 heralds a new epistemology of science for the public good', *History and Philosophy of the Life Sciences*, 43 (2021), pp. 1–6 (p. 2).

21 Caniglia and others, 'COVID-19 heralds a new epistemology', p. 1.

Bibliography

Adam, David, 'Special report: the simulations driving the world's response to COVID-19', *Nature*, 580 (2020), pp. 316–18.

Anderson, Chris, 'The End of Theory: The Data Deluge Makes the Scientific Method Obsolete', *Wired*, 23.06.2008, https://www.wired.com/2008/06/pb-theory/

Boyd, Danah, and Kate Crawford, 'Critical questions for big data', *Information, Communication and Society*, 15 (2012), pp. 662–79.

Caniglia, Guido, and others, 'COVID-19 heralds a new epistemology of science for the public good', *History and Philosophy of the Life Sciences*, 43 (2021), pp. 1–6.

Castiglione, Filippo, 'Agent based modelling', *Scholarpedia*, 1 (2006), p. 1562.

Cepelewicz, Jordana, 'The hard lessons of modeling the coronavirus pandemic', *Quanta Magazine* (2021), https://www.quantamagazine.org/the-hard-lessons-of-modeling-the-coronavirus-pandemic-20210128/

Douven, Igor, 'Covid-19, Induction and Social Epistemology', (2021), https://www.thebsps.org/short-reads/douven-socialepistemology/

Frigg, Roman, and Stephan Hartmann, 'Models in science', *The Stanford Encyclopedia of Philosophy*, 2020, https://plato.stanford.edu/archives/spr2020/entries/models-science/

Gelfert, Axel, *How to Do Science with Models: A Philosophical Primer* (Cham: Springer International Publishing, 2016).

Goldstein, Joshua R., and Serge Atherwood, 'Improved measurement of racial/ethnic disparities in COVID-19 mortality in the United States', *medRxiv* (2020) pp. 1–13, https://www.medrxiv.org/content/10.1101/2020.05.21.20109116v2.full-text

Hesse, Mary B., *Models and Analogies in Science* (London: Sheed and Ward, 1963).

Jewell, Nicholas P., and others, 'Predictive mathematical models of the COVID-19 pandemic: underlying principles and value of projections', *Journal of the American Medical Association*, 323(19) (2020), pp. 1893–94.

Jones, Martin R., 'Idealization and Abstraction: A Framework', in *Idealization XII: Correcting the Model*, ed. by Martin R. Jones and Nancy Cartwright (Poznań Studies in the Philosophy of the Sciences and the Humanities 86) (Amsterdam–New York: Rodopi, 2005), pp. 173–217.

Kitchin, Rob, 'Big Data, new epistemologies and paradigm shifts', *Big Data & Society*, (2014), pp. 1–12.

Lash, Timothy L., and others, 'Good practices for quantitative bias analysis', *International Journal of Epidemiology*, 43 (2014), pp. 1969–85.

Luczak, Joshua, 'Talk about Toy Models', *Studies in History and Philosophy of Science Part B: Studies in History and Philosophy of Modern Physics*, 57 (2017), pp. 1–7.

Luo, J., 'Predictive monitoring of COVID-19, Data-Driven Innovation Lab', (2020), https://www.newsbeast.gr/files/1/2020/05/COVID19PredictionPaper.pdf

McMullin, Ernan, 'Galilean Idealization', *Studies in History and Philosophy of Science Part A*, 16 (1985), pp. 247–73.

Potochnik, Angela, *Idealization and the Aims of Science* (Chicago: University of Chicago Press, 2017).

Reutlinger, Alexander, and others, 'Understanding (with) Toy Models', *The British Journal for the Philosophy of Science*, 69 (2018), pp. 1069–99.

Schurz, Gerhard, *Hume's Problem Solved: The Optimality of Meta-induction* (Cambridge, Mass.: MIT Press, 2019

PEJMAN ABDOLMOHAMMADI

13. The COVID-19 Pandemic

An Exogenous Shock into Political Systems in the Middle East and North Africa?[*]

▼ **ABSTRACT** This work will analyse in what extent the Covid-19 Pandemic has been influencing the Middle East and North African socio-political systems. It will focus on the economic, social, and political impacts by highlighting how the MENA countries are reacting to this exogenous shock. This chapter will also try to figure out how Covid-19 is influencing the ideological framework of middle eastern societies by highlighting the difficulties of the ruling elite in order to face this crisis. At last, the Omani case will be analysed in order to offer a more concrete example of how the pandemic has been triggering several socio-economic weak points in the MENA region.

1. Introduction

Democratic political systems have to face more procedures and bureaucracies in order to guarantee pluralism and representativeness. This is the price these systems are willing to pay in order to bring as much as possible the representativeness of every citizen into their political institution. Democracies have many benefits and advantages, but at the same time, the representative process, by nature, requires a series of procedural legal steps, which might influence the efficiency, and the effectiveness of decision-making. On the contrary, the one man in command model normally ignores the representative principles and the pluralism, but manages to be more rapid and efficient in the execution of policies. As much as the political systems are authoritarian, the chain of command become shorter and the decision makers are sharper in addressing their policies. However, these systems normally sacrifice the freedom and the pluralism of their citizens on behalf of efficiency and stability.

* This work has been accomplished with the support of my two PhD candidates Giulia Daga and David Marcel Sîp.

Epidemics and Pandemics, ed. by Michele Nicoletti and Alessandro Palazzo (Turnhout: Brepols, 2024), pp. 309–320
BREPOLS PUBLISHERS 10.1484/M.STPH-EB.5.136417

Both authoritarian and democratic systems are not a monolith. In other words, within the spectrum of political science, not everything is white and black. There are many grey zones to explore. The political science classifications of regimes define various levels of democracies and authoritarian systems by introducing categories such as hybrid regimes and semi-authoritarian political systems. Notable centres of research and agencies such as Freedom House and Polity 7 are continuously measuring the level of representativeness of states and making a classification of them.

According to the Economist Group's Democracy Index 2020 assessment, Israel is the sole democratic country in the Middle East (classified as a "flawed democracy" and rated 28th globally, while Tunisia [ranked 53rd globally] is the only democracy [also a "flawed democracy"]).[1] According to Freedom House, the Middle Eastern and North African countries with the highest rankings are Israel, Tunisia, Turkey, Lebanon, Morocco, Jordan, and Kuwait. Iran, Iraq, and Egypt have all been continually labelled as "not free" by Freedom House from 2017 to 2021. With their ratings continually declining, they have become increasingly hostile to the ideology of liberal democracy. Only Iraq, with a (partly free) score of 41/100, has preserved some amount of internet freedom among these countries. The remaining Middle Eastern nations are classified as authoritarian regimes, with Saudi Arabia and Yemen receiving the lowest rankings.

2. The COVID-19 in the MENA (Middle East and North Africa) Region

In such context, what are the main impacts of COVID-19 on these political regimes?[2]

The coronavirus has spread in the Middle East while the region has already struggled with a number of problems, including long-term conflicts, sectarian tensions, economic crises, and widespread political unrest. Some Middle Eastern countries paralyzed by conflict as well as political and economic crises, and above all millions of people living in overcrowded and unsanitary refugee camps, faced a terrible crisis with the coronavirus. The outlook for the fight against COVID-19 has been bleak due to a series of deep and long-standing crises across the region that have depleted the ability of governments. This situation will get worse with the economic collapse. Since the health infrastructure in some war-torn countries in the Middle East has been destroyed, the expansion of the coronavirus in these countries provoked a relevant humanitarian disaster, so the United Nations called for a ceasefire in all major conflicts on the planet. For example, the outbreak of COVID-19 disease led to the acceptance of a ceasefire by Russia and Turkey as the two main agents in the nine-year war in Syria. The situation in Syria before the outbreak of the disease

---

1 'Global democracy has another bad year But popular protests show potential for democratic renewal', *The Economist*, (2022) https://www.economist.com/graphic-detail/2020/01/22/global-democracy-has-another-bad-year (last accessed 25/03/22).

2 On the implications of the pandemic for politics and governance more generally, see chapter 9 of this volume.

was such that the 3 million people living in the Idlib region (the area subject to the ceasefire) had no hope of reaching an agreement. Thus, between 2020 and 2022, at least, some level of conflict decreased, even though, at the same time, the level of social control of the regimes increased.

For more than two years COVID-19 has occupied the minds of world leaders. The long-term effects of the pandemic are now gradually becoming clear. How will they affect the situation in the MENA region in terms of political and social systems?

Given the diversity of the situation in different states, rather than working through each country, this paper will instead attempt to broadly show how the pandemic will affect political regimes in the MENA region. The countries of the MENA region can roughly be classified as Arab monarchies (UAE, Saudi-Arabia, etc.), developing countries that are vulnerable to economic shocks but are generally considered stable (Jordan, Turkey, Iran, etc.) and countries devastated by war, poverty, and/or crisis (Lebanon, Syria, Yemen, and Afghanistan).

3. Economic Fallout

The world economy ground to a halt during the pandemic. These effects we see continuously to this day, with renewed lockdowns in China caused by new COVID-19 outbreaks halting production in many cities. The war in Ukraine will also exacerbate that fallout. But how concretely will this impact the MENA region?

One critical aspect is loss of income: when the global economy goes down, so does the economy in the MENA region.[3] Countries struggle and will continue to do so with reduced tax income.[4] This is problematic on two levels. The first level is the functioning of the state. Besides the Persian Gulf monarchies, most states in the MENA region struggle with budget problems. High population growth, increased urbanization, and repeated economic crises have led to higher demands for more welfare (UN 2020). At the same time, health care sectors were strained to the maximum.[5] Food and fuel subsidies will be harder to finance for countries that do not possess massive amounts of oil or gas wealth. There is a very real threat of a death spiral, whereby increased inflation and prices lead to higher corruption leading to even more reduced income. Bread revolts[6] were already seen during the 'Arab Spring'

---

3 Marek Dabrowski and Marta Domínguez-Jiménez, 'Economic Crisis in the Middle East and North Africa' (Bruegel, 2021) http://www.jstor.org/stable/resrep28495 (last accessed 25/03/2022).

4 Aziz Atamanov and Laura Rodriguez, 'The Islamic Republic of Iran: Battling Both Income Loss and Inflation', *MENA Development Report, Distributional Impacts of COVID-19 in the Middle East and North Africa Region*, 2021, December https://doi.org/10.1596/978–1-4648–1776-2_ch8 (last accessed 25/03/2022).

5 Itai Brun and Sarah Feuer, 'The Calm before the Storm?: Coping with Corona in the Middle East', *Institute for National Security Studies*, (2020) http://www.jstor.org/stable/resrep23535 (last accessed 25/03/2022).

6 Jane Kinninmont, 'Bread And Dignity', *The World Today* 67. 8/9 (2011), pp. 31–33.

and might appear again very soon. Furthermore, unemployment is a great source of recruitment for terrorist groups.[7]

The second level is internal regime stability. Generals, high bureaucrats, tribal elders, ruling family members, and many more all want to be paid for their continuous loyalty towards the regime, either directly or indirectly through control of the economy.[8] The economic crisis will stay with the world for the coming years, and this will therefore make it harder for political regimes to sustain themselves by buying the loyalty of the elite. This can lead to greater regime instability either through increased inter-elite competition or renewed outright power struggles, something that the regimes are seemingly aware of themselves.[9]

All three types of countries are affected by this, but the effect will be felt strongest in the developing countries. Rich oil and gas producing countries can mitigate the shocks of economic crises, while war-torn countries like Syria already had seen fighting in the past and an outflux of elites and middle-class people. They won't get damaged as much by another economic crisis, because simply put there is not much to damage. In countries like Iran and Turkey on the other hand, the economic crisis hits countries that had already previously struggled. Both countries have seen various protests over the last few years caused also by economic downturns and COVID-19 will only worsen the situation. For countries like Iran and Turkey where a well-educated population will continue to protest, the threat of a brain drain is even more severe. If protests won't change policy-making especially in regard to domestic policies, emigration will be the plan B for many. This will continue a trend across the MENA region which in general suffers from a brain drain.[10]

4. Increase in Violence

The most dangerous thing for any government is its people when they are hungry and angry. Lockdowns and economic downturns hurt in Europe; in the Middle East they are devastating. Many young men will slip into unemployment, which, given the already high numbers, they will be unable to escape from. Additionally, increased border regimes in Europe also make escape to the West a less and less feasible option.

---

7 Adesoji Adelaja and Justin George, 'Is Youth Unemployment Related to Domestic Terrorism?', *Perspectives on Terrorism*, 14. 5 (2020), pp. 41–62.

8 Raymond Hinnebusch, 'The Arab Uprisings and The MENA Regional States System', *Uluslararası İlişkiler / International Relations*, 11. 42 (2014), pp. 7–27.

9 Golnaz Esfandiari, ''State Of Explosion': Leaked IRGC Document Warns Of Rising Discontent In Iran', *Radio Free Europe / Radio Liberty* (2022) https://www.rferl.org/a/iran-irgc-leaked-document-discontent/31683642.html (last accessed 25/03/2022).

10 Mohammed Saïb Musette, 'Brain Drain from the Southern Mediterranean', *IEMed Mediterranean Yearbook 2016* (Barcelona: European Institute of the Mediterranean, 2016) https://www.iemed.org/publication/brain-drain-from-the-southern-mediterranean/ (last accessed 25/03/2022).

Combined with the still-rampant corruption[11] this makes for an ideal recruiting ground for terrorist organizations. The Islamic state (IS) is reorganizing across the Middle East,[12] while ethnic and sectarian tensions are also flaring up. Even relatively stable countries like Saudi Arabia[13] and Algeria[14] increasingly face minorities being willing to use violent means to achieve their rights and aspirations.

But beyond an increase in insurgents and terrorists, there is the everyday violence that undermines states and societies. Domestic violence and abuse rose across the West during the pandemic; the same will hold true for the Middle East, with the difference that the levels for normal times are already high.[15] Additionally, the added emotional pressure of having lost loved ones to the pandemic, increased prices, and dire economic prospects will see a general uptick in everyday violence, drug and alcohol abuse, and suicides. This will all further undermine the social and political order across the MENA region.

In the rich countries these effects can be mitigated with increased state spending, although decreased energy consumption during lockdowns and investments in renewables will also make this option increasingly less feasible.[16] Developing countries will face more dire prospects. An increase in violence and opposition will create more instability, instability which in turn will cause further economic struggles. Especially Turkey and Iran might face problems having to cut spending and tackle reduced growth at the same time. Both countries might face more widespread protest and an increase in insurgencies on the fringes, especially in the Kurdish areas which were especially hard hit during the pandemic, therefore destroying trust in the state.[17] Both Iran and Turkey are additionally host to large refugee populations of Afghans and Syrians respectively. Economic crises there will inevitably lead to an increase in xenophobia and violence.

---

11 Dina Talaat Badr Elsayed, 'Causes of Corruption in the MENA Region: A Cross-National Comparative Study' (Duisburg–Essen: Universität Duisburg Essen, 2019) https://duepublico2.uni-due.de/receive/duepublico_mods_00070009 (last accessed 25/03/2022).

12 Anthony H. Cordesman and Abdullah Toukan, 'The Return of ISIS in Iraq, Syria, and the Middle East', Center for Strategic & International Studies (2019) https://www.csis.org/analysis/return-isis-iraq-syria-and-middle-east (last accessed 25/03/2022).

13 Cenap Çakmak, 'The Arab Spring and the Shiite Crescent: Does Ongoing Change Serve Iranian Interests?', *The Review of Faith & International Affairs*, 13. 2 (2015), pp. 52–63. https://doi.org/DOI: 10.1080/15570274.2015.1039299 (last accessed 25/03/2022).

14 Anouar Boukhars, 'The Paranoid Neighbor: Algeria and the Conflict in Mali', (Washington D.C., USA: Carnegie Endowment for International Peace, 2012) https://www.jstor.org/stable/resrep12737 (last accessed 25/03/2022).

15 Shereen El Feki, 'MENA Men under Pressure', *The World Today*, 73, 6 (2017), pp. 18–20.

16 Jo. Harper, 'Riyadh Slashes Welfare as Oil and Coronavirus Effects Kick In.' *Business. Deutsche Welle*, (2020) https://www.dw.com/en/riyadh-slashes-welfare-as-oil-and-coronavirus-effects-kick-in/a-53391229 (last accessed 25/03/2022).

17 Philip Kowalski, 'COVID-19 Is Amplifying the Plight of Turkish and Iranian Kurds', *Geopolitical monitor* (2020) https://www.geopoliticalmonitor.com/covid-19-is-amplifying-the-plight-of-turkish-and-iranian-kurds/ (last accessed 25/03/2022).

Countries devastated by war, crisis, and chaos might slip further. Yemen for example is acutely threatened by famine.[18] The remaining institutions from Syria, Lebanon, Yemen, and Afghanistan might collapse further. In these countries there is a very real danger of renewed fighting and civil war, or an escalation of such.

5. Ideological Damage

Never let a good crisis go to waste is a saying attributed to Winston Churchill. It is something that was witnessed in the MENA region throughout the pandemic. As in the West, quacks were trying to use the pandemic and debates around vaccines for their own political goals. Ayatollah Hashem Bathaie Golpayegani declared in 2020 that he had cured himself from COVID-19 using Islamic medicine, only to die of COVID shortly afterwards.[19] Instances of theological hubris aside, the pandemic challenged states on multiple levels. For many deeply religious people the pandemic might very well be perceived as divine punishment, while it might also have the opposite effect in other people. Seeing all the 'righteous' but old religious leaders die and seeing states that legitimize themselves through Quran and Hadith not being able to tackle the pandemic might lead some to question official theological narratives. Broadly speaking cynical attitudes towards modernity narratives as well as traditional religious narratives might increase in the aftermath of the pandemic.

Lockdowns also hit the middle classes in countries like Iran, Turkey, and those in North Africa hard. The social contract between them and the ruling elite might be damaged through the policies implemented during the pandemic and the economic turmoil afterwards. Especially those whose wealth depends on trade — the Bazaaris in Iran[20] and the Anatolian Tigers in Turkey[21] — might feel betrayed and reevaluate their relationship with the current system.

6. Critical Discussion of the Findings

There are several intellectuals and thinkers who have expressed their views on the impact of COVID-19 on Middle Eastern societies and political processes in the region.

Rami Khouri, Director of Global Engagement and senior public policy fellow at the American University of Beirut, wrote that COVID-19 has revealed the

18 Daniel Byman, 'Yemen's Disastrous War', *Survival*, 60. 5 (2018), pp. 141–58.

19 Alijani Ershad, 'Prophet's Perfume and Flower Oil: How Islamic Medicine Has Made Iran's Covid-19 Outbreak Worse' *France24*, March 30, 2020 https://observers.france24.com/en/20200330-iran-coronavirus-islamic-medicine-covid-19-worse (last accessed 25/03/2022).

20 Sussan Siavoshi, 'Factionalism and Iranian Politics: The Post-Khomeini Experience', *Iranian Studies*, 25. 3–4 (1992), pp. 27–49.

21 Ömer Demir, 'Anatolian Tigers or Islamic Capital: Prospects and Challenges', *Middle Eastern Studies*, 40. 6 (2004), pp. 166–188.

shortcomings of health systems and government institutions in the Middle East. According to Khouri, the pandemic has also highlighted the importance of international cooperation and highlighted the need for political and socio-economic reforms to address the region's challenges. Khoui states that incompetent or uncaring Arab governments that cannot meet and protect citizens' basic rights now grapple unsuccessfully with simultaneous crises of governance, economy, environment, health, warfare, citizenship, and even state integrity. It's unlikely they can respond effectively to the new menaces that are upon us, and we should anticipate larger-scale human suffering and displacement in the years ahead.[22]

Marwan Muasher, the Vice President for Studies at the Carnegie Endowment for International Peace, said that COVID-19 has challenged the Middle East's model of economic and social development, based on oil and government revenues. Muasher stressed the importance of greater economic diversification and reform of the political system to meet the challenges of the future.[23]

Gerges Fawaz, Professor of International Relations of Middle East at the London School of Economics and Political Sciences, highlighted how COVID-19 has exacerbated political and social tensions in the Middle East, with an increase in protests and political grievances. Gerges also stressed the importance of regional cooperation to address the pandemic and other common challenges.[24]

Sari Hanafi: Hanafi, a Lebanese sociologist and philosopher, argues that the pandemic has exposed the weaknesses of neoliberal economic policies in the region. He writes: 'COVID-19 has laid bare the inadequacies of neoliberal economic policies in the Arab world, which have prioritized market efficiency over social welfare and left many vulnerable to economic shocks and crises'.[25]

The above mentioned reflections have been putting light how the COVID-19 became a new source of argumentation within the public debate of the Middle Eastern thought.

7. The Omani Example

A last interesting example to focus in this paper is Oman, the most neutral country of the Middle East. The Omani government reacted to the outbreak of the COVID-19 pandemic with similar measures to those implemented in the other states of the

22 Rami G. Khouri, 'Alrab leaders were already incompetent, then came coronavirus', *The New Arab*, March 20, 2020 https://www.newarab.com/opinion/arab-leaders-were-already-incompetent-then-came-coronavirus (last accessed 26/02/2023).

23 https://newlinesinstitute.org/events/covid-19-and-arab-regimes-a-conversation-with-dr-marwan-muasher/ (last accessed 26/02/2023).

24 A. Gerges Fawaz, 'Morning in the Middle East', *The Jordan Times*, August 4, 2021 https://jordantimes.com/opinion/fawaz-gerges/morning-middle-east (last accessed 26/02/2023).

25 Sari Hanafi, 'Toward a post-COVID-19 Sociology', *Journal du MAUSS* https://journaldumauss.net/?Toward-a-post-COVID-19-Sociology (last accessed 26/02/2023).

Gulf Cooperation Council.[26] In March 2020, a national Supreme Committee was established to coordinate governmental responses.[27] Restrictions to freedom of movement, sanitary precautions, e-learning, and smart-working solutions were introduced. With the deteriorating worldwide situation, the Omani government implemented lockdowns in different areas of the country, differentiating the intensity of the measures based on the number of cases. Muscat governorate, for example, experienced a lockdown from April 2020 — when the first death was registered — to the end of May 2020.[28]

New measures were introduced from the end of March to mid-August 2021. Curfews replaced lockdowns as the most restrictive measures, which changed weekly in length and intensity based on the government's considerations. The curfews restricted the movement and gathering of individuals, as well as the opening hours of commercial activities. Both during Ramadan 2020 and 2021, private gatherings were not allowed. In 2021, restaurants could stay open for *iftar* gatherings — which started at around 6:30 pm — until the curfew, which was set at 9 pm during the month of April. The limitations to freedom of movement in Oman were rigid, even compared to those implemented in EU countries. For example, the compulsory quarantine for infected people and incoming foreign travelers was coupled with the obligation to wear an electronic bracelet to guarantee isolation and contact tracing.[29]

While the implementation of preventive measures was strict, the vaccination campaign obtained much lesser results. At the end of May 2021, only 1.5% of the population was fully vaccinated, and 2.6% had received a partial dose. In August 2021, 41% had received a vaccination, of which 26% received a partial vaccination and 15% were fully vaccinated.[30] Since summer 2021, the vaccination rate has started to increase. As of March 2022, 64% of the population has been vaccinated — of which only 6.9% with a partial dose. However, Oman remains the country with the lowest vaccination rate in the GCC.[31]

The COVID-19 frustrations exacerbated popular discontent with the deteriorating economic conditions, and especially unemployment, leading in May 2021 to the first public protests since 2011. The increase in oil prices in Fall 2021 and the

---

26 Chris Alden and Charles Dunst, 'COVID-19: Gulf States and the Gulf Cooperation Council (GCC)', *The London School of Economics and Political Science*, (2022) https://www.lse.ac.uk/international-relations/centres-and-units/global-south-unit/COVID-19-regional-responses/Gulf-States-and-COVID-19 (last accessed 25/03/2022).

27 Amhed Al-Saidi (Minister of Health), *Sultanate of Oman Preparedness and Response to Covid19 Pandemic* https://apps.who.int/gb/COVID-19/pdf_files/11_06/Oman.pdf (last accessed 25/03/2022).

28 Tommy Hilton, 'Coronavirus: Oman to end Muscat lockdown on May 29', *Alarabiya News* (May 2020) https://english.alarabiya.net/coronavirus/2020/05/27/Coronavirus-Oman-to-end-Muscat-lockdown (last accessed 25/03/2022).

29 http://www.emro.who.int/fr/health-topics/corona-virus/using-technology-to-contain-covod-19-in-oman.html (last accessed 25/03/2022).

30 https://ourworldindata.org/covid-vaccinations (last accessed 25/03/2022).

31 https://ourworldindata.org/covid-vaccinations (last accessed 25/03/2022).

implementation of reforms supported a partial economic recovery.[32] The Sultan and private institutions provided additional funds to cope with the effects of the pandemic and the restrictions.[33]

8. Conclusion

The effects of COVID-19 will not be fully felt and understood in the short term. But over time their cumulative effect will for the most part be negative. Turkey, Jordan, Lebanon, Syria, Iran, and Iraq all were already struggling in economic terms when the new crisis hit. The economic crisis might easily translate into a political crisis in the years to come and this could provoke an uptick in violence and a decrease in stability, in a situation where unresolved violent conflicts from Palestine to Afghanistan frame the regional outlook already. This instability in turn will make countries less attractive to investors, increasing the economic crisis. There is a very real threat that the social contracts that keep most states, if not stable, at least functioning, might rip under the increased pressure. Countries that have been seeing protests already like Iran and Turkey might slip further into economic crisis and instability. All these factors increase the potential for separatism, sectarianism, and an overall increase in violence, weakening already weakened states further. It should be also highlighted that, at least in short term, the COVID-19 has managed to increase the authoritarianism of the MENA regimes which had managed to socially and politically control the unrest of the citizens.

However, the key strategic role of the MENA cannot be ignored within the new global 'Cold War' between the so called 'western coalition forces' and the 'oriental forces' such as China and Russia. In such a context, the MENA, such as the Pacific and the sub-Saharan Africa, will be influencing the new global balance of power. Both authoritarian ruling elite and pro-democracy citizens will be influenced, in their political struggle, by this new upcoming order.

32 Giulia Daga, 'EU and Oman: Small Steps Toward a Stronger Partnership?', *The Arab Gulf States Institute in Washington*, (2022) https://agsiw.org/eu-and-oman-small-steps-toward-a-stronger-partnership/ (last accessed 25/03/2022).

33 Marc J. Sievers, 'Oman's handling of the coronavirus', *Atlantic Council* (2020) https://www.atlanticcouncil.org/blogs/menasource/omans-handling-of-the-coronavirus/ (last accessed 25/03/2022).

Bibliography

Adelaja, Adesoji, and Justin George, 'Is Youth Unemployment Related to Domestic Terrorism?', *Perspectives on Terrorism*, 14. 5 (2020), pp. 41–62.

Alden, Chris, and Charles Dunst, 'COVID-19: Gulf States and the Gulf Co-operation Council (GCC)', *The London School of Economics and Political Science*, (2022), https://www.lse.ac.uk/international-relations/centres-and-units/global-south-unit/COVID-19-regional-responses/Gulf-States-and-COVID-19

Atamanov, Aziz, and Laura Rodriguez, 'The Islamic Republic of Iran: Battling Both Income Loss and Inflation', MENA Development Report, Distributional Impacts of COVID-19 in the Middle East and North Africa Region, 2021, December, https://doi.org/10.1596/978–1-4648–1776-2_ch8

Boukhars, Anouar, 'The Paranoid Neighbor: Algeria and the Conflict in Mali', (Washington D.C., USA: Carnegie Endowment for International Peace, 2012), https://carnegieendowment.org/2012/10/22/paranoid-neighbor-algeria-and-conflict-in-mali-pub-49756

Brun, Itai, and Sarah Feuer, 'The Calm before the Storm?: Coping with Corona in the Middle East', *Institute for National Security Studies*, (2020), http://www.jstor.org/stable/resrep23535

Byman, Daniel, 'Yemen's Disastrous War', *Survival*, 60. 5 (2018), pp. 141–58.

Çakmak, Cenap, 'The Arab Spring and the Shiite Crescent: Does Ongoing Change Serve Iranian Interests?', *The Review of Faith & International Affairs*, 13. 2 (2015), pp. 52–63, https://doi.org/DOI: 10.1080/15570274.2015.1039299

Cordesman, Anthony H., and Abdullah Toukan, 'The Return of ISIS in Iraq, Syria, and the Middle East', Center for Strategic & International Studies (2019), https://www.csis.org/analysis/return-isis-iraq-syria-and-middle-east

Dabrowski, Marek, and Marta Domínguez-Jiménez, 'Economic Crisis in the Middle East and North Africa' (Bruegel, 2021), http://www.jstor.org/stable/resrep28495

Daga, Giulia, 'EU and Oman: Small Steps Toward a Stronger Partnership?', *The Arab Gulf States Institute in Washington*, (2022), https://agsiw.org/eu-and-oman-small-steps-toward-a-stronger-partnership/

Demir, Ömer, 'Anatolian Tigers or Islamic Capital: Prospects and Challenges', *Middle Eastern Studies*, 40. 6 (2004), pp. 166–188.

Ershad, Alijani, 'Prophet's Perfume and Flower Oil: How Islamic Medicine Has Made Iran's Covid-19 Outbreak Worse' *France24*, March 30, 2020, https://observers.france24.com/en/20200330-iran-coronavirus-islamic-medicine-covid-19-worse

Esfandiari, Golnaz, ''State Of Explosion': Leaked IRGC Document Warns Of Rising Discontent In Iran', *Radio Free Europe / Radio Liberty*, (2022), https://www.rferl.org/a/iran-irgc-leaked-document-discontent/31683642.html

Fawaz, A. Gerges, 'Morning in the Middle East', *The Jordan Times*, August 4, 2021, https://jordantimes.com/opinion/fawaz-gerges/morning-middle-east

Feki, Shereen El, 'MENA Men under Pressure', *The World Today*, 73, 6 (2017), pp. 18–20.

Hanafi, Sari, 'Toward a post-COVID-19 Sociology', *Journal du MAUSS*, https://journaldu-mauss.net/?Toward-a-post-COVID-19-Sociology

Harper, Jo., 'Riyadh Slashes Welfare as Oil and Coronavirus Effects Kick In.' *Business. Deutsche Welle,* (2020), https://www.dw.com/en/riyadh-slashes-welfare-as-oil-and-coronavirus-effects-kick-in/a-53391229

Hilton, Tommy, 'Coronavirus: Oman to end Muscat lockdown on May 29', *Alarabiya News* (May 2020), https://english.alarabiya.net/coronavirus/2020/05/27/Coronavirus-Oman-to-end-Muscat-lockdown

Hinnebusch, Raymond, 'The Arab Uprisings and The MENA Regional States System', *Uluslararası İlişkiler / International Relations,* 11. 42 (2014), pp. 7–27.

'Global democracy has another bad year But popular protests show potential for democratic renewal', *The Economist,* (2022), https://www.economist.com/graphic-detail/2020/01/22/global-democracy-has-another-bad-year

Kinninmont, Jane, 'Bread And Dignity', *The World Today* 67. 8/9 (2011), pp. 31–33.

Khouri, Rami G., 'Alrab leaders were already incompetent, then came coronavirus', *The New Arab,* March 20, 2020, https://www.newarab.com/opinion/arab-leaders-were-already-incompetent-then-came-coronavirus

Kowalski, Philip, 'COVID-19 Is Amplifying the Plight of Turkish and Iranian Kurds', *Geopolitical monitor* (2020), https://www.geopoliticalmonitor.com/covid-19-is-amplifying-the-plight-of-turkish-and-iranian-kurds/

Musette, Mohammed Saïb, 'Brain Drain from the Southern Mediterranean', *IEMed Mediterranean Yearbook 2016* (Barcelona: European Institute of the Mediterranean, 2016),
https://www.iemed.org/publication/brain-drain-from-the-southern-mediterranean/

Siavoshi, Sussan, 'Factionalism and Iranian Politics: The Post-Khomeini Experience', *Iranian Studies,* 25. 3–4 (1992), pp. 27–49.

Sievers, Marc J., 'Oman's handling of the coronavirus', *Atlantic Council* (2020), https://www.atlanticcouncil.org/blogs/menasource/omans-handling-of-the-coronavirus/

Talaat Badr Elsayed, Dina, 'Causes of Corruption in the MENA Region: A Cross-National Comparative Study' (Duisburg–Essen: Universität Duisburg Essen, 2019), https://duepublico2.uni-due.de/receive/duepublico_mods_00070009

***

http://www.emro.who.int/fr/health-topics/corona-virus/using-technology-to-contain-covod-19-in-oman.html

https://newlinesinstitute.org/events/covid-19-and-arab-regimes-a-conversation-with-dr-marwan-muasher/

https://ourworldindata.org/covid-vaccinations

MICHELE NICOLETTI, ALESSANDRO PALAZZO

Conclusion

These concluding remarks will attempt to outline possible future lines of inquiry stemming from the analyses in this volume. As said in the introduction, pandemics and epidemics are complex phenomena. Even though they first and foremost involve medical issues, pandemics and epidemics cannot be viewed only from the perspective of biomedical management of disease (cure, prevention, diagnosis, prognosis, etc.). As they are general health crises, they affect human life on many levels (psychological, ecological, religious, social, economic, political, etc.). Accordingly, to adequately understand these phenomena, a multi-perspective and interdisciplinary approach is required that makes use of the methods and concepts of the most important human and social sciences. The papers collected in this volume show that philosophy, with the variety of its fields, styles, and notions, can also make a decisive contribution to this analysis. As such, this volume signals the need for new comprehensive, multidisciplinary, and cross-cultural studies with a strong philosophical background.

Due to their catastrophic nature and devastating effects, epidemics, pandemics, and other health crises have stimulated — and still stimulate, as the COVID-19 pandemic revealed — philosophical reflections on the relationship between man and God, the interplay between the human world and the natural ecosystem, the mechanisms of individual psychology, the reactions of masses, the nature and processes of political institutions, etc.

According to Mauro Bonazzi, Thucydides' account of the epidemic that ravaged Athens in the fifth century BCE goes far beyond the chronicle of those events. The Greek historian interprets the epidemic from a broader anthropological perspective as a collapse of the fabric of society. Comparing epidemics/pandemics with other emergencies (wars, revolutions, natural disasters, such as earthquakes, floods, fires, etc.) can help establish the specific characters of health crises at a social level and their similarities with and differences from natural calamities.[1] From a strictly philosophical

1 Significantly, in the literature on natural catastrophes, epidemics and pandemics are given limited attention, a sign that they are perceived as having specific traits: see, e.g., Michael Matheus, Gabriella Piccinni, Giuliano Pinto, Gian Maria Varanini (eds.), *Le calamità ambientali nel tardo medioevo europeo: realtà, percezioni, reazioni*. Atti del XII convegno del Centro di Studi sulla civiltà del tardo Medioevo. S. Miniato, 31 maggio — 2 giugno 2008 (Firenze: Firenze University Press, 2010); Thomas Labbé, *Les catastrophes naturelles au Moyen Âge: XIIe-XVe siècle* (Paris: CNRS éditions, 2017).

Epidemics and Pandemics, ed. by Michele Nicoletti and Alessandro Palazzo (Turnhout: Brepols, 2024), pp. 321–328
BREPOLS PUBLISHERS 10.1484/M.STPH-EB.5.136418

point of view, it would be interesting to analyze how epidemics/pandemics relate to the concept of state of emergency from both a theoretical and a historical perspective: in other words, does the social devastation triggered by epidemics/pandemics fall into the conceptual category of state of emergency? And in theorizing this concept, have philosophers also been influenced by their experience or knowledge of the social impact of epidemics and pandemics? By focusing on fear and dispossession as two widespread psychological effects of the COVID-19 crisis, Michele Nicoletti's paper can be read as an attempt to interpret the recent pandemic outbreak and its social impact through the framework of the state of emergency.

The social impact and political management of epidemics/pandemics have been the focus of philosophical investigations in the past. In one of his courses at the Collège de France (*Les anormaux*), Michel Foucault theorized the existence of two antithetical social dispositives of power and control of individuals devised in the Middle Ages to manage the emergencies posed by epidemics: the 'leprosy model', based on the isolation of lepers from the rest of society and their physical seclusion outside the city, and the 'plague model', based on the inclusion of plague-stricken people through a pervasive system of checks and control of their lives.[2] Foucault's analyses prove insightful and pave the way for further research into the ways in which, over the centuries, epidemics and pandemics and the processes elicited by health crises have impacted political thinking by contributing to the formation of new conceptual models.

The papers in the historical section of the volume, which revolve around the problem of the etiology of epidemics (especially plague pandemics) and the mechanisms of transmission, contribute to problematizing the simplifying commonplace view that the Galenic miasma theory was the only explanation of the pathogenesis of the epidemics advanced in the Antiquity and the Middle Ages up until the bacteriological breakthrough of the nineteenth century. As a matter of fact, the intellectual landscape was much more diverse, with contagionist models being already adopted in ancient and medieval sources. Explanations based on contagion were sometimes variously mixed with miasma theories. Future research should seek to provide a systematic analysis of the actual role played by contagion in ancient and medieval medical, historical, and literary sources.

Marco di Branco highlights the importance of the fideistic understanding of the plague outbreak in medieval Islamic circles. Many studies have already clarified the complexity of leprosy, a disease which was in the past profoundly shaped by religious preconceptions. Further investigation should consider the cultural and religious aspects involved in other epidemic diseases. It will then become clear that cultural contexts had a strong impact on the ancient and medieval scientific explanations of epidemics and contagious diseases, which were strongly conditioned by theological and religious assumptions.

---

2 Michel Foucault, *Les anormaux. Cours au Collège de France 1974–1975* (Paris: Seuil–Gallimard, 1999), lecture 15 January 1975.

Alessandro Palazzo's study on Albert the Great's views on pestilences and contagious diseases and their aftermath stimulates further research on the medical views of other medieval intellectuals who were not masters at the Faculty of Medicine or professional physicians. On the other hand, the extensive literature on plague produced from 1347–1348 onward for at least two centuries deserves careful re-examination today. The first pioneering studies of Karl Sudhoff, who in the first decades of the twentieth century provided editions, transcriptions, and descriptions of manuscripts of many late medieval and early modern plague treatises have been followed in the course of the century to the present by numerous studies dealing with the characters, sources, and contents of this literature. Special attention has been paid, above all, to the earliest treatises written between 1347 and 1351. New research should be conducted on the individual treatises in an attempt to clarify similarities and differences among them, to establish lines of development and discontinuities in this tradition, to study the relationship with coeval literary, historical, and philosophical sources.

Diana Di Segni's study of medieval Hebrew plague treatises and Hebrew translations of Latin plague treatises contributes to a deeper understanding of the more general issue of the circulation of scientific learning among different linguistic, cultural, and religious civilizations in the medieval world. This study opens a largely unexplored field of research where new analyses will both address specific questions (authorship, dating, nature of these texts) and elucidate the conceptual transformations that the scientific theories about plague underwent through the process of transposition from the medieval Latin university milieu into Hebrew-speaking contexts.

Although from different points of view, all the last three papers in the historical section confirm that contagion remains a crucial point in the philosophical-medical debates about epidemics and pandemics throughout the modern era. In addition to addressing medical theories on plague, Concetta Pennuto explores this phenomenon from an ethical-practical perspective, reflecting on patient care and physicians' ethical commitment. Future studies should shed light on the intertwining of theory and practice, examining, on the one hand, the ways in which scientific theories about plague and epidemics in the Middle Ages and modern era influenced concrete forms of treatment of the sick and, on the other, how clinical activity contributed to changing theoretical conceptions and reshaping physicians' deontology and self-perception.

Mariangela Priarolo explains why and how the Galenic miasmatic explanation of the plague was able to survive and even predominate until the nineteenth century, despite the fact that mechanism had become the new dominant scientific paradigm in the seventeenth century. Her hypothesis that the Galenic model was made compatible with mechanism through a reinterpretation of Fracastoro's notion of seeds of contagion needs to be tested against a larger body of texts.

Fabrizio Meroi examines some examples of philosophical reinterpretation of the concept of contagion. His view that this notion can be traced, explicitly or implicitly — behind the concepts of influence, diffusion, propagation, and transmission — in the works of philosophers and intellectuals of the nineteenth and twentieth centuries and that in these contexts contagion is not merely a metaphor, but a real conceptual category tool is inspiring and innovative. Even though several attempts have recently been made to study the pervasive dissemination of the notion of contagion outside the medical field across other disciplinary areas,[3] no systematic study has been carried out on the philosophical recategorization of contagion by modern philosophers. Meroi's line of research, therefore, deserves further investigation, including a wider range of works and authors from the nineteenth to the present.

The historical analysis contained in the first part of the volume highlighted the set of words, concepts, and theories that, over the centuries, philosophy has elaborated to describe and interpret the phenomenon of epidemics and pandemics. This impressive linguistic, conceptual, and theoretical armamentarium has been able to sediment itself over the centuries and survive the vitality of the scientific theories that were intended to explain these phenomena. The extraordinary development of medical and epidemiological science has falsified a large number of past hypotheses, but the vocabulary of the pandemic has demonstrated, in the crisis produced by the worldwide spread of COVID-19, its incredible resilience.

Not only that. As the analysis of nineteenth- and twentieth-century culture already showed, this vocabulary has remained alive in the medical sciences, but has also found application in the most diverse sectors of social and cultural life. The concepts of 'contagion' and 'immunisation', to take two examples already mentioned, are the clearest demonstration of this. Not only do descriptions of natural and social reality make ample use of it, but also the vocabularies of virtual reality amply attest to it.

In short, the language of the pandemic has gone 'viral' and it would certainly be interesting to understand to what this vitality can be attributed. It certainly depends on at least two factors. Firstly, medicine has progressively become the 'spiritual' centre of reference of the contemporary era, a new religion bringing salvation, whose prescriptions have been able to impose themselves — as the COVID experience has shown — over the prescriptions of traditional religions. Secondly, the pandemic is an incredibly intense and widespread experience of fear, and it is not surprising that its vocabulary remains engraved in human consciousness through the ages and retains a formidable evocative power.

In this sense, the essays in the second part of the volume also open up fascinating avenues of research. The theme of zoonosis — the focus of Carlo Brentari's essay — evokes the very ancient and topical issue of the relationship between human beings and other living beings, particularly those in the animal world. The clash with the pandemic not only evokes the conflict between life and death, but also that between human life and other life forms. The virus is a living being, itself living in other living beings and carried by other living beings. In the age of the anthropocene, of the unchallenged dominance of the human species over other living forms, the dialectic between human and non-human life is reopened. The fear of the 'beasts' that has accompanied human life for millennia and inhabited its imagination, pushing human

3 *Tracés. Revue de Sciences humaines*, 21 (2011) (*Contagions*); Thomas Rütten and Martina King (eds.), *Contagionism and Contagious Diseases. Medicine and Literature 1880–1933* (Berlin–Boston: De Gruyter, 2014); Béatrice Delaurenti, Thomas Le Roux, *De la contagion* (Paris: Vendemiaire, 2020) (Engl. transl. *Cultures of Contagion* [Cambridge, Mass.: MIT Press, 2021]).

beings to conceive of themselves as 'other' than the animal being, seen in turn as a past and as a limit to be overcome, is once again taking shape.

Alongside this, another dialectic is reopened, that between 'wild' life and domestication, calling into question the agricultural model that emerged from the Neolithic period and forged the food and daily life of the past millennia. All this forces the human being to rethink not only his relations with other life, but also with his own life: the human being as a 'species' and his self-understanding, i.e., the relationship with his biological identity. The pandemic not only reopens the game of relations between living species, but also the game of the environment, since an overly humanised environment can be a relevant element in the spread of contagion. The conceptual constellations of miasma theory and germ theory intertwine again in the present.

This anthropological dimension called into question by COVID not only concerns the human being's relationship with nature and the animal sphere but also its social dimension, which — in Michele Nicoletti's reconstruction of it — is radically challenged by the emergence of the pandemic. The fear of contagion is part of a broader universe of fears that seems to characterize the present age and which are traced back to the fear of self-dispossession. COVID threatens not only the position of untouchable superiority that human being seems to have gained over the rest of the natural world, but it also threatens the goal that the development of Western culture seems to have handed over to every human individual, namely the conquest of the self. The great themes of fear, of uncertainty, but also of the dispossession of the self by the other and thus of alienation, of 'mutual affliction', return overbearingly to the scene. And the question re-emerges as to what is the proper role of the politician: that of creating ever stronger protective networks by establishing new 'states' of existence in order to escape the state of nature, or that of creating more advanced conditions of freedom in which everyone has an equal chance to be herself and to belong to herself and not to others.

The theme of the equality of human beings, called into question by COVID and its management, is also touched upon by Nidesh Lawtoo's essay, which reinterprets the issue of contagion on the basis of a reinterpretation of mimetic theory in the digital age. If on the one hand the experience of the pandemic unites the entire human species because everyone can be affected by it ('the eternal ethos of the plague'), on the other hand it is clear that it can trigger new processes of discrimination, particularly through unequal access to health care and vaccines. Moreover, the spread of the virus has brought with it profound transformations in the public arena. If this — with the advent of the masses in the twentieth century — was already marked by the 'metaphorical' dynamic of the contagion of crowds and the spread of conspiracy theories, now, because of the 'real' contagion, these phenomena are also amplified thanks to the power of the new media. This opens up the question of how to react to false theories and pathological practices. Is it sufficient to reaffirm the role of rationality and scientific knowledge or is a new 'pathos' of human coexistence needed?

It is difficult to underestimate the importance of the transformations of human communication in the pandemic and the questions they bring. Starting with interpersonal communication, COVID was a dramatic experience. The practices of estrangement and forced distancing marked personal existences. The compulsory wearing of masks altered non-verbal communication, which is a fundamental element of human interaction. The explosion of distant communication practices thanks to digital technologies has altered personal communication, but also social communication. Schools, universities, parliaments, and governments have replaced personal transmission of information, content, and in-person discussion, animated by physical immediacy, with communication at a distance. As Ľudmila Lacková shows in her essay, all communication has become 'mediated' and she thus asks how this hegemony of mediation will affect the crisis of the subject.

But not only personal and social communication have been affected. Scientific communication too has opened up radical questions about its own nature, its foundations, and its relationship with society. Questioning the 'model' of scientific knowledge, Federico Laudisa wonders whether the COVID experience has challenged traditional descriptive and predictive models, also starting from the characteristic of the present age that is the age of Big Data. Considering the fact that critical events can recur, it is necessary to develop an epistemology in a time of systemic crisis for the public good. The search for this new epistemology should be based on a number of elements: a solid scientific basis that is nonetheless aware of the need to support urgent decisions; awareness of the social importance of science and therefore the appropriateness of scientific communication within the public discourse; the need, in a liberal and democratic society, to guarantee equal access and freedom to the plurality and diversity of voices; and the ability to counter the manipulation of information and the fabrication of lies so as not to weaken the freedom of research.

The reflections in this volume mainly concern the Western world, but this is only one part of the world, as Pejman Abdolmohammadi reminds us in his contribution on the Middle East and North Africa. Here, too, there are similar dynamics to those in Western countries, and the same questions for future research arise. But alongside the similarities, there are also differences that have to do with religious and cultural traditions, economic and social contexts, and different political and institutional dynamics. And above all, given the 'anthropological' depth of the crisis, this dimension should be properly investigated in the different areas of the world in order to get a complete picture of what the pandemic has brought with it.

Here too, philosophy and the history of philosophy could contribute original perspectives to understanding the phenomenon and open up new avenues of research, as we hope this volume can do in the area we examined.

Bibliography

Delaurenti, Béatrice, and Thomas Le Roux (eds.), *De la contagion* (Paris: Vendemiaire, 2020).

———, and ——— (eds.), *Cultures of Contagion* [Cambridge, Mass.: MIT Press, 2021]).

Foucault, Michel, *Les anormaux. Cours au Collège de France 1974–1975* (Paris: Seuil–Gallimard, 1999).

Labbé, Thomas, *Les catastrophes naturelles au Moyen Âge: XIIe-XVe siècle* (Paris: CNRS éditions, 2017).

Matheus, Michael, and (eds.), *Le calamità ambientali nel tardo medioevo europeo: realtà, percezioni, reazioni.* Atti del XII convegno del Centro di Studi sulla civiltà del tardo Medioevo. S. Miniato, 31 maggio – 2 giugno 2008 (Firenze: Firenze University Press, 2010).

Rütten, Thomas, and Martina King (eds.), *Contagionism and Contagious Diseases. Medicine and Literature 1880–1933* (Berlin–Boston: De Gruyter, 2014).

Tracés. Revue de Sciences humaines, 21 (2011) (Contagions).